Green Biotechnology

— *Editors* —

Dr Anjani Singh Tomar

Dr Bindu Vijay

Dr Viralkumar B. Mandaliya

2019

Daya Publishing House®

A Division of

Astral International Pvt. Ltd.

New Delhi – 110 002

ISBN: 9789388173926 (Int. Edition)

Published by : **Daya Publishing House®**
A Division of
Astral International Pvt. Ltd.
– ISO 9001:2015 Certified Company –
4736/23, Ansari Road, Darya Ganj
New Delhi-110 002
Ph. 011-43549197, 23278134
E-mail: info@astralint.com
Website: www.astralint.com

Digitally Printed at : Replika Press Pvt. Ltd.

Green Biotechnology

The Editors

Dr Anjani Singh Tomar is Associate Professor of Law at GNLU. She is recipient of 5 Gold medals from Devi Ahilya Vishwavidyalaya, (DAVV) Indore, for holding merit positions in LL.B. (Hons) & LL.M. exams. She is also holder of M.Sc. degree in Clinical Bio-Chemistry from Holkar Science College, DAVV, Indore. She passed her NET (Law) exam in 2008 & received Ph.D. degree in 2010. She has an experience of more than 11 years as a faculty in Law. She has written books on variety of subjects including labor law, information technology, taxation laws, intellectual property laws etc. She is editor of leading journal of the country, The GNLU Law Review. She has published the papers in leading journals of the country as well. She has also worked as faculty of law at Indore Institute of Law, Indore, & University of Petroleum & Energy Studies, Dehradun.

Dr Bindu Vijay, MSc PhD., serves as Assistant Professor of Science and Technology, at Gujarat National Law University (GNLU). She also serves as member of Centre for Environment and Sustainable Development at GNLU. She has nearly 15 years of experience in teaching Science and Law. She teaches Genetics, Biotechnology, and Bioethics to law students both for undergraduate and postgraduate program. She has designed and offered a certificate course in "Genetics and Law". Her areas of interest include Bioethics, Genetics and Biotechnology. She frequently delivers lectures on "Biotechnology, Bioethics and Law" at various forums. She has several publications to her credit.

Dr Viralkumar B. Mandaliya is an Assistant Professor – Research at Gujarat National Law University, Gandhinagar. He was awarded with "Bharat Shiksha Ratan" by Global Society for Health and Educational Growth, Delhi, and "Young Scientist" by Venus International Foundation, India. He hold numerous member positions of Scientific and Educational Society and Council. He has pursued several short term courses from WIPO, Geneva; agMOOCs, Ministry of HRD, GOI; EUIPO, Spain. He has numerous publications (national and international), book and book chapters, paper-presentations to his credit.

Acknowledgements

Team members would like to acknowledge the Government of Gujarat for graciously accepting the research project "The Key Development in Biotechnology and its Impact on the Society, and Creation of Techno-legal Awareness towards the Recent Trends in Biotechnology" to be conducted by GNLU. We are equally obliged & thankful to Director, Gujarat National Law University, Prof. (Dr.) Bimal N Patel, Professor of Law, who have posed his confidence & trust in our team and have given us this opportunity to bring our research into success. We are also thankful to Dean, Research division, Prof. (Dr.) Ranita Nagar, who has been a source of encouragement to us. We would like to thank all the members of Research Division, with special reference to Mr. Rahul B. Pandya, who has been instrumental in the completion of the research project and this book. We would also like to acknowledge the administrative support given to us by the Registrar's office, GNLU.

The entire project and the book could not take up the shape without the hard efforts put in by our Project Assistant, Ms. Urvi Vacchheta. She, being the active support to us, has really worked very hard to bring our project into reality. We are very thankful to her whole hearted contribution, in every aspect of our project.

We express our sincere thanks to all the contributing authors for their contributions that resulted in this book. We also express our sincere thanks to Astral Publishers especially Mr. Kanav for his support and suggestion to bring it in a form of book.

We would also like to thank all our friends and family members who have directly and indirectly supported us to bring out this book.

Contents

Preface

Biotechnology is a broad area and its development is dependent on relationship with various disciplines of science. The term "Biotechnology" derives from three Greek words: *bios* - life; *techno* – technology and *logos* - thinking. There exist a vast variety of definitions of Biotechnology. Presumably the most general one is given by the United Nations Convention on Biological Diversity, 1992, which states that "Any technological application that uses biological systems, living organisms, or derivatives thereof, to make or modify products or processes for specific use." Biotechnology has diverse applications. From producing food to designing baby, biotech today is considered as million dollar industry. Today industry and researchers use biotechnology as a tool in their process to a greater extent in a diverse manner.

This diversity has, in turn, brought about the need for a system to classify biotechnology uses based on common features or final purpose. As a result, nowadays there exist **five** main groups in biotechnological applications, which have been identified by a color system.

Red Biotechnology brings together all those biotechnology uses connected to medicine which includes producing vaccines and antibiotics, developing new drugs, molecular diagnostics techniques, regenerative therapies and the development of genetic engineering to cure diseases through genetic manipulation. It also includes reproductive technologies.

White Biotechnology comprises all the biotechnology uses related to industrial processes - that is why it is also called "industrial biotechnology". It includes the use of microorganisms in chemicals production, the design and production of new materials for daily use (plastics, textiles, etc.) and the development of new sustainable energy resources such as biofuels.

Green Biotechnology is focused on agriculture as working field. It includes creating hybrid varieties, new plant varieties and transgenic plants of agricultural interest using modern biotechnology, producing biofertilizers and biopesticides etc.

Purple Biotechnology deals with different domains of Intellectual Property such as Patents, Trademarks, Copyrights and Geographical Indications. It is connected with inventions and trade in biotechnology, especially in an economically globalised scenario, where technology transfers by way of intellectual property protection is now part of global trade.

Blue Biotechnology is based on the exploitation of aquatic and marine resources to create products and applications of industrial interest. Sea has covered ¾ of the planet where diversity of sea creatures is enormous. The researcher has explored a huge portion of the ocean and a lot of species, yet many mysteries are waiting to be discovered.

The present book on the topic **"Green Biotechnology"** aimed at finding out the issues and challenges in plant and agriculture field and how they can be addressed. The contributions were invited from the people involved in plant and agriculture field as well as people involved in regulatory framework of issues pertaining to plant and agriculture biotechnology. The articles have covered the substantive matter from India and abroad. We believe that this edited book will be useful not only to scientific community but also to others who are involved in policy making.

Editors

Chapter 1

Genetically Modified Crops: Issues and Challenges with Special Reference to IPR and Farmers' Rights

Ruchi Tiwari and Archana Gadekar

Faculty of Law, The Maharaja Sayajirao University of Baroda, Vadodara, Gujarat - 390 002

e-mail: rtiwar@gmail.com, gadekararchana@gmail.com

ABSTRACT

Intellectual property rights are globalizing in the age of information technology, so association can be identified between intellectual property protection and environmental conservation and their use. The development of biotechnology and its capacity to create Genetically Modified Organisms (GMOs) has posed a threat to environment protection. Patents are the fresh generation's defensive projectile. More or less everyone agrees that patent have helped the developers to invent new technologies and enjoy monopoly for several years. Patent protections have encouraged the scientist and inventors to invent new technologies to recover the development money with the improved inventions on various sectors like pesticides, irrigation, fertilizers and even in seeds. In relation to biotechnology for agriculture, TRIPS allow patent to be granted for plant varieties, but not plants.

One of the most fascinating and important issues surrounding GM crops is perhaps the question of intellectual property rights in relation to trade and technology transfer. The IPRs that are associated with the flow of private research in biotechnology may, if not properly managed, block access to new developments by the public sector and non-profit research. This is particularly true for developing countries.

Countries like India have being governing with agriculture. However, it is equally important to note that because of its land, skilled and unskilled laborers, the developed countries are eyeing towards it. Developed countries rule the world in agriculture technologies and they dominate the developing countries through them. Transformation and the gene-transfer techniques have influenced the development of new technologies. Majority of the farmers still follow the traditional old methods of farming, irrigation and all. Granting of patent will create dependencies of the farmers which will create certain issues like monopoly of seed companies which is to be taken proper care off. Is this coming technology is blessing is disguise or is need of the coming hour.

With the more emphasis on Genetically Modified Crops the use of intellectual property poses some research questions:

- Does patent of seed affect the free trade of farmers?
- Does coming of terminator seeds increase the dependency of farmer of packed seed?
- Issues and challenges faced by Genetically Modified Crops?
- Does IPRs represent the legal framework to insure that the use of biotechnology is properly governed?
- Finally, is R&D capacity real the key of a country and its consumers are to make informed choices about the adoption and development of genetic technology?

The focus of this chapter is to examine the above questions **and study the Issues and Challenges of Genetically Modified Crops and their impact on seed patenting with reference to IPR and Farmers Rights related contemporary issues.** Further the chapter traces the development in the era of genetically modified seeds with reference to the issues of the farmers.

Introduction

Intellectual property rights (IPRs) have never been more economically and politically important and controversial than they are today. This is due to rapid introduction of high standards of protections of Intellectual Property Rights in most of the developing countries under the aegis of the WTO Agreement on Trade related aspects of the Intellectual Property rights (TRIPS Agreement). This issue is frequently mentioned in discussions and debates on such diverse topics as relating to biological resources, biotechnology, traditional knowledge, biopiracy, access and benefit sharing, transfer of technology, agriculture, food security and Public health. So IPRs have a number of socio-economic impacts which require the adoption of a broader perspective, which sees intellectual property protection within the context of sustainable development rather than purely in terms of economic development.

The increasing economic importance of biological resources and the question of the ownership of these biological resources have made the allocation of Property Rights, as one of the most contentious issues in the debate concerning biodiversity management at the national and international level. IPRs are often granted to individuals of one country over genetic resources oBTained from another country. These new developments have led to the emergence of new conflicts concerning the ownership of biodiversity and related knowledge, and have forced states to rethink intellectual property rights regimes in a fundamental way.

IPR in Connection with Traditional Knowledge, Biodiversity and Agriculture

The introduction of IPRs in agriculture is of special significance because agriculture and food security are closely interlinked. It can only be justified if

IPRs foster food security or in other words the realization of the human right to food. Food security remains an overwhelming concern for developing countries. Existing IPR systems such as patents may increase the risk of misappropriation of traditional knowledge. The relationship between intellectual property rights and environmental management is one of the specific issues which call for attention. The development of biotechnology and its capacity to create Genetically Modified Organisms (GMOs) has posed a threat to environment protection. The need for transfer of environmentally sound technology (EST) to developing countries has for a long time been seen as one of the major aspects of the process of sustainable development.

The question of access and benefits sharing clearly illustrate the close links between intellectual property protection and sustainable development. The assertion of IPRs and the resulting private monopolies over biological resources have direct implications on the state of India's biodiversity, the protection of traditional knowledge, food security, right to health and sustainable development in overall. India being a member of the various international conventions and agreements is bound to enact/amend relevant domestic Laws to gear up and face the challenges of globalization

Intellectual Property Rights and Traditional Knowledge

Traditional knowledge is now widely recognised as having played and as still playing crucial role in economic, social and cultural life and development, not only in traditional societies but also in modern societies. The recent increased awareness of the value of biodiversity, the need for its conservation and sustainable use for present and future generation has highlighted the importance of traditional knowledge (TK).[1] Developing countries find themselves with most traditional knowledge and developed countries are keen to use the traditional knowledge in further applications. The increased economic value of TK has led to the search for better ways to access the knowledge through legal mechanism to assert claims.

The term "traditional knowledge" is a very broad concept, which encompasses within itself indigenous knowledge related to various categories like agricultural knowledge, medicinal knowledge; bio diversity related knowledge as well as expressions of folklore in the form of music, dance, songs, handicraft, designs *etc.* It has played and still plays an important role in the lifestyle of indigenous communities. The knowledge of local communities, farmers and indigenous peoples, for instance plant varieties locally developed, wild and domesticated biological resources, knowledge of healers regarding medicinal and therapeutic properties of plants as well as on how to conserve these resources is now recognised precious for future development or even survival of mankind.[2]

Traditional knowledge makes valuable contribution in the conservation of biodiversity, environment and fulfilment of human need for sustainable

---

1 Intellectual Property Rights, Biodiversity and sustainable development, Martin Khor, p. 15.

2 Mulhausler 2001, p. 143.

development.[3] Indigenous people have an immense understanding about their complex ecosystems, properties of plants and animals and regarding the techniques of using them based on their living close with nature for centuries[4]. TK in agriculture has been affected in many developing countries by conversion from biodiversity based farming system to monocultures promoted through IPRs. Another factor that calls for protection of TK is to maintain the practices and knowledge derived from traditional life styles. Preservation of TK is intended to provide self identification to these indigenous communities and thereby provide continuous existence of indigenous people.[5]

The protection of diverse knowledge systems requires a diversity of IPR systems, including systems which do not reduce knowledge and innovation to private property for monopolistic profits. Systems of common property in knowledge need to be evolved for preserving the integrity of indigenous knowledge systems on the basis of which our every day survival is based.

Despite the growing body of literature and the involvement of several international and nongovernmental organizations in the study and debate of issues relating to the protection of TK, slow progress has being made at the national level for the design of specific regimes on the matter. The problems at stake are very complex and any legal solution should respond to the real needs of the intended beneficiaries.

Intellectual Property Rights and Biodiversity

IPRs are awarded to individuals or organizations mainly for inventions and creative works, giving the creator/inventor the incentive of a right to prevent others from unauthorized use for a limited time period. Biological diversity or biodiversity refers to the variety of life forms: the different plants, animals and microorganisms, the genes they contain and the ecosystems they form. This living wealth is the product of hundreds of millions of years of evolutionary history. The concept emphasizes the interrelated nature of the living world and its processes.

Biological Diversity Act, 2002

India drafted, (after a long period of intense debates) as a follow-up to the Convention on Biological Diversity, the Biological Diversity Act, 2002. Consequently, it addresses social concerns regarding the conservation and sustainable use of bio-resources including habitat and species protection. The following are some of the main features of the Act:

- ✰ Recognition of conservation of biodiversity, sustainable use of biological resources, and equitable sharing of benefits arising from such use;
- ✰ Provision for setting up of a National Biodiversity Authority (NBA), State Biodiversity Boards (SBBs) and Biodiversity Management Committees

3 World commission on environment and sustainable development (WCED) report, Bruttland (1987).

4 RAFI 1997,p vii.

5 see correa carlos M, *Traditional Knowledge and intellectual property*, pages 6 and 7, available @ www.geneva.quno.info.

(BMCs) in local bodies; NBA and SBB to consult BMCs in decisions relating to use of biological resources/related knowledge within their jurisdiction and BMCs to promote conservation, sustainable use and documentation of biodiversity;

- Need for foreign nationals/organizations to seek prior approval of NBA for oBTaining biological resources and/or associated knowledge for any use;
- Approval of NBA for Indian individuals/entities for transferring results of research with respect to any biological resources to foreign nationals/organizations;
- Levy of appropriate fees and royalties on such transfers and IPRs;
- Sharing of benefits to all concerned parties;
- Measures to conserve and sustainably use biological resources, including habitat and species protection, conservation in gene banks, environmental impact assessments of all projects which could harm biodiversity *etc.*;
- Decision-making power to local communities regarding the use of resources and knowledge within their jurisdiction, and negotiations with parties who want to use these resources and knowledge;
- Development of an appropriate legislation or administrative steps, including registration, to protect indigenous and community knowledge;
- Governments to declare Biodiversity Heritage Sites, as areas for special measures for conservation and sustainable use of biological resources, and notification of threatened species to control their collection and use; risk associated with biotechnology (including the use of GMOs), to be regulated or controlled through appropriate means;
- Designation of repositories of biological resources, at national and other levels;
- Creation of Funds at local, state, and national levels, to be generated from fees, royalties, donations *etc.*

However, the notification of the Biological Diversity Rules, 2004 under the Biological Diversity Act, 2002 has attracted vitriolic criticisms from the NGOs that the role of local communities in safeguarding biodiversity and traditional knowledge has become diminutive, and thus, the spirit and letter of the Act, has been totally watered down.

Intellectual Property Rights and Agriculture

Agro biodiversity which is a subset of biological diversity is a major concern for the world food and livelihood security and the issues of conservation and management of agro biodiversity are one of the high priorities for a diversity-rich country like India. Agriculture is a way of life, a tradition, which, for centuries, has shaped the thought, the outlook, the culture and economic life of the people. India is bound by all the provisions of TRIPS Agreement, which oblige the country to enact/amend relevant domestic laws. Further, with such shifts in legal provisions and also national policies, increased private participation in agricultural R&D and far more public-private relationships, including both competition and cooperation in relevant areas, are imminent.

Agriculture and biodiversity management are linked inextricably. Biodiversity resources constitute a primary input to agricultural production system and evolved through selection and collection of plant varieties which depends on ecosystem products and services.[6] Agro biodiversity contributes directly to the livelihood of a large segment of humankind and is the basis for all human food consumption for world food security and sustainable agriculture. Farmers have traditionally played pivotal role in conserving and enhancing agro biodiversity. They have developed crop varieties and domestic animals breeds specifically suited to their diverse local environment which is today undertaken on a larger scale and has become a major industrial activity.[7]

In a country like India where the farming community provides for the country's annual requirements of seed, it is fundamentally important for the farmer to sell seed. If a farmer does not have the right to sell seed, it implies that each time the farmer wishes to grow a new crop, he or she has to turn to the market to buy seeds. Such dependence on the market for seeds is not economically feasible for farmers in India and hence will have hindrance in agricultural growth of the country.

New inputs derived from biotechnology, especially those coming from the private sector, are finding wide utility in agriculture. Therefore, it is considered important to identify and develop various national policy options for addressing the emerging areas of IPR in agriculture, including the access to various protected technologies to the Indian farmers, entrepreneurs and users. It is high time that a critical analysis of the system is undertaken for its strengths, weaknesses, opportunities and threats (SWOT), to convert threats into opportunities and mitigate weaknesses through timely action.

Genetically Modified (GM) Seeds Development in India

Genetically Modified Meaning

Genetic modification involves altering an organism's DNA. This can be done by altering an existing section of DNA, or by adding a new gene altogether. A gene is a code that governs how we appear and what characteristics we have. Genetic modification allows selected individual genes discovered in one organism to be inserted directly into other. This can be related or unrelated species. The transferred genes called the transgene. Thus, genetically modified crops are produced by genetic engineering. In these plants a foreign gene is introduced, that is, a gene alien to the plant species. This creates plants that never be created naturally. For example, fish genes can be introduced into tomato or pig genes can be inserted into rice.

---

6 Pagiola, mainstreaming Biodiversity in agricultural development (WDC: AAAS 1930). p. xix.

7 CM Correa, access to genetic resources, world completion-I Econ Rev 57 (1997).

Procedure and Classification of GM Crops

For many years plant breeding entailed the selection of the finest plants to get the best crops. In those days variations occurred through induced mutation or hybridization where two or more plants were crossed. Today scientist can not only select, but also create crops by inserting genes to make a seed bare any trait desired. In order to make a transgenic crop, there are four main steps,extracting DNA, cloning a gene of interest, designing the gene for plant infiltration, and finally plant breeding.

The first generation application of genetic engineering to crop agriculture has been targeted towards the generation of plants expressing foreign genes that confer resistance to virus, insects, herbicides or pest harvest deterioration and accumulation of useful modified storage product.

The Classification of GM Crops has been discussed below

1. Resistance to biotic (that is living: used to describe the features of a natural system that are living) stresses. Resistance to biotech stress includes the following:

   a) Insect Resistance

   Insect resistance crops-mainly maize and cotton have been engineered with a gene from the soil bacterium, Bacillus thuringiensis (BT). This gives the plants themselves insecticide properties. They express a toxin which kills certain target pests such as the corn and cotton bollworm.

   b) Disease Resistance and Virus Resistance.

   Genes that provide resistance against plants virus has been introduced into such crops plants as tobaccos, tomatoes and potatoes.Tomato plants infected with tobacco mosaic virus (which attaches tomato plants as well as tobacco).

2. Herbicide resistance;

   An herbicide tolerant plant is a genetically modified plant that contains genes that enable it to resist chemicals that are sprayed to destroy weeds. For example, Roundup Ready corn is an herbicide tolerant maize variety that will survive the application of an herbicide called Roundup, when all other plants will die after its application.

3. Resistance to abiotic stresses

   Almost all the abiotic stresses such as drought, low temperature, salinity and alkalinity. There are number of genes which have been inserted in different plants to reduce abiotic stresses and improve quality of crops such as transgenic plant of tobacco have shown increase salt resistance (Transgenics - Genetic Manipulation).[8]

---

8 Transgenics - Genetic Manipulation*http://users.rcn.com/jkimball.ma.ultranet/BiologyPages/T/TransgenicPlant s.html*

Development of GM Seed in India

Agriculture is the backbone of Indian economy contributing approximately 17.32 per cent of the national GDP[9]. Enhancement of yields on small farms which tends to increase the demand and hence rewards for poor labors addresses this problem. This is only possible through new technology of agriculture. The Government of India realized the need for creating a separate institutional framework to strengthen biology and biotechnology research during 1980s. Modern biological research is supported by the government agencies such as Council of Scientific and Industrial Research, Indian Council for Agricultural Research, Indian Council of Medical Research, and the funding agencies like the Department of Biotechnology, Department of Science and Technology and the University Grants Commission. Biotechnology was given a boost in 1982 with the establishment of the National Biotechnology Board. The success and impact of the National Biotechnology Board prompted the Government to establish a separate Department of Biotechnology (DBT) in 1986. The first transgenic BT cotton underwent field testing in 1995.

Adoption of GM Crops among Indian Farmers

The preference of Indian farmers for BT cotton or genetically modified crops has been assessed by direct and indirect ways. The word 'direct way' itself explains that the farmers straight forward are accepting the technology, and indirect way involves the evaluation and benefit of the crop, trend of cultivation and demand for packet of seed sold by seed producing companies to the farmers

Legal Framework for the Regulation of GM Crops

The government regulates the seed industry and the seed trade in various respects. The Seed Act of 1966, the Seeds Control Order of 1983, and the Seeds Policy of 1988 are the major components of policy specific to the industry. The Seed Act of 1966 and the Seeds Control Order of 1983 provide statutory backing to the system of variety release, seed certification and seed testing.

Cartegena Protocol

The Cartagena Protocol on Biosafety under the Convention on Biological Diversity (CBD), a multilateral agreement covering the movement across national boundaries of living modified organisms (LMOs) that might have an adverse effect on biological diversity.

The Protocol contains procedures rather than substantive measures, relating to the provision of information and the carrying out of tests to assess the safety of GMOs such as GM crops. Some of the main procedures introduced by the Protocol are as follows:

a) **Advanced Informed Agreement Procedure (AIA):** Before exporting GMOs which are intended for release in the environment, the recipient country

9 Statistics times March 2017 http://statisticstimes.com/economy/sectorwise-gdp-contribution-of-india.php.

must be notified. The notification must include a detailed description of the GMO, including reference to existing risk assessment reports. The export may take place only upon the consent of the recipient county.

b) **Risk assessment:** Parties to the Protocol decide whether or not to accept GMOs primarily on the basis of scientific risk assessment procedures. Parties may decide to apply a precautionary approach and refuse the import of GMOs if the available scientific evidence is considered insufficient. Parties may also take into account socio-economic implications likely to result from the import of GMOs. Article 15 of 'Cartagena Protocol on Biosafety' enables a potential recipient to require the exporter to carry out a risk assessment. It may also charge the exporting country the full cost of the regulatory approval.

c) **Capacity-building and involvement of the public:** Article 22 expects the parties to the Protocol to cooperate in the development and/or strengthening of human resources and institutional capacities. Article 23 requires the involvement of the public in the decision making process.

d) **Biosafety clearing house:** In order to assist parties of the Protocol in its implementation and in order to facilitate the exchange of scientific, technical, environmental and legal information on, and experience with, GMOs, the Protocol established the Biosafety Clearing House as a central source of reference.

e) **GMOs intended for direct use as food or feed:** Parties in developing countries can declare through the Biosafety clearing house that they wish to take a decision based on risk assessment information before agreeing to accept an import.

Regulation in India

The government regulates the seed industry and the seed trade in various respects. The Seed Act of 1966, the Seeds Control Order of 1983, and the Seeds Policy of 1988 are the major components of policy specific to the industry. The Seed Act of 1966 and the Seeds Control Order of 1983 provide statutory backing to the system of variety release, seed certification and seed testing. Varieties are released after evaluation at multi-location trials for a minimum of three years. Varieties approved are "notified" which is an obligatory for certification. While all public sector varieties go through this process, it is not compulsory for private varieties (Guidelines for Research in Transgenic Plants, 1998).[10]

Major changes in this system of regulation are proposed in the National Seeds Policy of 2002. Under this policy, variety registration (*i.e.*, notification) is mandatory for all varieties, new and extant. The evaluation is done over three seasons of field trials. Besides regulating quality, the government has also controlled imports and exports of seed. The Seed Policy of 1988 allowed limited imports of commercial

10 Guidelines for Research in Transgenic Plants, 1998, DBT, Government of India *http://www.dbtindia.nic.in.*

seed. The proposed new Seed Policy of 2002 allows imports and exports of seeds of all crops. However, all imported seed is also required to go through the process of registration. The emphasis on registration in the new seeds policy ties in with the demands of the Plant Variety Protection and Farmer's Rights Act passed in 2001. This Act provides for plant breeder's rights, which requires extant and new plant varieties to be registered on the basis of characteristics relating to novelty, distinctiveness, uniformity and stability.

The other major change in intellectual property protection has been the change in patent laws. The Trade Related Aspects of Intellectual Property Rights (TRIPs) Agreement came into force in WTO member countries in 1995. This requires member countries to comply with fixed minimum standards for intellectual property rights protection. As a result, India has amended its Patent Act in 1999, 2002 and 2005. The major impact of these provisions has been to provide product patents in the area of pharmaceuticals. However, the changes have implications for biotechnology innovations as well. The TRIPs agreement requires that patents be provided for micro-organisms. It is unclear, however, to what extent the Indian law is consistent with this provision. It is also not known how the Indian patent office will choose to define micro-organisms.

The Seeds Bill, 2004 was taken up after a decade in 2014 is proposed as a replacement for the existing Seeds Act, 1966. The stated objective of the proposed law is to regulate the seed market and ensure seeds of "quality". With the proposed changes the seed law would be harmonised with other seed laws around the world and ensure the Indian seed market is open to big business. The rationale for a new act can be traced back to the relatively rapid changes that have been taking place in the seed sector in the past couple of decades. These include in particular the growing role of private seed companies and the progressive introduction of transgenic seeds. It was enacted to confirm stipulation in the TRIPS Agreement which authorized the seed growers to get their seeds patented. The farmers will not be allowed to exchange their seed without patents. The provisions of this act are really a cause of concern.[11]

GM Seeds: Issues and Challenges

A new technology represents both its positive and negative sides. But it is always better to minimize harmful effects and improve welfare of the technology. Any farmer in the world would continue to grow, save and breed the transgenic and non-transgenic crops that provide benefits to them. Genetically-modified foods have the potential to solve many of theworld's hunger and malnutrition problems, and to help, protect and preserve the environment by increasing yield and reducing reliance upon chemical pesticides and herbicides. Yet, there are many challenges ahead for governments, especially in the areas of safety testing, regulation, international policy and food labeling. Many people feel that genetic engineering is the inevitable motive of the future and that we cannot afford to

---

11 Vandana Shiva 2005.

ignore a technology that has such enormous potential benefits. However, we must proceed with caution to avoid causing unintended harm to human health and the environment from this powerful technology (WHO/EURO, 2000)[12]

The perceived negative forms and problems of the new technology in India may be grouped in the following categories:

(i) Illegal seeds, illiteracy and lack of awareness of the BT technology;
(ii) Lack of regulatory system in India;
(iii) Terminator seeds;
(iv) Refuge problems in India;
(v) Lack of Infrastructure;
(vi) Difference in expenditure of private sector and public sector
(vii) Food and human safety problems;
(viii) Problems of safe genetically modified food;
(ix) Religious factor in GM food; and
(x) Problems of labeling of genetically modified crops.

Perceived disadvantages of genetically modified crops may also include exchange of genetic material between the transgenic crop and related plant species and selection for resistance among populations of the target pests as well as other problems related to cultivation of genetically modified crops.

Conclusion

Global food demand is forecasted to be at least double by the year 2050 and the world population is expected to reach from the current 6.3 billion to 9.3 billion, of which about 90 per cent will reside in Asia, Africa and Latin America. The jump in the price of global food grains, naturally posed challenges to food security in India. Food grains production in India has not kept pace with the growth in population and demand. There are some reasons because of which the farmers in India failed to get optimum benefit from genetically modified crops, BT cotton. There is lack of irrigation, limited awareness of BT cotton, higher cost of BT cotton, illegal adoption of the genetically modified, old method of production *etc.* For failure of BT cotton cultivation, not only the farmers are responsible but also the authority of both states and Central government which are not providing adequate information and facility to the farmers so as the technology is new for them.

12 World Health Organization and Europe European Centre for Environment and Health (2000) "Release of Genetically Modified Organisms in the Environment: is it a Health Hazard?" *Report of a Joint WHO/EURO* – ANPA Seminar, Rome, Italy, 7-9 September.

Chapter 2

Plant Growth Promoting Rhizobacteria: Mechanism, Application, Advantages and Disadvantages

Anjali U. Joshi, Kavan N. Andharia, Priyank A. Patel, Rohit J. Kotadiya and Ramesh K. Kothari

UGC-CAS Department of Biosciences, Saurashtra University, Rajkot – 360005, Gujarat, India
e-mail: anjy021@gmail.com

ABSTRACT

Rhizobacteria are the bacteria found in rhizosphere which has positive effect on plants. These bacteria which can either be free-living or in symbiosis with plant roots stimulate the growth and health of the plants and termed as Plant Growth Promoting Rhizobacteria (PGPR). The major role of these bacteria is: (a) to supply nutrients to crops (b) to stimulate plant growth (c) to supress or inhibit the activity of plant pathogens (d) to improve soil structure (e) bioaccumulation or microbial leaching of inorganic compounds. The rhizobacteria promote the plant growth by two mechanisms: (i) Direct mechanism (Production of plant hormones, nitrogen fixation, phosphorous solubilization, and sequestering) (ii) Indirect Mechanism (Antibiotics and lytic enzymes, Induced resistance, HCN production and competition). PGPR have also been reported to aid in plant growth against stressed conditions like elevated salt concentration, petroleum hydrocarbon or trace metal level as well as other factors like drought condition, by enhancing the tolerance of plant. PGPR have gained acceptance as beneficial bacteria globally. They promote the plant growth when used as biofertilizer as well as biocontrol agents. When added as biofertilizers, PGPR increase the soil natural nutrient cycle and help in building soil organic matter and maintain the soil fertility. They have advantages over the use of chemical pesticides viz. they are cheaper and safer. However, when it comes to field application the use of PGPR is hindered because of incomplete understanding of mechanism of plant growth enhancement. Natural variation in the behaviour of the bacteria and sensitivity of the bacteria to environmental and soil conditions is another issue. PGPR have a narrow spectrum of biocontrol activity compared with synthetic pesticides and often exhibit inconsistent performance in practical agriculture. Selection, Mechanism, Application, Advantages of these bacteria would be the main focus of this chapter.

Keywords: Plant Growth Promoting Rhizobacteria, Biofertilizers, Biocontrol agent, Plant hormones, Bioleaching

The portion of soil in the close vicinity of roots, characterized by high microbial activity due to exudate nutrients, is defined as the rhizosphere [1]. According to Vessey [2], bacteria living in the rhizosphere, in or around the plant tissues and enhance the plant growth are collectively known as PGPR (plant growth promoting rhizobacteria). PGPR should possess the following inherent characteristics:

(i) They must be able to colonize the root surface
(ii) They must survive, multiply and compete with another microbiota
(iii) They must enhance plant growth (Kloepper, 1994).

Based on their functions, PGPR can be classified as (i) biofertilizers (increasing the availability of nutrients to plant), (ii) phytostimulators (plant growth promotion, generally through phytohormones), (iii) rhizoremediators (degrading organic pollutants) and (iv) biopesticides (controlling diseases, mainly by the production of antibiotics and antifungal metabolites) [3,4]. Based on the type of associations of PGPR with the roots, they can be separated into extracellular (ePGPR), existing in the rhizosphere, on the rhizoplane, or in the spaces between cells of the root cortex [5] and intracellular (iPGPR), which exist inside root cells, generally in specialized nodular structures (Table 2.1) [6].

Table 2.1: Types of PGPR based on their Association with Plant Roots

PGPR	*Examples*	*Reference*
ePGPR	*Agrobacterium*, *Arthrobacter*, *Azotobacter*, *Azospirillum*, *Bacillus*, *Burkholderia*, *Caulobacter*, *Chromobacterium*, *Erwinia*, *Flavobacterium*, *Micrococcous*, *Pseudomonas* and *Serratia etc.*	[7]
iPGPR	*Allorhizobium*, *Azorhizobium*, *Bradyrhizobium*, *Mesorhizobium* and *Rhizobium*	

Apart from the above bacteria, many researchers have reported actinomycetes as one of the major rhizospheric microorganisms giving magnificent benefits to plant growth [7, 8]. Giving few examples, *Micromonospora* sp., *Streptomyces* sp., *Streptosporangium* sp., and *Thermobifida* sp., have displayed great potential as biocontrol agents against different root fungal pathogens [7, 9]. PGPR exhibit some plant growth promotion (PGP) traits like biological nitrogen fixation, phosphate solubilization, ACC deaminase activity, and production of siderophores and phytohormones. Plant roots release various compounds, termed as root exudates, that attract microorganisms and the resulting association can be either beneficial or neutral or detrimental to plants [10, 11]. There can be a symbiotic, endophytic or associative interaction between the plants and bacteria with different degrees of proximity with the roots and surrounding soil as depicted in Figure 2.1. Type

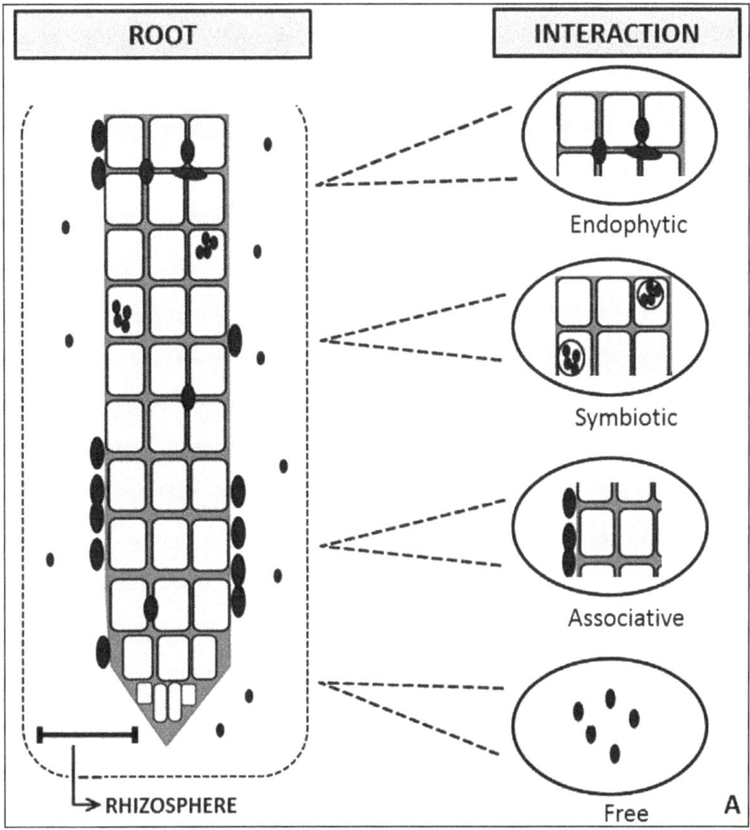

Figure 2.1: Interactions between Plants and Bacteria (Adapted from [16].

of root exudates, soil health and ability of the bacteria to colonize the plant roots decide the success and efficiency of PGPB as inoculants for agricultural crops. Only those bacteria who survive the microbial competition in the rhizosphere and are efficient in expression of several genes and cell-cell communication via quorum sensing can emerge as potential PGPR [12, 13, 14, 15].

Mechanisms of Plant Growth Promotion

According to Kloepper and Schroth [17], whole microbial community in rhizosphere niche needs to be altered to mediate the plant growth promotion by PGPR. Figure 2.2 shows various mechanisms of PGPR to promote plant growth directly or indirectly. PGPR promote the plant growth by either facilitating procurement of nitrogen, phosphorus and essential minerals or by controlling plant hormone levels, or indirectly by decreasing the inhibitory effects of various pathogens on plant growth and development in the forms of biocontrol agents [18].

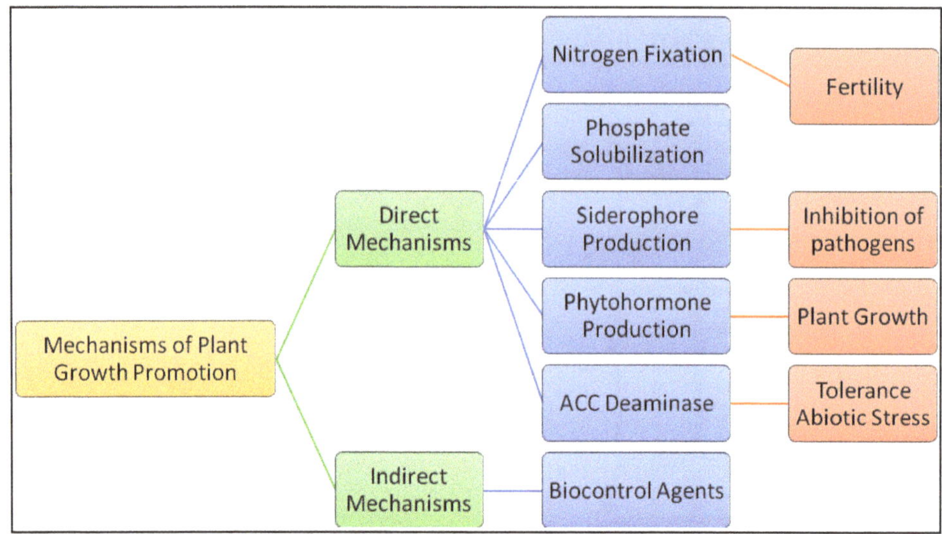

Figure 2.2: Mechanisms of Plant Growth Promotion.

Direct Mechanisms

1. Biological Nitrogen Fixation

Nitrogen (N) is the most vital nutrient for plant growth and productivity. The inorganic nitrogen (N_2) present in the atmosphere (78 per cent) cannot be utilized by plants for growth. Reduction of N_2 to ammonia (NH_3) is termed as Biological nitrogen fixation (BNF) performed in nitrogen fixing microorganisms, particularly bacteria and archaea [19] using a complex enzyme system known as nitrogenase [20]. Approximately, two-thirds of the nitrogen fixed globally occurs by BNF, while the rest of the nitrogen is industrially synthesized by the Haber–Bosch process [21]. N_2 fixers are widely distributed in nature and this ability of microorganisms can be economically beneficial alternative to chemical fertilizers [22, 23]. These microorganisms can be classified into two main groups named as (i) symbiotic

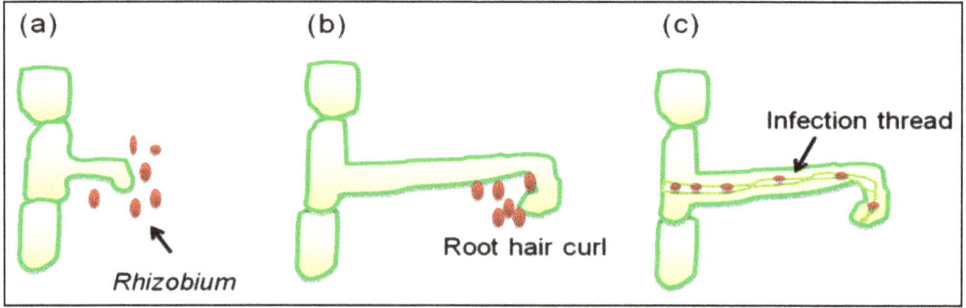

Figure 2.3: The Nodulation Process (a) Interaction and Attachment of *Rhizobium* with Root Cells of Host (b) Excretion of Nod Factors by Rhizobia Causes Root Hair Curling (c) Formation of Infection Thread and Nodule Formation (Adapted from [31]).

(symbiosis with leguminous plants and non-leguminous trees) and (ii) non-symbiotic, *i.e.*, free living, associative and endophytic nitrogen fixing organisms [7, 24, 25]. *Rhizobium* and *Frankia* are symbiotic nitrogen fixers whereas cyanobacteria *Anabaena, Nostoc, Azospirillum, Azotobacter, Gluconoacetobacter diazotrophicus* and *Azocarus etc.* are non-symbiotic nitrogen fixers. However, non-symbiotic N_2 fixers fix very small amount of nitrogen, but, enough to fulfil the requirement of the associated host plants [18]. Symbiosis of nitrogen fixing rhizobia (Family: Rhizobeaceae, Group: α-proteobacteria) and the roots of leguminous plants occur by formation of nodules where a complex process of infection and establishment takes place between the host and symbiont [26] (Figure 2.3). The diazotrophs, PGPR capable of fixing N_2 in non-leguminous plants form a non-obligate interaction with the host plants [27]. Dean and Jacobson [28] elucidated the structure of nitrogenaseas a two-component metalloenzyme consisting of (i) dinitrogenase reductase which is the iron protein and (ii) dinitrogenase which has a metal cofactor. The function of dinitrogenase reductase is to provide electrons with high reducing power while dinitrogenase uses these electrons to reduce N_2 to NH_3. N_2-fixing system varies among different bacterial genera in terms of structure. On the basis of metal cofactor, three different nitrogen fixing systems have been identified (a) Mo-nitrogenase, (b) V-nitrogenase and (c) Fe-nitrogenase. All diazotrophs use the molybdenum nitrogenase for nitrogen fixation [29]. The genes responsible for nitrogen fixation are *nif* genes present in both symbiotic and free-living systems [20]. Nitrogenase (*nif*) genes consist of structural genes, genes involved in activation of the Fe protein, iron molybdenum cofactor biosynthesis, electron donation, and regulatory genes. In diazotrophs, *nif* genes are typically found in a cluster of around 20–24 kb with seven operons encoding 20 different proteins [18]. The structure of molybdenum nitrogenase enzyme complex consist of two component proteins encoded by the *nifDK* and the *nifH* genes. The NifDK component is a hetero tetrameric (α2β2) protein formed by two ab dimers related by a twofold symmetry. NifDK carries one iron molybdenum cofactor (Fe Mo-co) within the active site in each α-subunit (NifD) [21]. In *Rhizobium,* activation of *nif*-genes is dependent on low oxygen concentration, which in turn is regulated by *fix*-genes found in both symbiotic and free-living nitrogen fixation systems [20, 28]. Table 2.2 indicates a brief list of all the rhizobial genes known to be involved in N fixation [30]. Nitrogen fixation process is a very energy demanding process, requiring at least 16 moles of ATP for each mole of reduced nitrogen.

Table 2.2: Rhizobial Genes involved in N Fixation

Genes	*Predicted Function*
nifA	Nif- specific regulatory protein, transcriptional activator
nifB	Fe - Mo cofactor biosynthesis protein
nifD	Nitrogenase molybdenum -iron protein, alpha chain
nifE	Nitrogenase molybdenum cofactor synthesis protein
nifH	Nitrogenase protein
nifK	Nitrogenase molybdenum - iron protein, beta chain
nifN	Nitrogenase Fe - Mo molybdenum cofactor biosynthesis protein
nifQ	Nitrogen fixation protein, molybdenum - iron binding

Genes	Predicted Function
nifR	Nitrogen regulation protein
nifS	Nitrogenase metallocluster biosynthesis protein, Cysteine desulfurase
nifU	Iron - sulphur cluster scaffold protein
nifW	Nitrogenase stabilizer
nifV	Homocitrate synthase
nifX	Iron - molybdenum cluster binding protein protein
nifZ	Nitrogen fixation protein
fixA	Nitrogen fixation protein, electron transfer flavo protein beta chain
fixB	Nitrogen fixation protein, electron transfer flavoprotein alpha chain
fixC	Nitrogen fixation protein, oxidoreductase
fixG	Iron sulphur binding domain
fixH	Nitrogen fixation cation transport protein
fixI	Transmembrane copper transport ATPase protein
fixJ	Two component nitrogen fixation regulatory protein
fixK	Ferrodoxin like protein, FNR/CRP transcriptional regulator
fixL	Two component nitrogen fixation oxygen regulated sensory histidine kinase
fixN	Cytochrome c oxidase
fixO	Cytochrome c oxidase
fixP	Cytochrome c oxidase membrane anchored subunit
fixQ	Cbb3 Cytochrome oxidase
fixR	Short chain dehydrogenase, oxidoreductase
fixS	Nitrogen fixation protein
fixU	Nitrogen fixation protein
fixX	Ferredoxin like protein

2. Phosphate Solubilization

Phosphorus (P) is the second important plant growth-limiting nutrient after nitrogen which is abundantly available in soils in both organic and inorganic forms (Figure 2.4) [32]. However, the available forms of P for plant uptake is very low. The plants absorb P only in two soluble forms, the monobasic ($H_2PO^-_4$) and the diabasic (HPO_4^{2-}) ions [7]. Insoluble forms of P available in soil include apatite (inorganic), inositol phosphate or soil phytate, phosphor monoesters, and phosphor triesters (organic) [18]. The phosphatic fertilizers applied to soil to overcome the P deficiency is costly and harmful to environment. Hence, it is important to explore for an ecologically safe and economically reasonable option for making P available in soil for plant growth. Phosphate solubilizing microorganisms (PSM) coupled with phosphate solubilizing activity may provide the available forms of P to the plants [33]. Phosphate-solubilizing bacteria (PSB) can be promising biofertilizers since they can supply plants with P by various mechanisms (Figure 2.5) [34]. Bhattacharyya and Jha [7] have reported *Azotobacter*, *Bacillus*, *Beijerinckia*, *Burkholderia*, *Enterobacter*, *Erwinia*, *Flavobacterium*, *Microbacterium*, *Pseudomonas*, *Rhizobium* and *Serratia*as the

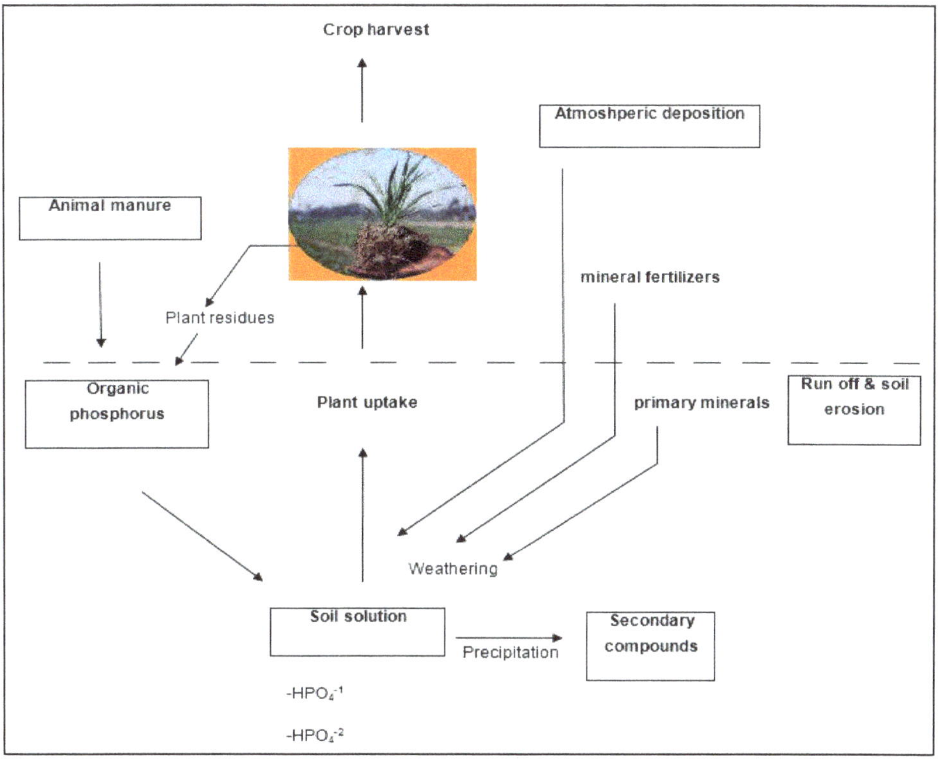

Crop harvest
Atmoshperic deposition
Animal manure
mineral fertilizers
Plant residues
Organic phosphorus
Plant uptake
primary minerals
Run off & soil erosion
Weathering
Soil solution
Precipitation
Secondary compounds
-HPO4-1
-HPO4-2

Figure 2.4: Phosphorous Mobilization is Soil (Adapted from [31]).

EPS produced by PSB hold free P from insoluble phosphate in the medium
Indirect dissolution of Ca-P compounds (organic P compounds)
Exo-polysaccharides
P Assimilation
Various molecules produced by PSB to solubilize P
Phytases
Inorganic Acids
Mineralization of organic P by bacterial enzymes
H+ excretion accompanying the decrease in pH
Acid Phosphatases
H+, (H+ + NH4+), (NH4+ - N), H2CO3, H2S
Organic Acids
Excretion of organic acids which chelate mineral ions or drop the pH to bring P into solution

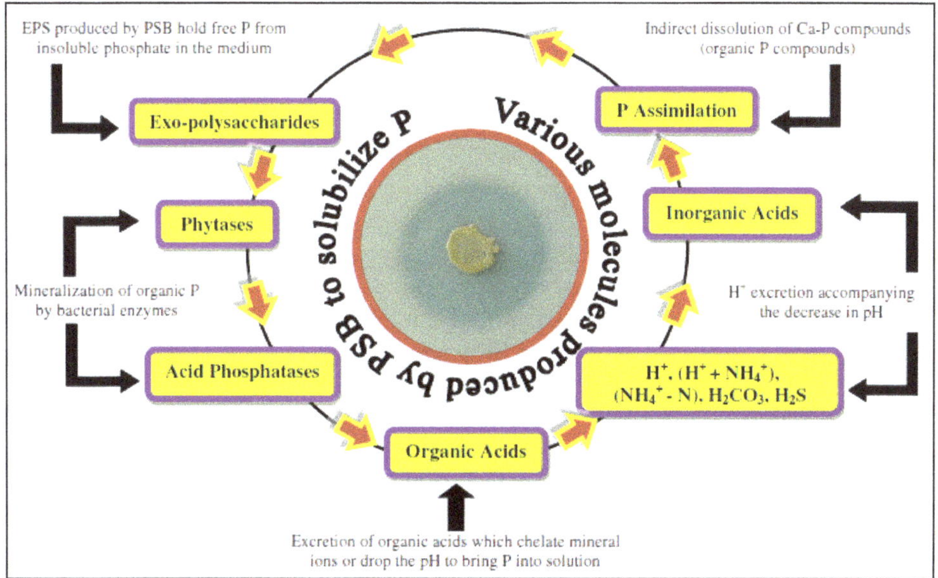

Figure 2.5: Various Mechanisms of PSB (Phosphate Solubilizing Bacteria) for Providing P to Plants (Adapted from [31]).

most significant phosphate solubilizing bacteria. Most of the soil bacteria including actinobacteria solubilize inorganic phosphate by secreting low molecular weight organic acids [34, 35] whereas mineralization of organic phosphorus occurs through the synthesis of a variety of different phosphatases, catalysing the hydrolysis of phosphoric esters [18]. Tao *et al.* [36] reported that phosphate solubilization and mineralization can coexist in the same bacteria. However, establishment and performance of PSB are affected by environmental factors [37, 38]. The beneficial effects of the inoculation with PSB used alone [39, 40] or in combination with other rhizospheric microbes have been reported [41, 42]. Apart from providing P to the plants, PSB enhance plant growth by stimulating the efficiency of BNF and also help providing other trace elements by synthesizing PGP hormones [34, 43, 44].

3. Siderophore Production

Iron is a vital nutrient for almost all forms of life. All microorganisms known hitherto, except certain lactobacilli, essentially require iron [45]. Iron is present as ferric ion (Fe^{3+}) in the aerobic environment and tends to form insoluble hydroxides and oxyhydroxides, which are inaccessible to plants and microorganisms [46]. Most of the bacteria acquire iron by the secretion of low-molecular mass iron chelators, siderophores. Siderophores are water-soluble present extracellularly or intracellularly. Some rhizobacteria are proficient in using siderophores of the same genus (homologous siderophores) while others could utilize those produced by other rhizobacteria of different genera heterologous siderophores [32]. In rhizobacteria, reduction of ferric Iron (Fe^{3+}) in Fe^{3+}-siderophore complex on bacterial membrane to ferrous iron (Fe^{2+}) takes place and ferrous iron is released into the cell from the siderophore using a gating mechanism linking the inner and outer membranes. In this process, the siderophore may be destroyed/recycled [45, 46]. Siderophores perform as solubilizing agents for iron from minerals or organic compounds under conditions of iron limitation [47]. Siderophores also form stable complexes with other heavy metals such as Al, Cd, Cu, Ga, In, Pb and Zn, as well as with radionuclides including U and Np that are of environmental concern, [48, 49]. Schmidt [50] concluded that bacterial siderophores help to ease the stresses imposed on plants by high levels of heavy metals in soil. Plants assimilate iron from bacterial siderophores by means of different mechanisms, *i.e.*, chelate and release of iron, the direct uptake of siderophore-Fe complexes, or by a ligand exchange reaction. Siderophore producing rhizobacterial inoculations help in the plant growth promotion via siderophore-mediated Fe-upake [46]. For instance, Crowley and Kraemer [51] studied that oat plant uses a siderophore mediated iron transport system for uptake of iron under iron-limited conditions. Similarly, *Pseudomonas fluorescens* C7 synthesized Fe-pyoverdine complex which was taken up by *Arabidopsis thaliana* plants, resulting in increase of iron inside plant tissues and hence plant growth was enhanced [52]. Similar study was carried out by Sharma *et al.*, [53] where the role of the siderophore-producing *Pseudomonas* strain GRP3 on iron nutrition of *Vigna radiate* was assessed. After 45 days, the plants showed a decline in chlorotic symptoms and iron, chlorophyll a and chlorophyll b content increased in strain GRP3 inoculated plants compared to control.

4. Phytohormone Production

Microorganisms possess the ability to synthesize and release a phytohormone auxin (indole-3-acetic acid/indole acetic acid/IAA) as the secondary metabolite [54]. Various soil bacteria secrete IAA which may alter the endogenous pool of plant IAA affecting the plant's developmental process [18, 55]. Evidently, IAA performs the function of a reciprocal signalling molecule affecting gene expression in several rhizobacteria. It can be concluded that IAA plays a very important role in rhizobacteria-plant interactions. As a signalling molecule, IAA also take part in plant defence mechanism by fighting against a variety of plant pathogens when applied exogenously. Thus, rhizobacterial IAA takes part in both pathogenesis and phytostimulation [56]. Santner *et al.*, [57] reported diversity of function is due to extraordinary complexity of IAA biosynthetic, transport and signalling pathways. IAA plays multifunctional role in plants for instance, IAA affects cell division, extension, and differentiation; stimulates seed and tuber germination; increases the rate of xylem and root development; controls processes of vegetative growth; initiates lateral and adventitious root formation; mediates responses to light, gravity and florescence; affects photosynthesis, pigment formation, biosynthesis of various metabolites, and resistance to stressful conditions. Apart from the above functions, bacterial IAA increases root surface area and length providing a greater access to soil nutrients. Also, rhizobacterial IAA loosens plant cell walls and facilitates an increasing amount of root exudation thus providing additional nutrients to support the growth of rhizosphere bacteria [18]. Amino acid tryptophan is the main precursor of IAA and is responsible for modulating the level of IAA synthesis [34]. It is a strange fact that tryptophan stimulates IAA production but, anthranilate, a precursor for tryptophan, reduces IAA synthesis. This mechanism is an advantage for IAA biosynthesis because tryptophan inhibits anthranilate formation by a negative feedback regulation on the anthranilate synthase, resulting in a fine-tuned IAA production [55]. When the culture media of rhizobacteria is supplemented with tryptophan, IAA production increases. Biosynthesis of tryptophan starts from the metabolic node chorismate in a five-step reaction encoded by the *trp* genes. The branch point compound chorismate is synthesized starting from phosphoenolpyruvate and erythrose4-phosphate in the shikimate pathway, a common pathway for the biosynthesis of aromatic amino acids and many secondary metabolites [54, 56]. Five different pathways starting from tryptophan have been reported: (1) IAA formation via indole-3-pyruvic acid and indole-3-acetic aldehyde is found in a majority of bacteria like, *Erwiniaherbicola;* saprophytic species of the genera *Agrobacterium* and *Pseudomonas;* certain representatives of *Bradyrhizobium, Rhizobium, Azospirillum, Klebsiella,* and *Enterobacter,* (2) The conversion of tryptophan into indole-3-acetic aldehyde may involve an alternative pathway in which tryptamine is formed as in pseudomonads and azospirilla, (3) IAA biosynthesis via indole-3-acetamide formation is reported for phytopathogenic bacteria *Agrobacterium tumefaciens, Pseudomonas syringae,* and *E. herbicola;* saprophytic pseudomonads like (*e.g. Pseudomonas putida* and *P. fluorescens*), (4) IAA biosynthesis that involves tryptophan conversion into indole-3-acetonitrile is found in the cyanobacterium (*Synechocystis* sp.), (5) The tryptophan-independent pathway, more common in plants, is also found in azospirilla and cyanobacteria (Figure 2.6) [55].

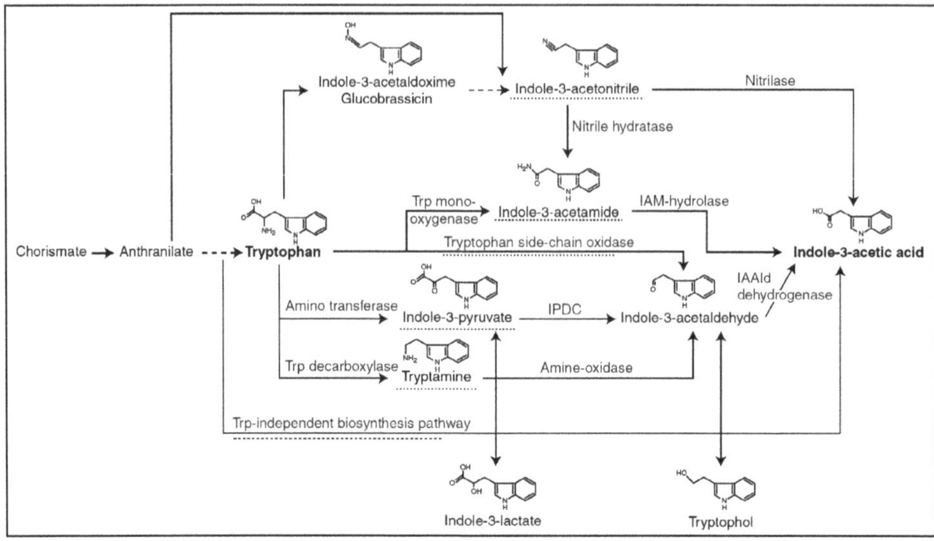

Figure 2.6: Overview of different Pathways for IAA Synthesis (Adapted from [55]).

Almost all *Rhizobium* species produce IAA [24, 58, 59]. Nodule formation involves cell division, differentiation and vascular bundle formation in which IAA is involved which in turn implies the fact that auxin levels in the host legume plants are necessary for nodule formation [18, 55]. For instance, inoculation with *Rhizobium leguminosarum bv. viciae* wherein the IAA biosynthetic pathway had been introduced, 60- fold more IAA containing root nodules were produced than nodules formed by the wild-type counterpart in *Vicia hirsute* [60]. Acidic pH, osmotic and matrix stress and carbon limitation are some environmental stress factors which modulate the IAA biosynthesis in different bacteria. Location of auxin biosynthesis genes (either plasmid or chromosomal) and the mode of expression (constitutive vs. induced) are the genetic factors affecting the level of IAA production [55, 56].

5. ACC Deaminase

Ethylene is an essential metabolite for the normal growth and development of plants and is produced endogenously by all plants and is also produced by different biotic and abiotic processes in soils and is important in inducing diverse physiological changes in plants [61]. Apart from being a plant growth regulator, ethylene is also recognized as a stress hormone as it negatively affects the plant growth by its increased level under stress conditions like those generated by salinity, drought, water logging, heavy metals and pathogenicity. For instance, the high concentration of ethylene induces defoliation and other cellular processes that may lead to reduced crop performance [7, 62]. The enzyme 1-aminocyclopropane-1-carboxylate (ACC) deaminase present in plant growth promoting rhizobacteria facilitate plant growth and development by decreasing ethylene levels and making the plants salt tolerant and drought resistant [63]. ACC deaminase activity have been exhibited by a wide range of bacteria such as *Acinetobacter, Achromobacter, Agrobacterium, Alcaligenes,*

Azospirillum, Bacillus, Burkholderia, Enterobacter, Pseudomonas, Ralstonia, Serratia and *Rhizobium etc.* [64, 65, 66, 67].

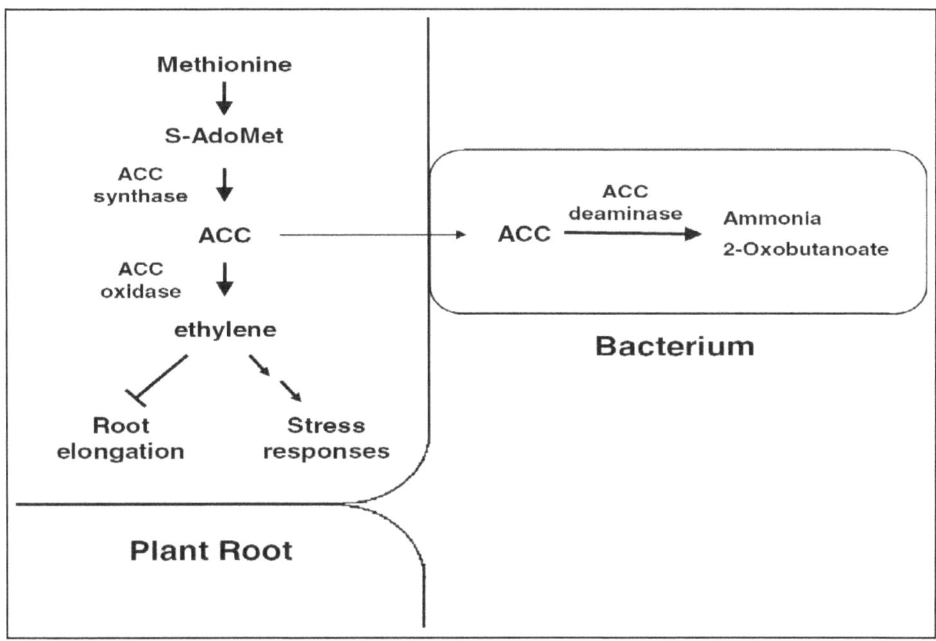

Figure 6.7: A Possible Mechanism of How Stress Controller Bacteria Reduce Ethylene Levels in the Plant Root using Bacterial ACC Deaminase (Adapted from [67]).

Figure 2.7 shows the uptake of ethylene precursor ACC by rhizobacteria which is converted into 2-oxobutanoate and NH_3 [68]. ACC deaminase producers relieves the plants from effects of phytopathogenic microorganisms (viruses, bacteria, and fungi *etc.*), and also protects the plants from the stress caused by polyaromatic hydrocarbons, heavy metals, radiation, wounding, insect predation, high salt concentration, extremes of temperature, high light intensity, and flooding [18, 69]. Consequently, ACC deaminase producing rhizobacteria enhance the plant growth by root elongation, promotion of shoot growth, and uptake of N, P and K as well as mycorrhizal colonization in various crops when inoculated as root or seed inoculant [18, 70].

Indirect Mechanisms

The major indirect mechanism of plant growth promotion in rhizobacteria is through acting as biocontrol agents (18). HCN, phenazines, pyrrolnitrin, 2, 4-diacetylphloroglucinol, pyoluteorin, viscosinamide and tensin are some of the antifungal metabolites produced by PGPR [7]. Modes of action of biocontrol in PGPR are competition for nutrients, niche exclusion, induced systemic resistance and antifungal metabolites production. Interaction of some rhizobacteria with the plant roots can result in plant resistance against some pathogenic bacteria, fungi, and viruses. This phenomenon is called induced systemic resistance (ISR) [69]. ISR

Table 2.3: Effects of PGPR on Various Plant Species to Fight against Adverse Environmental Conditions (Adapted from [71])

Sl.No.	Plants	Types of PGPR	Effect
1	*Prosopis juliflora* *Lolium multiflorum*	*Bacillus,* *Staphylococcus,* *Aerococcus*	Improved efficiency of phytoremediation of Chromium, Copper, Lead and Zinc
2	*Brassica napus*	*Bacillus megaterium*	Decreased Lead pollution in soil and increase in total yield of plant.
3	*Solanum lycopersicum*	*Bacillus,* *Amyloliquefaciens,* *Bacillus subtilis*	Resistance against Fusarium wilt, increase in lycopence content and improved texture of fruits
4	*Piper nigrum* *Cucumis sativus*	*Bacillus spp.*	P and K solubilisation, increase infertility of soil planted with cucumber and pepper
5	*Bacillus licheniformis*	*Arachis hypogaea*	Increased saline stress tolerace, increased biomass, increased root length and total length of plant.
6	*Helianthus annus* *Triticum aestivum*	*Bradyrhizobium* *Japonicum*	Excess plant biomass and organic matter in soil and growth promotion in high arsenic concentration

encompasses jasmonate and ethylene signalling inside the plant stimulating the host plant's defence responses against a wide variety of plant pathogens [18]. ISR can be induced by lipo-polysaccharides (LPS), flagella, siderophores, cyclic lipopeptides, 2, 4-diacetylphloroglucinol, homoserine lactones, and volatiles like, acetoin and 2, 3-butanediol [69].

Applications and Advantages

Plant growth promoting bacteria can have impact on plant growth by direct or indirect way. Synthesizing and providing a compound necessary for plant growth or facilitating the uptake of nutrient from the environment; can be considered as direct mechanism for plant growth promotion. While suppressing toxic effect of external non-native chemical compound, either of biological or chemical (men made) origin, or decreasing or preventing phytopathogenic effect of other microorganisms by one or more mechanisms; can be considered as indirect mechanism for promotion of plant growth and health. Besides soil, PGPR is also proved to promote the activities of bioremediation and biodegradation of hazardous substances present in air or water. Thus, Plant Growth Promoting Rhizobacteria (PGPR) technology can be widely recognized, offering the use of soil microorganisms in practicing sustainable and climate resilient agriculture, eliminating the use of chemical fertilizers and pesticides. Activity of PGPR is thus advantageous in two ways: 1) as biofertilizer 2) as biocontrol agent (Table 2.3) [71].

a) PGPR as Biofertilizers

Biofertilizers are the products, constituting living microorganisms, which, when applied to the seeds or plant surfaces adjacent to soil, can colonize rhizosphere or the interior parts of the plants and thereby promotes root growth. The PGPR functional as biofertilizer can be categorized into two groups, according to their mode of interaction with their host: (1) rhizospheric and (2) endophytic. In rhizospheric relationship, the PGPRs can colonize the rhizosphere or the surface of the root superficially [72]. Colonizing properties of rhizobacteria depends on soil pH, water potential and partial pressure of O_2 and plant exudation [73]. The endophytic PGPR are found to be settled in the apoplastic spaces of the host plants. In sugarcane plant, Dong *et al.*, reported presence of *Acetobacter diazotrophicus* as endophyte existing in the intercellular spaces of parenchyma tissue [74] while James *et al.*, reported the massive presence of *Gluconacetobacter diazotrophicus* in xylem vessel of the lower stem [75]. Thus, the attribute of the PGPR acting as biofertilizers, and thus enhancing the nutrient status of host plant, can be categorized into five distinct areas by mechanisms:

1. Biological N_2 fixation
2. Increasing the availability of nutrients in rhizosphere
3. Increase in root surface area
4. Enhancing beneficial symbioses of the host
5. Combinations of all the above modes of action

Some PGPR are reported to promote plant growth by acting as both; biofertilizer and biopesticide. For example, *Burkholderia cepacia* can stimulate growth of maize under iron-stress conditions via siderophore production as well as it has shown the biocontrol or antifungal activity against *Fusarium* spp. [76]. *Allorhizobium, Azorhizobium, Bradyrhizobium, Mesorhizobium, Rhizobium* and *Sinorhizobium* are the known potent PGPR strains for their ability to act as biofertilizers [2].

b) Rhizoremediation

Rhizoremediation is a process in which microorganisms degrade soil contaminants present in the rhizosphere region. Soil pollutants that are degraded by rhizospheric microbes are the organic compounds which cannot enter the plant because of their high hydrophobicity. PGPRs in rhizoremediation are of considerable importance, as inoculation with PGPRs can aid in enhancement in plant growth and development on contaminated soils. PGPR strains like *Pseudomonads* sp. and *Acinetobacter* sp. enhance uptake of Fe, Zn, Mg, Ca, K and P by crop plants [77] and PGPR in combination with AM fungi can be utilized in the solubilization of the heavy metals in contaminated soils and thereby increasing the chances of success in rhizoremediation, detoxifying chemicals, as well as crop succession [78].

c) Growth Enhancement

PGPRs have been used to support the plant growth, seed germination and overall yield of crop plants [79]. Plant growth characters like area of leaf, chlorophyll content and as a result total biomass have been reported to be increased; one such observation is made by Baset *et al.*, [80] in the musa plantlets as compared to the uninoculated control. Another observation was made by Dobbelaere *et al.*, [81]; when inoculated with *Azospirillum* sp., the growth of some agriculturally important plants and considerable increase in the dry weight of the root system and aerial parts of the plants were observed, which further resulted in better development and flowering. PGPR strains namely *Achromobacter xylosoxidans, Bacillus subtilis, B. licheniformis, B. pumilus, Brevibacterium halotolerans* and *Pseudomonas putida* are known for their role in plant growth promotion by cell elongation and increasing ACC deaminase activity [82]. Wheat crop depends on various factors like plant genotype, nature of PGPR inoculants as well as environmental conditions. Rice crops inoculated with arbuscular mycorrhizal fungi *Glomus* sp. and PGPR *Azotobacter chroococcum* showed maximum shoot biomass, shoot phosphorus and nitrogen content [83]. Thus, overall results of various research prove the influence of microbial inoculants in reducing the inorganic fertilizer demand approximately by 50 per cent.

d) Effects of PGPR on Root Growth

Auxins are the hormones responsible for plant cell division, cell growth and cell differentiation; overall one can say body development of plants. According to the tissue, auxins can promote lateral expansion in root, axial elongation in shoots and isodiametric expansion in fruits. Inoculation of seeds or cuttings of plants with PGPRs like *Agrobacterium, Alcaligenes, Bacillus, Pseudomonas,* and *Streptomyces* are reported to induce root formation [84]. As well as PGPRs have been reported for increasing the elongation rate of lateral roots, resulting in more branched root system formation in growing plants [85] which can be correlated to the production of auxin and inhibition of ethylene synthesis by PGPRs [86]. Erturk *et al.,* [87] investigated the effect of PGPRs on rooting and root growth of *Actinidia deliciosa* (kiwifruit) stem cuttings. *Bacillus* RC23, *Bacillus* RC03, *B. megaterium* RC01, *B. subtilis* OSU142, *B. simplex* RC19, *Comamonas acidovorans* RC41 and *Paenibacillus polymyxa* RC05 were the PGPRs under study. All the bacteria were found to be IAA producers. They concluded from the results that the highest rooting was obtained at 47.50 per cent for semihardwood stem cuttings from *Bacillus* RC03 and *B. simplex* RC19 treatments and 42.50 per cent for hardwood stem cuttings from *Bacillus* RC03. This observation can considerably support the usage of PGPR system for plant root development, rather using synthetic auxins.

e) PGPR as Biotic Elicitors

Elicitors are chemicals or bio factors of various sources that can trigger physiological and morphological responses in plants. It may be abiotic elicitors such as metal ions or inorganic compounds and biotic elicitors. It has now been observed that the treatment of plants with biotic elicitors can cause a sequence of defence reactions including the accumulation of a range of plant defensive bioactive molecules such as phytoalexins. Thus, elicitation is being used to induce the expression of genes responsible for the synthesis of antimicrobial metabolites. Rhizosphere microbes are best known to act as biotic elicitors, which can induce the synthesis of secondary products in plants [88]. Ajmalicine, serpentine, picrocrocin, crocetin, hyoscyamine and scopolamine, safranal compounds and tanshinone are recorded as the important metabolites produced by PGPR species in eliciting the physiological and morphological responses in crop plants.

f) Production of Volatile Organic Compounds

A few strains of PGPR can produce volatile organic compounds (VOCs), which can be an aiding mechanism in plant growth promotion. Synthesis of VOCs is a strain-specific phenomenon. During study with *Arabidopsis thaliana*, they reported *Bacillus subtilis* GB03, *Bacillus amyloliquefaciens* IN937a and *Enterobacter cloacae* JM22 releasing a mixture of volatile compounds like 2, 3-butanediol and acetoin. It's also been observed that VOCs produced by PGPR act as signalling molecules for plant-microbe (PGPR) interaction; only if they are produced in enough quantities to induce plant response [89]. Other VOCs reported are terpenes, jasmonates by Farmer [90] identified low-molecular weight plant volatiles such as and green leaf components as potent signal molecules for living organisms in different trophic levels. However, more focused investigation on plant-PGPR interactions is necessary for understanding the VOCs as signalling molecules in various plant responses.

g) Induction of Systemic Disease Resistance

Non-pathogenic strains of PGPR can induce systemic disease resistance in plants against broad spectrum phytopathogens [91, 92]. Different PGPR strains when blend in proper mixture and applied to the seeds or seedlings of certain plants; can result in increased efficiency of induced systemic resistance (ISR) against several pathogens [93]. Elbadry *et al.*, [92] treated seeds of fava bean (*Vicia faba L.*) with *Pseudomonas fluorescens* and *Rhizobium leguminosarum* and noted the systemic disease resistance against bean yellow mosaic potyvirus (BYMV) [92]. They isolated PGPR strains from the roots of fava bean; and examined singly or in combination for the induction of resistance in fava bean against BYMV, and reported significant reduction in disease incidence (PDI) compared to the non-bacterized plants. Bean seeds when treated with *Pseudomonas fluorescens* protected the plant against the halo blight disease caused by *Pseudomonas syringae pv. phaseolicola*. Similarly, Liu *et al.*, [94] studied induction of systemic resistance by *Pseudomonas putida* strain 89B-27 and *Serratia marcescens* strain 90–166 against Fusarium wilt of cucumber caused by *Fusarium oxysporum* sp. *cucumerinum*. Kloepper *et al.*, [95] treated cucumber seeds with rhizobacterial strains like *Pseudomonas putida* 89B-27 and *Serratia marcescens* 90–166 and recorded decrease in incidence of bacterial wilt.

As one more evidence we can consider investigations of Wei *et al.*, [96]. They treated cucumber seeds with a large number of PGPR strains such as *Pseudomonas putida* 89B-27, *Flavomonas oryzihabitans* INR-5, *Serratia marcescens* 90–166 and *Bacillus pumilus* INR-7 to induce systemic disease resistance against angular leaf spot disease caused by *Pseudomonas syringae pv. lachrymans*.

Several enzymes like chitinases, β-1, 3-glucanase, peroxidise (PO) and polyphenol oxidase (PPO) are reported to be synthesized by PGPR strains which can induce systemic resistance in plants [97]. Several strains of Bacillus like *B. amyloliquefaciens*, *B. subtilis*, *B. pasteurii*, *B. cereus*, *B. pumilus*, *B. mycoides* and *B. sphaericus* are recorded to elicit significant reduction in disease incidence on diversity of hosts in green house and field trials [98].

h) Resistance to Water Stress

Drought stress is one of the plant growth limiting environmental factor which affects productivity of agricultural crops. Inoculating the seeds or plants with PGPR can enhance the drought tolerance; which is possibly be regulated by the production of IAA, cytokinins, antioxidants and ACC deaminase. Inoculation with PGPR helps growth of the plants like tomatoes and peppers growing on water deficit soils [99]. More investigations on the mechanisms by which PGPR inducing tolerance to stress factors can be a useful piece of information to use these rhizobacteria in agriculture of arid and semi-arid area.

i) Quorum Sensing Signal Interference and Inhibition of Biofilm Formation

Quorum sensing (QS) is a genetic regulation mechanism at community level that controls microbiological functions of agricultural importance. Microbial Quorum sensing signalling in rhizospheric bacteria led to identification of numerous enzymatic and non-enzymatic signal interference mechanisms that could inhibit biofilm formation [100]. Quorum sensing responsible for cell–cell communication and the coordinated action in PGPR is mediated by an auto-inducer molecule. Most commonly reported auto inducer signal molecules are N- acyl homoserine lactones (AHLs) [101]; with a few more reported to be responsible for density-dependent signalling. Thus, in depth study of QS signal interference mechanisms in PGPR communication and succession in interactions is a possible scope of research in agricultural biotechnology.

j) Antagonistic Activity of PGPR

Rhizobacteria can suppress the growth of phytopathogens by various mechanisms like competing for nutrients and space, producing growth limiting factors like lytic enzymes and antibiotics, limiting the availability of iron (Fe) through producing siderophores [102]. Fluorescent *pseudomonads* are one of the most reported PGPR for its antagonistic activity against number of phytopathogens.

Delftia tsuruhatensis HR4 suppresses the growth of various plant pathogens like *Xanthomonas oryzae, Pyricularia oryzae*. Inoculating the soil with antagonist microbe, delivered in agricultural waste system are best way for supressing the root pathogens [103]. Pathogen, *Macrophomina phaseolina*, causing agent of charcoal rot of groundnut, is reported to be supressed by PGPR strains of *Rhizobium meliloti*; producing siderophores [104].

k) PGPR as Biocontrol Agent

PGPRs act as biocontrol agent by competitng for nutrients and niche, inducing systemic resistance and production of anti-fungal metabolites (AFMs) [105]. Commonly the PGPRs are reported to produce AFMs, of which phenazines, pyrrolnitrin, 2, 4-diacetylphloroglucinol (DAPG), pyoluteorin, viscosinamide and tensin are the frequently detected classes.

Pseudomonas fluorescens WCS374 has been reported to have genes phzO and phzH, responsible for the presence of functional group on phenazine compound, suppresses Fusarium wilt in radish leading to an overall 40 per cent of yield increase [106, 107]. Other strains, *Pseudomonas fluorescens* Pf-5 and *P. fluorescens* Q2-87 are able to produce pyoluteorin and 2, 4-diacetylphloroglucinol respectively [108]. *Azospirillum, Azotobacter, Bacillus, Enterobacter, Paenibacillus, Pseudomonas* and *Streptomyces* are the potent genera of PGPRs acting as biocontrol agent against tomato mottle virus, tobacco necrosis virus, *Rhizoctonia bataticola* and *Fusarium avenaceum etc.*

Experiments on the dual effect of PGPR and AM fungi led to a new inoculation preparation known as composite inoculation. Composite inoculums exhibited much better efficiency in disease suppression with the increase in chlorophyll content, total number of leaves, shoot height and overall crop yield. However, the PGPR strains used in composite inoculum did not affect populations of beneficial indigenous rhizosphere bacteria including the fluorescent pseudomonads and the siderophore-producing bacterial strains [7].

Disadvantages

a) Challenges in Selection and Characterization of PGPR

Developing PGPR based products for commercial application, one of the challenges is assurance of the effective selection and screening procedure, so as to bring forward the most promising organisms. Considering the host plant adaptation to a particular soil, climate conditions or pathogen can be useful for selection the isolation conditions, and screening [109, 110]. Approaches like spermosphere model, an enrichment technique in which seed exudates is used as the nutrient source, should be used for selection and isolation of PGPRs, like one used to screen promising N_2-fixing rhizosphere bacteria from rice [111]. Similarly for selection of organisms with the potential to control soil-borne phytopathogens, the isolate should be obtained from soils that are suppressive to that pathogen [112]. Other approaches involve selection based on attributes known to be associated with PGPR [113] like ACC deaminase activity [114, 115] and antibiotic [116] and siderophore production [114]. Development of high throughput assay systems and effective bioassays might help selecting the superior strains of PGPR [117, 118].

b) Challenges in Field Application of PGPR

The application of PGPR as biocontrol agent against fungal pathogens showed promising results in greenhouse systems [119]. But the environmental conditions in greenhouse are consistent throughout the season of crop plant. Achieving such consistent environmental conditions in the field is not possible, where variability of abiotic and biotic factors is higher and competition with indigenous organisms is more stressful.

Knowledge regarding these factors can help determining optimal timing of inoculation, type and concentration of PGPR strain and soil and crop management strategies to support the survival and proliferation of the PGPR [109, 118]. Thus, the concept of rhizosphere engineering to enhance PGPR function is gaining increasing attention [109, 120]. Developing better formulations or composite formulations to ensure the survival, proliferation and activity of PGPR in the field practices and to focus on compatibility with chemical seed treatments is another area of concern to overcome the limitations of PGPR to field application; approaches include optimization of growth conditions prior to formulation and development of improved carriers and application technology [121, 109, 122, 117, 123].

c) Challenges in Commercialization of PGPR

Prior to registration of commercialize PGPR products, a number of hurdles must be overcome [124, 117, 118] including scale up of fermentation conditions and commercial production of the organism while maintaining quality, stability, and efficacy of the product. During formulation development factors like shelf life, compatibility, cost, and ease of application should be taken into account. Toxigenicity, allergenicity and pathogenicity studies, as well as persistence in environment and horizontal gene transfer potential studies are required to improvise the health and safety measures of the products. Claiming the product under proper category is important, whether a biofertilizer or a biological control agent. Capitalization costs and potential markets must be studied in the decision to commercialize.

Future Prospects/Conclusion

Understanding the complexity of the rhizosphere environment, the mode of action of PGPR, and practical aspects about inoculants formulation and delivery systems, one can expect new PGPR products becoming available. The success of these products depends on our ability to manage and engineering the rhizosphere to support the survival and competitiveness of these microorganisms [109]. Rhizosphere management includes consideration of soil structure and composition and crop cultural practices, as well as inoculant formulation and delivery systems [109, 118]. Genetic manipulation techniques can aid to enhance colonization and effectiveness of PGPR strains; an attribute associated with plant growth promotion [105, 115, 125]. However, regulatory issues and public acceptance of genetically engineered organisms may delay their commercialization.

The use of multi-strain inoculums or composite inoculum of PGPR with known functions is important as these formulations may increase performance consistency in the field [126, 127]. PGPR technology offers an environmentally sustainable approach in agricultural production and health. The application of molecular tools helps precisely understanding and managing the rhizosphere; that may lead to new products with improved effectiveness.

References

1. Hiltner, L. (1904). Uber neuereerfahrungen und probleme auf demgebiet der bodenbakteriologie und unterbesondererberucksichtigung der grundungung und brache. Arb DtschLandwirtschGes 98, 59–78.
2. Vessey, J. K. (2003). Plant growth promoting rhizobacteria as biofertilizers. *Plant and soil, 255*(2), 571-586.
3. Somers, E., Vanderleyden, J., Srinivasan, M., 2004. Rhizosphere bacterial signalling: a love parade beneath our feet. Crit. Rev. Microbiol. 30, 205–240.

4. Antoun, H., Pre´vost, D., 2005. Ecology of plant growth promoting rhizobacteria. In: Siddiqui, Z.A. (Ed.), PGPR: biocontrol and biofertilization, Springer, Dordrecht, pp. 1–38.
5. Gray EJ and Smith DL (2005) Intracellular and extracellular PGPR: Commonalities and distinctions in the plant bacterium signaling processes. Soil BiolBiochem 37:395-412.
6. Figueiredo, M.V.B., Seldin, L., Araujo, F.F., Mariano, R.L.R., 2011. Plant growth promoting rhizobacteria:fundamentals and applications. In: Maheshwari, D.K. (Ed.), Plant Growth and Health Promoting Bacteria. Springer-Verlag, Berlin, Heidelberg, pp. 21–42.
7. Bhattacharyya, P. N., and Jha, D. K. (2012). Plant growth-promoting rhizobacteria (PGPR): emergence in agriculture. *World Journal of Microbiology and Biotechnology*, *28*(4), 1327-1350.
8. Merzaeva, O.V., Shirokikh, I.G., 2006. Colonization of plant rhizosphere by actinomycetes of different genera. Microbiology 75, 226–230.
9. Franco-Correa, M., Quintana, A., Duque, C., Suarez, C., Rodrý´guez, M.X., Barea, J.M., 2010. Evaluation of actinomycete strains for key traits related with plant growth promotion and mycorrhiza helping activities. Appl. Soil Ecol. 45, 209–217.
10. Lynch JM (1990) The rhizosphere. Wiley-Interscience, Chichester, 458 p.
11. Badri DV and Vivanco JM (2009) Regulation and function of root exudates. Plant Cell Environ 32:666-681.
12. Danhorn T and Fuqua C (2007) Biofilm formation by plant associated bacteria. Annu Rev Microbiol 61:401-422.
13. Meneses CH, Rouws LF, Simões-Araújo JL, Vidal MS and Baldani JI (2011) Exopolysaccharide production is required for biofilm formation and plant colonization by the nitrogen fixing endophyte *Gluconacetobacterdiazotrophicus*. Mol Plant-Microbe Interact 24:1448-1458
14. Alquéres S, Meneses C, Rouws L, Rothballer M, Baldani I, SchmidMand Hartmann A (2013) The bacterial superoxide dismutase and glutathione reductase are crucial for endophytic colonization of rice roots by *Gluconacetobacterdiazotrophicus*PAL5. Mol Plant-Microbe Interact 26:937- 945.
15. Beauregard PB, Chai Y, Vlamakis H, Losick R and Kolter R (2013) *Bacillus subtilis* biofilm induction by plant polysaccharides. Proc Natl AcadSci USA 110:E1621-E1630.
16. Souza, R.D., Ambrosini, A. and Passaglia, L.M., 2015. Plant growth-promoting bacteria as inoculants in agricultural soils. Genetics and molecular biology, 38(4), pp.401-419.
17. Kloepper, J.W., Schroth, M.N., 1981. Relationship of in vitro antibiosis of plant growth promoting rhizobacteria to plant growth and the displacement of root microflora. Phytopathology 71, 1020–1024.

18. Glick, B.R., 2012. Plant Growth-Promoting Bacteria: Mechanisms and Applications. Hindawi Publishing Corporation, Scientifica.

19. Dixon R and Kahn D (2004) Genetic regulation of biological nitrogen fixation. Nat Rev Microbiol 2:621-631.

20. Kim, J., Rees, D.C., 1994. Nitrogenase and biological nitrogen fixation. Biochemistry 33, 389–397.

21. Rubio, L.M., Ludden, P.W., 2008. Biosynthesis of the iron-molybdenummcofactor of nitrogenase. Annu. Rev. Microbiol. 62, 93–111.

22. Ladha, J.K., de Bruijn, F.J., Malik, K.A., 1997. Introduction: assessing opportunities for nitrogen fixation in rice-a frontier project. Plant Soil 124, 1–10.

23. Raymond, J., Siefert, J.L., Staples, C.R., Blankenship, R.E., 2004. The natural history of nitrogen fixation. Mol. Biol. Evol. 21, 541–554.

24. Ahemad, M., Khan, M.S., 2012d. Effects of pesticides on plant growth promoting traits of Mesorhizobium strain MRC4. J. Saudi Soc. Agric. Sci. 11, 63–71.

25. Zahran, H.H., 2001. Rhizobia from wild legumes: diversity, taxonomy, ecology, nitrogen fixation and biotechnology. J. Biotechnol.91, 143–153.

26. Giordano, W., Hirsch, A.M., 2004. The expression of MaEXP1, a Melilotusalbaexpansin gene, is upregulated during the sweet clover-Sinorhizobiummeliloti interaction. MPMI 17, 613–622.

27. Glick, B.R., Patten, C.L., Holguin, G., Penrose, G.M., 1999. Biochemical and Genetic Mechanisms Used by Plant Growth Promoting Bacteria. Imperial College Press, London.

28. Dean, D.R., Jacobson, M.R., 1992. Biochemical genetics of nitrogenase. In: Stacey, G., Burris, R.H., Evans, H.J. (Eds.), Biological Nitrogen Fixation. Chapman and Hall, New York, pp. 763–834.

29. Bishop, P.E., Jorerger, R.D., 1990. Genetics and molecular biology of an alternative nitrogen fixation system. Plant Mol. Biol. 41, 109–125.

30. Iyer, B. and Rajkumar, S., 2017. Host specificity and plant growth promotion by bacterial endophytes. Current Research in Microbiology and Biotechnology. 5(2), 1018-1030.

31. Ahemad, M. and Kibret, M., 2014. Mechanisms and applications of plant growth promoting rhizobacteria: current perspective. Journal of King Saud University-Science. *26*(1), 1-20.

32. Khan, M.S., Zaidi, A., Wani, P.A., Oves, M., 2009. Role of plant growth promoting rhizobacteria in the remediation of metal contaminated soils. Environ. Chem. Lett. 7, 1–19.

33. Khan, M.S., Zaidi, A., Wani, P.A., 2006. Role of phosphatesolubilizing microorganisms in sustainable agriculture – a review. Agron. Sustain. Dev. 27, 29–43.

34. Zaidi, A., Khan, M.S., Ahemad, M., Oves, M., 2009. Plant growth promotion by phosphate solubilizing bacteria. ActaMicrobiol. Immunol. Hung. 56, 263–284.

35. Jog, R., Pandya, M., Nareshkumar, G. and Rajkumar, S., 2014. Mechanism of phosphate solubilization and antifungal activity of Streptomyces spp. isolated from wheat roots and rhizosphere and their application in improving plant growth. Microbiology. *160*(4), 778-788.

36. Tao, G.C., Tian, S.J., Cai, M.Y., Xie, G.H., 2008. Phosphate solubilizing and -mineralizing abilities of bacteria isolated from. Pedosphere 18, 515–523.

37. Ahemad, M., Khan, M.S., 2012a. Effect of fungicides on plant growth promoting activities of phosphate solubilizing Pseudomonas putida isolated from mustard (Brassica compestris) rhizosphere. Chemosphere 86, 945–950.

38. Ahemad, M., Khan, M.S., 2012e. Alleviation of fungicide-induced phytotoxicity in greengram [Vignaradiata(L.) Wilczek] using fungicide-tolerant and plant growth promoting Pseudomonas strain. Saudi J. Biol. Sci. 19, 451–459.

39. Poonguzhali, S., Madhaiyan, M., Sa, T., 2008. Isolation and identification of phosphate solubilizing bacteria from Chinese cabbage and their effect on growth and phosphorus utilization of plants. J. Microbiol. Biotechnol. 18, 773–777.

40. Chen, Z., Ma, S., Liu, L.L., 2008. Studies on phosphorus solubilizing activity of a strain of phosphobacteria isolated from chestnut type soil in China. Biores. Technol. 99, 6702–6707.

41. Zaidi, A., Khan, M.S., 2005. Interactive effect of rhizospheric microorganisms on growth, yield and nutrient uptake of wheat. J. Plant Nutr. 28, 2079–2092.

42. Vikram, A., Hamzehzarghani, H., 2008. Effect of phosphate solubilizing bacteria on nodulation and growth parameters of greengram (Vigna radiate L. Wilczec). Res. J. Microbiol. 3, 62–72.

43. Suman, A., Shasany, A.K., Singh, M., Shahi, H.N., Gaur, A., Khanuja, S.P.S., 2001. Molecular assessment of diversity among endophytic diazotrophs isolated from subtropical Indian sugarcane. World J. Microbiol. Biotechnol. 17, 39–45.

44. Ahmad, F., Ahmad, I., Khan, M.S., 2008. Screening of free-living rhizospheric bacteria for their multiple plant growth promoting activities. Microbiol. Res. 163, 173–181.

45. Neilands, J.B., 1995. Siderophores: structure and function of microbial iron transport compounds. J. Biol. Chem. 270, 26723–26726.

46. Rajkumar, M., Ae, N., Prasad, M.N.V., Freitas, H., 2010. Potential of siderophore-producing bacteria for improving heavy metal phytoextraction. Trends Biotechnol. 28, 142–149.

47. Indiragandhi, P., Anandham, R., Madhaiyan, M., Sa, T.M., 2008. Characterization of plant growth-promoting traits of bacteria isolated from larval guts of diamondback moth Plutellaxylostella(Lepidoptera: Plutellidae). Curr. Microbiol. 56, 327–333.

48. Kiss, T., Farkas, E., 1998. Metal-binding ability of desferrioxamine B. J. Inclusion Phenom. Mol. Recognit. Chem. 32, 385–403.

49. Neubauer, U., Furrer, G., Kayser, A., Schulin, R., 2000. Siderophores, NTA, and citrate: potential soil amendments to enhance heavy metal mobility in phytoremediation. Int. J. Phytoremediation 2, 353–368.

50. Schmidt, W., 1999. Mechanisms and regulation of reduction-based iron uptake in plants. New Phytol. 141, 1–26.

51. Crowley, D.E., Kraemer, S.M., 2007. Function of siderophores in the plant rhizosphere. In: Pinton, R. *et al.* (Eds.), The Rhizosphere, Biochemistry and Organic Substances at the Soil-Plant Interface. CRC Press, pp. 73–109.

52. Vansuyt, G., Robin, A., Briat, J.F., Curie, C., Lemanceau, P., 2007. Iron acquisition from Fe-pyoverdine by Arabidopsis thaliana. Mol. Plant Microbe Interact. 20, 441–447.

53. Sharma, A., Johri, B.N., Sharma, A.K., Glick, B.R., 2003. Plant growth-promoting bacterium Pseudomonas sp. strain GRP3 influences iron acquisition in mung bean (VignaradiataL. Wilzeck). Soil Biol. Biochem. 35, 887–894.

54. Patten, C.L., Glick, B.R., 1996. Bacterial biosynthesis of indole-3- acetic acid. Can. J. Microbiol. 42, 207–220.

55. Spaepen, S., Vanderleyden, J., Remans, R., 2007. Indole- 3-acetic acid in microbial and microorganism-plant signaling. FEMS Microbiol. Rev. 31, 425–448.

56. Spaepen, S., Vanderleyden, J., 2011. Auxin and plant-microbe interactions. Cold Spring Harb. Perspect. Biol. http://dx.doi.org/10.1101/cshperspect.a001438.

57. Santner, A., Calderon-Villalobos, L.I.A., Estelle, M., 2009. Plant hormones are versatile chemical regulators of plant growth. Nature Chem. Biol. 5, 301–307.

58. Ahemad, M., Khan, M.S., 2012b. Ecological assessment of biotoxicity of pesticides towards plant growth promoting activities of pea (Pisumsativum)-specific Rhizobium sp. strain MRP1. Emirates J. Food Agric. 24, 334–343.

59. Ahemad, M., Khan, M.S., 2012f. Productivity of greengram in tebuconazole-stressed soil, by using a tolerant and plant growthpromotingBradyrhizobiumsp. MRM6 strain. Acta Physiol. Plant.34, 245–254.

60. Camerini, S., Senatore, B., Lonardo, E., Imperlini, E., Bianco, C., Moschetti, G., Rotino, G.L., Campion, B., Defez, R., 2008. Introduction of a novel pathway for IAA biosynthesis to rhizobia alters vetch root nodule development. Arch. Microbiol. 190, 67–77.

61. Khalid, A., Akhtar, M.J., Mahmood, M.H., Arshad, M., 2006. Effect of substrate-dependent microbial ethylene production on plant growth. Microbiology 75, 231–236.

62. Saleem, M., Arshad, M., Hussain, S., Bhatti, A.S., 2007. Perspective of plant growth promoting rhizobacteria (PGPR) containing ACC deaminase in stress agriculture. J. Indian Microbiol. Biotechnol. 34, 635–648.

63. Nadeem, S.M., Zahir, Z.A., Naveed, M., Arshad, M., 2007. Preliminary investigations on inducing salt tolerance in maize through inoculation with rhizobacteria containing ACC deaminase activity. Can. J. Microbiol. 53, 1141–1149.
64. Shaharoona, B., Arshad, M., Khalid, A., 2007a. Differential response of etiolated pea seedlings to inoculation with rhizobacteria capable of utilizing 1-aminocyclopropane-1-carboxylate or L-methionine. J. Microbiol. 45, 15–20.
65. Shaharoona, B., Jamro, G.M., Zahir, Z.A., Arshad, M., Memon, K.S., 2007b. Effectiveness of various Pseudomonas spp. And Burkholderiacaryophylli containing ACC-deaminase for improving growth and yield of wheat (TriticumaestivumL.). J. Microbiol. Biotechnol. 17, 1300–1307.
66. Zahir, Z.A., Ghani, U., Naveed, M., Nadeem, S.M., Asghar, H.N., 2009. Comparative effectiveness of Pseudomonas and Serratiasp. containing ACC-deaminase for improving growth and yield of wheat (TriticumaestivumL.) under salt-stressed conditions. Arch. Microbiol. 191, 415–424.
67. Kang, B.G., Kim, W.T., Yun, H.S., Chang, S.C., 2010. Use of plant growth-promoting rhizobacteria to control stress responses of plant roots. Plant Biotechnol. Rep. 4, 179–183.
68. Arshad, M., Saleem, M., Hussain, S., 2007. Perspectives of bacterial ACC deaminase in phytoremediation. Trends Biotechnol. 25, 356–362.
69. Lugtenberg, B., Kamilova, F., 2009. Plant-growth-promoting rhizobacteria. Annu. Rev. Microbiol. 63, 541–556.
70. Shaharoona, B., Naveed, M., Arshad, M., Zahir, Z.A., 2008. Fertilizer-dependent efficiency of Pseudomonads for improving growth, yield, and nutrient use efficiency of wheat (TriticumaestivumL.). Appl. Microbiol. Biotechnol. 79, 147–155.
71. Srivastava, R. (2017). Plant Growth Promoting Rhizobacteria (PGPR) for Sustainable Agriculture. International Journal of Agricultural Science and Research,7(4), 505-510.
72. McCully, M. E. (2001). Niches for bacterial endophytes in crop plants: a plant biologist's view. *Functional Plant Biology, 28*(9), 983-990.
73. Griffiths, B. S., Ritz, K., Ebblewhite, N., and Dobson, G. (1998). Soil microbial community structure: effects of substrate loading rates. *Soil Biology and Biochemistry, 31*(1), 145-153.
74. Dong, Z., McCully, M. E., and Canny, M. J. (1997). Does Acetobacter diazotrophicus live and move in the xylem of sugarcane stems? Anatomical and physiological data. *Annals of Botany, 80*(2), 147-158
75. James, E. K., Olivares, F. L., de Oliveira, A. L., dos Reis Jr, F. B., da Silva, L. G., and Reis, V. M. (2001). Further observations on the interaction between sugar cane and Gluconacetobacter diazotrophicus under laboratory and greenhouse conditions. *Journal of Experimental Botany, 52*(357), 747-760.

76. Bevivino, A., Sarrocco, S., Dalmastri, C., Tabacchioni, S., Cantale, C., and Chiarini, L. (1998). Characterization of a free-living maize-rhizosphere population of Burkholderia cepacia: effect of seed treatment on disease suppression and growth promotion of maize. *FEMS Microbiology Ecology*, *27*(3), 225-237.

77. Esitken, A., Pirlak, L., Turan, M., and Sahin, F. (2006). Effects of floral and foliar application of plant growth promoting rhizobacteria (PGPR) on yield, growth and nutrition of sweet cherry. *Scientia Horticulturae*, *110*(4), 324-327.

78. Denton, B. P. (2007). Advances in phytoremediation of heavy metals using plant growth promoting bacteria and fungi. *MMG 445 Basic Biotechnology eJournal*, *3*(1), 1-5.

79. Minorsky, P. V. (2008). On the inside. *Plant Physiology*, *146*(3), 1020-1021.

80. Baset, M., Shamsuddin, Z. H., Wahab, Z., and Marziah, M. (2010). Effect of Plant Growth Promoting Rhizobacterial (PGPR) Inoculation on Growth and Nitrogen Incorporation of Tissue-cultured'Musa'Plantlets under Nitrogen-free Hydroponics Condition. *Australian Journal of Crop Science*, *4*(2), 85.

81. Dobbelaere, S., Croonenborghs, A., Thys, A., Ptacek, D., Vanderleyden, J., Dutto, P., Labandera-Gonzalez, C., Caballero-Mellado, J., Aguirre, J.F., Kapulnik, Y. and Brener, S. (2001). Responses of agronomically important crops to inoculation with Azospirillum. *Functional Plant Biology*, *28*(9), 871-879.

82. Sgroy, V., Cassán, F., Masciarelli, O., Del Papa, M. F., Lagares, A., and Luna, V. (2009). Isolation and characterization of endophytic plant growth-promoting (PGPB) or stress homeostasis-regulating (PSHB) bacteria associated to the halophyte Prosopis strombulifera. *ApplIed microbiology and Biotechnology*, *85*(2), 371-381.

83. Ahanthem, S., and Jha, D. K. (2007). Response of rice crop inoculated with arbuscular mycorrhizal fungi and plant growth promoting rhizobacteria to different soil nitrogen concentrations. *Mycorrhiza News*, *18*(4), 15-20.

84. Esitken, A., Karlidag, H., Ercisli, S., Turan, M., and Sahin, F. (2003). The effect of spraying a growth promoting bacterium on the yield, growth and nutrient element composition of leaves of apricot (Prunus armeniaca L. cv. Hacihaliloglu). *Australian Journal of Agricultural Research*, *54*(4), 377-380.

85. Kapulnik, Y., Okon, Y., and Henis, Y. (1985). Changes in root morphology of wheat caused by Azospirillum inoculation. *Canadian Journal of Microbiology*, *31*(10), 881-887.

86. Steenhoudt, O., and Vanderleyden, J. (2000). Azospirillum, a free-living nitrogen-fixing bacterium closely associated with grasses: genetic, biochemical and ecological aspects. *FEMS microbiology reviews*, *24*(4), 487-506.

87. Erturk, Y., Ercisli, S., Haznedar, A., and Cakmakci, R. (2010). Effects of plant growth promoting rhizobacteria (PGPR) on rooting and root growth of kiwifruit (Actinidia deliciosa) stem cuttings. *Biological research*, *43*(1), 91-98.

88. Sekar, S., and Kandavel, D. (2010). Interaction of plant growth promoting rhizobacteria (PGPR) and endophytes with medicinal plants–new avenues for phytochemicals. *Journal of Phytology, 2*(7).

89. Ryu, C. M., Farag, M. A., Hu, C. H., Reddy, M. S., Wei, H. X., Paré, P. W., and Kloepper, J. W. (2003). Bacterial volatiles promote growth in Arabidopsis. *Proceedings of the National Academy of Sciences, 100*(8), 4927-4932.

90. Farmer, E. E. (2001). Surface-to-air signals. *Nature, 411*(6839), 854-856.

91. Kloepper, J. W., Ryu, C. M., and Zhang, S. (2004). Induced systemic resistance and promotion of plant growth by Bacillus spp. *Phytopathology, 94*(11), 1259-1266.

92. Elbadry, M., Taha, R. M., Eldougdoug, K. A., and Gamal-Eldin, H. (2006). Induction of systemic resistance in faba bean (Vicia faba L.) to bean yellow mosaic potyvirus (BYMV) via seed bacterization with plant growth promoting rhizobacteria *Journal of plant diseases and protection*, 247-251.

93. Ramamoorthy, V., Viswanathan, R., Raguchander, T., Prakasam, V., and Samiyappan, R. (2001). Induction of systemic resistance by plant growth promoting rhizobacteria in crop plants against pests and diseases. *Crop protection, 20*(1), 1-11.

94. Liu, L., Kloepper, J. W., and Tuzun, S. (1995). Induction of systemic resistance in cucumber against Fusarium wilt by plant growth-promoting rhizobacteria. *Phytopathology, 85*(6), 695-698.

95. Kloepper, J. W., Tuzun, S., Liu, L., and Wei, G. (1993). Plant growth-promoting rhizobacteria as inducers of systemic disease resistance. *Pest management: biologically based technologies. American Chemical Society Books, Washington, DC*, 156-165.

96. Wei, G., Kloepper, J. W., and Tuzun, S. (1996). Induced systemic resistance to cucumber diseases and increased plant growth by plant growth-promoting rhizobacteria under field conditions. *Phytopathology, 86*(2), 221-224.

97. Bharathi, S. (2004). *Developing botanical formulations for the management of major fungal diseases of tomato and onion* (Doctoral Dissertation, Tamil nadu Agricultural University Coimbatore).

98. Ryu, C. M., Farag, M. A., Hu, C. H., Reddy, M. S., Kloepper, J. W., and Paré, P. W. (2004). Bacterial volatiles induce systemic resistance in Arabidopsis. *Plant physiology, 134*(3), 1017-1026.

99. Aroca, R., and Ruiz-Lozano, J. M. (2009). Induction of plant tolerance to semi-arid environments by beneficial soil microorganisms–a review. In *Climate change, intercropping, pest control and beneficial microorganisms* (pp. 121-135). Springer Netherlands.

100. Ren, D., Sims, J. J., and Wood, T. K. (2001). Inhibition of biofilm formation and swarming of Escherichia coli by (5Z) 4 bromo 5 (bromomethylene) 3 butyl 2 (5H) furanone. *Environmental Microbiology, 3*(11), 731-736.

101. von Bodman, S. B., Bauer, W. D., and Coplin, D. L. (2003). Quorum sensing in plant-pathogenic bacteria. *Annual review of phytopathology*, *41*(1), 455-482.

102. Jing, Y.D., He, Z.L., and Yang, X.E. (2007). Role of soil rhizobacteria in phytoremediation of heavy metal contaminated soils. Journal of Zhejiang University SCIENCE B, 8(3), 192-207.

103. Sultana, V., Ara, J., Parveen, G., Ehteshamul-Haque, S., and Ahmad, V. U. (2006). Role of crustacean chitin, fungicides and fungal antagonist on the efficacy of Pseudomonas aeruginosa in protecting chilli from root rot. *Pakistan Journal of Botany*, *38*(4), 1323.

104. Arora, N. K., Kang, S. C., and Maheshwari, D. K. (2001). Isolation of siderophore-producing strains of Rhizobium meliloti and their biocontrol potential against Macrophomina phaseolina that causes charcoal rot of groundnut. *Current Science*, 673-677.

105. Bloemberg, G. V., and Lugtenberg, B. J. (2001). Molecular basis of plant growth promotion and biocontrol by rhizobacteria. *Current opinion in plant biology*, 4(4), 343-350.

106. Bakker, P. A., Pieterse, C. M., and Van Loon, L. C. (2007). Induced systemic resistance by fluorescent Pseudomonas spp. *Phytopathology*, *97*(2), 239-243.

107. Chin-A-Woeng, T. F., Thomas-Oates, J. E., Lugtenberg, B. J., and Bloemberg, G. V. (2001). Introduction of the phzH gene of Pseudomonas chlororaphis PCL1391 extends the range of biocontrol ability of phenazine-1-carboxylic acid-producing *Pseudomonas* spp. strains. *Molecular plant-microbe interactions*, *14*(8), 1006-1015.

108. Kidarsa, T. A., Goebel, N. C., Zabriskie, T. M., and Loper, J. E. (2011). Phloroglucinol mediates cross talk between the pyoluteorin and 2, 4 diacetylphloroglucinol biosynthetic pathways in Pseudomonas fluorescens Pf 5. *Molecular microbiology*, *81*(2), 395-414.

109. Bowen, G. D., and Rovira, A. D. (1999). The rhizosphere and its management to improve plant growth. *Advances in agronomy*, *66*, 1-102.

110. Chanway, C. P., Nelson, L. M., and Holl, F. B. (1988). Cultivar-specific growth promotion of spring wheat (Triticum aestivum L.) by coexistent Bacillus species. *Canadian journal of microbiology*, *34*(7), 925-929.

111. Thomas-Bauzon, D., Weinhard, P., Villecourt, P., and Balandreau, J. (1982). The spermosphere model. I. Its use in growing, counting, and isolating N2-fixing bacteria from the rhizosphere of rice. *Canadian Journal of Microbiology*, *28*(8), 922-928.

112. Weller, D. M., Raaijmakers, J. M., Gardener, B. B. M., and Thomashow, L. S. (2002). Microbial populations responsible for specific soil suppressiveness to plant pathogens. *Annual review of phytopathology*, *40*(1), 309-348.

113. Silva, H. S. A., Romeiro, R. D. S., and Mounteer, A. (2003). Development of a root colonization bioassay for rapid screening of rhizobacteria for potential biocontrol agents. *Journal of Phytopathology*, *151*(1), 42-46.

114. Cattelan, A. J., Hartel, P. G., and Fuhrmann, J. J. (1999). Screening for plant growth–promoting rhizobacteria to promote early soybean growth. *Soil Science Society of America Journal*, *63*(6), 1670-1680.

115. Glick, B. R. (1995). The enhancement of plant growth by free-living bacteria. *Canadian Journal of Microbiology*, *41*(2), 109-117.

116. Giacomodonato, M. N., Pettinari, M. J., Souto, G. I., Méndez, B. S., and López, N. I. (2001). A PCR-based method for the screening of bacterial strains with antifungal activity in suppressive soybean rhizosphere. *World Journal of Microbiology and Biotechnology*, *17*(1), 51-55.

117. Mathre, D. E., Cook, R. J., and Callan, N. W. (1999). From discovery to use: traversing the world of commercializing biocontrol agents for plant disease control. *Plant Disease*, *83*(11), 972-983.

118. McSpadden Gardener, B. B., and Fravel, D. R. (2002). Biological control of plant pathogens: research, commercialization, and application in the USA. *Plant Health Progress*, *10*(10.1094).

119. Paulitz, T. C., and Bélanger, R. R. (2001). Biological control in greenhouse systems. *Annual review of phytopathology*, *39*(1), 103-133.

120. Mansouri, H., Petit, A., Oger, P., and Dessaux, Y. (2002). Engineered rhizosphere: the trophic bias generated by opine-producing plants is independent of the opine type, the soil origin, and the plant species. *Applied and environmental microbiology*, *68*(5), 2562-2566.

121. Bashan, Y. (1998). Inoculants of plant growth-promoting bacteria for use in agriculture. *Biotechnology advances*, *16*(4), 729-770.

122. Date, R. A. (2001). Advances in inoculant technology: a brief review. *Australian Journal of Experimental Agriculture*, *41*(3), 321-325.

123. Yardin, M. R., Kennedy, I. R., and Thies, J. E. (2000). Development of high quality carrier materials for field delivery of key microorganisms used as bio-fertilisers and bio-pesticides. *Radiation Physics and Chemistry*, *57*(3), 565-568.

124. Fravel, D. R., Rhodes, D. J., and Larkin, R. P. (1999). Production and commercialization of biocontrol products. In *Integrated pest and disease management in greenhouse crops* (pp. 365-376). Springer, Dordrecht.

125. Lübeck, P. S., Hansen, M., and Sørensen, J. (2000). Simultaneous detection of the establishment of seed-inoculated Pseudomonas fluorescens strain DR54 and native soil bacteria on sugar beet root surfaces using fluorescence antibody and in situ hybridization techniques. *FEMS microbiology ecology*, *33*(1), 11-19.

126. Jetiyanon, K., and Kloepper, J. W. (2002). Mixtures of plant growth-promoting rhizobacteria for induction of systemic resistance against multiple plant diseases. *Biological control*, *24*(3), 285-291.

127. Siddiqui, I. A., and Shaukat, S. S. (2002). Resistance against the damping off fungus Rhizoctonia solani systemically induced by the plant growth promoting rhizobacteria Pseudomonas aeruginosa (IE 6S+) and P. fluorescens (CHA0). *Journal of Phytopathology*, *150*(8 9), 500-506.

Chapter 3

Integrating the Role of Computational and Imaging Methods in Crop Protection and Management: Insights in a New Age of Precision Agriculture

Gayatri Dave

Department of Biotechnology, P D Patel Institute of Applied Sciences
Charotar University of Science and Technology, Changa, Gujarat - 388421
e-mail: gayatridave.bt@charusat.ac.in

ABSTRACT

Precision farming integrates the technologies like remote sensing, global positioning system and geographical information system with traditional agriculture practices. It can be define as the location specific, time-specific and plant specific agriculture practice for sustainable development of agriculture. It works through obtaining the images from satellites, these images are further transformed to geographical coordinates and subsequently used to guide the farmers. It is more than simple image processing practice, the cameras are allied with variety of sensors that captures the sensor-guided images. This allows the real-time monitoring of the dynamic field condition through sensors. Proximal and non- proximal sensors are common types of sensors that usually used in precision agriculture. Principally, it detects the difference between the absorbed and reflected light for object under study. In further advancement, these sensors can be mounted on farming vehicles that embarks the access to the larger field. It provides the real time information on plant pathogens, weeds distribution and location, nutrient stress, nutrient burden, water stress and other soil parameters such as soil salinity. This precision farming practice is an eco-friendly way that reduce the burden on environment through reducing the nutrient and pesticide over-load.

Keywords: *Precision agriculture, Global positioning system, Sensors.*

Introduction

Plant cultivation is an ancient practice dates back to 14000 BC[1] that advances with evolution in human races. Presently, the traditional plant breeding practices requiring the huge land have shifted to miniature scale laboratory flasks. This progress of in-vitro culturing techniques has reduced the burden of environmental stress on growing plants. On other hand through the advances in gene editing tools and recombinant DNA technology transgenic plant varieties have been introduced, BT-cotton and herbicide-resistant plants are household tale. Drought-tolerant and abiotic-stress tolerant plant varieties are introduced in commercial farming practice as an outcome of transgenic plant technology. These biotechnological advances are uplifting the quality of agricultural products and traditional agronomy practices.

The sustainable agriculture is a heart of economy that drives the country and eventually touches the life of each countryman. Increasing population and subsequent food crisis have limited the flow of resources in agriculture, the crops is susceptible to environmental factors, pathogens and other uncanny. The biotechnological advances are focused around the better crop production but provide limited solution towards the crop protection and management.

The monitoring of crop field, prediction of weather fluctuations and its impact on crop, even distribution of crop protecting agents like herbicides and pesticides are other agronomy practices that have huge impact on agriculture.

Recently, the remote sensing and near-range imaging techniques have demonstrated great potential in monitoring the abiotic factors and detecting the plant disease. These can be achieved through integrating the sensor obtained data into the designed algorithm that predicts and analyse the impact of these factors. This approach has incorporated the technological advances for the sustainable farming practice (Figure 3.1), known as **precision farming** or **precision agriculture** (PA). As cited by Mcbratney *et al.*[2] a generic definition for precision agriculture could be "that kind of agriculture that increases the number of (correct) decisions per unit area of land per unit time with associated net benefits".

PA is a management concept related to detecting, computing and responding to intra-field variability in crops[3]. This practice facilitates the real time detection of the fields and also optimizes the treatments with a precision. PA and the use of digital tools and smartphones are almost inseparable. The tiny mobile applications have gain momentum through giving the accessibility to common man. Although this advances are promising the bright future of agriculture the lack of awareness towards this practice limits its application on large scale. PA practices is an amalgamation of diverse technological tools depicted through Figure 3.1.

Smallholder agriculture still dominates the rural economy in developing countries. In particular, a Precision Agriculture (PA) technology holds great potential for farmers in this regard. However this practice is more famous among the farmer who holds the larger farms. This chapter focuses on the technologies that involved in PA, it limitations and future.

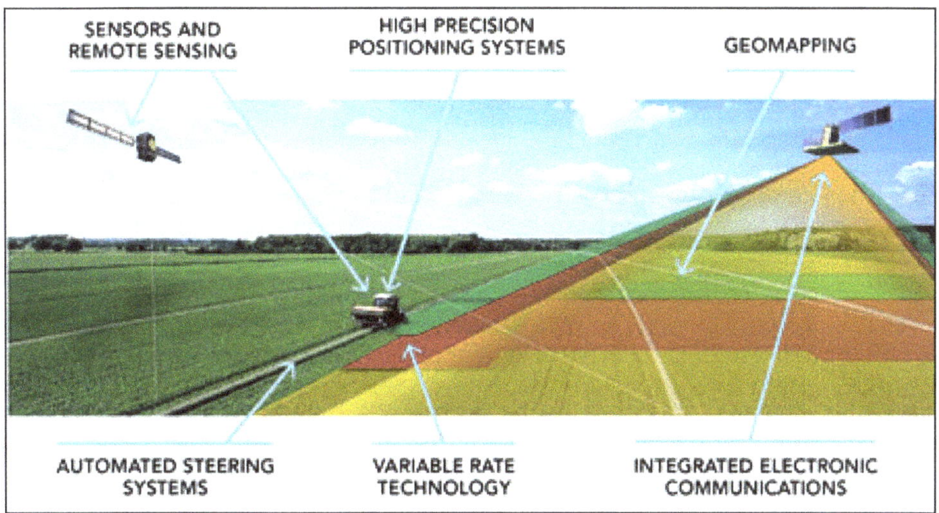

Figure 3.1: Basic Techniques Involved in Precision Farming Practice[4].

Technologies for PA

In last 25 years image processing technologies have taken great leap, from simple silver halide photographic film to liquid crystal display of computer screen. Furthermore, the improved precision in spatial information technology such as global positioning systems and GIS software have introduced the new techniques like variable-rate technology, yield monitoring devices. The advances in chemical, physical and biological sensing technologies gave variety of soil, plant and pest sensors. Incorporation of these sensors with satellite based remote sensing has changed the traditional agriculture practice to large extent[6]. In this section, the role of technological advances are summarised.

Remote Sensing and its Role in PA

Remote sensing is the technique for gathering the information about an object, at a certain distance, usually without touching the object. The public understanding about the remote sensing method refers to the simple photographic images of an object taken through camera. Amid these assumptions, remote sensing has evolved far ahead than looking at objects with our eyes. Each objects on earth adsorbs the light of different wavelength and according to its characteristic it reflects back in to the environment. The remote sensing devices works with this this absorption-reflection wavelengths of sunlight and subsequently develops images from that. The application of remote sensing for assessing crop condition is based on the relationship between multispectral reflectance, temperature of crop canopy, photosynthesis, and evapotranspiration[7]. The devices that are used for these measurements include satellites, aircraft, tractors and hand-held sensors. Jackson (1984)[8] suggested the following roles for remote sensing in farm management:

I. It provides frequent coverage
II. It rapidly delivers the spatial data
III. It provides resolution of 5 – 25 m,
IV. Integration with meteorological and agronomic data into expert systems.

The Remote sensing images are acquired through various types of sensors that can be grouped according to the number of bands and the frequency range of those bands that the sensor can detect. Common categories of remote sensors include panchromatic, multispectral and hyperspectral. Multispectral remote sensing systems use parallel sensor array, which detect radiation in a broad wavelength bands that often used in the fields of agriculture and food production. Hyperspectral remote sensing imagers acquire many, very narrow, adjoining spectral bands across the visible, near-infrared, mid-infrared, and thermal infrared portions of the electromagnetic spectrum. It has several applications in field of water-resource monitoring, and environment monitoring[9]. Principally, these spectral sensors detects the amount of light reflected from plant, this reflected amount is inversely proportional to the amount of light absorbed by particular plant. Plant pigments like chlorophyll a, chlorophyll b, carotenoids and anthocyanin absorbs the light of different wavelengths. Collectively, these various types of spectral indices are used to assess various attributes of plant canopies, such as leaf area index (LAI), biomass, chlorophyll content or N content[8–9].

Remote sensing applications in agriculture are based on the interaction of electromagnetic radiation with soil or plant material. In remote sensing, sensors typically measure the amount of reflected radiations from particular region[10].

Soil Sensing

Earlier the two practices were very familiar among the farmers. One that involves the "farming by soil" approach, in which manually collected soil samples are tested in to the soil mapping units. Whilst in another approach known as Soil Sampling Management Zone in which the farm specific customized treatments are practiced for specific locations. In PA, sensors mounted on tractor like multiple light emitting diodes (LED) or NIR can be applied for testing of soil organic matters and soil moistures. In early 20th century, a method using near infrared reflectance spectroscopy (NIRS) was developed for the measuring of attributes like soil moisture, soil pH, soil carbon and soil phosphorus, potassium, and calcium[10].The sensing technology further advanced through the introduction of non-proximal sensors like Geonics EM-38[11] for measurement of soil electrical conductivity, soil salinity and soil clay content.

The concept of proximal sensing is based on the direct contact with soil or plants. Proximal remote sensing implicates sensors mounted on tractors, spreaders, sprayers or irrigation booms. Proximal sensing allows real time site specific management of fertiliser, pesticides or irrigation[8–12]. It measures the leaf greenness and thereby predicts the level of Nitrogen stress on growing plants. Similarly, these sensors can be applied for measuring the soil conductance and thereby the soil moisture and soil salinity.

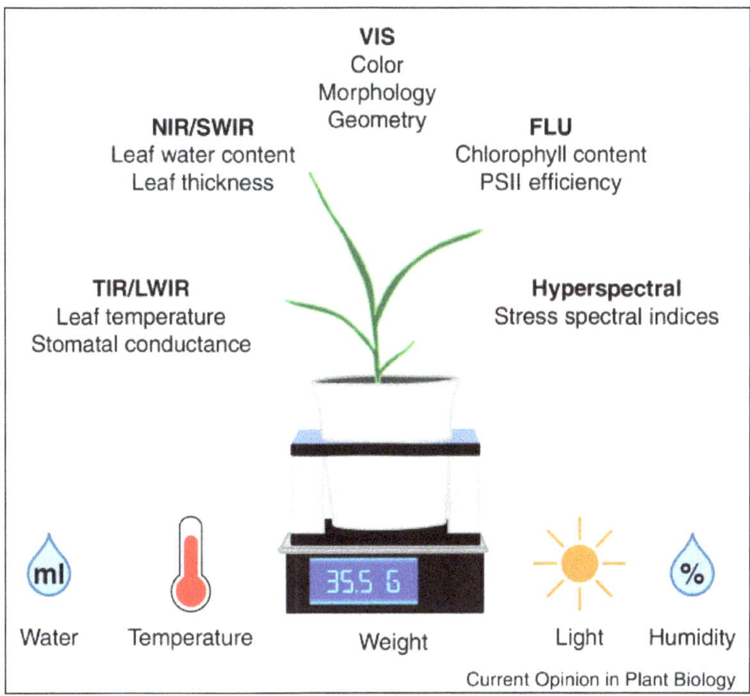

Figure 3.2: Various Types of Sensors and its Application in PA (*Source*: Figure is obtained from current pinion in plant biology).

Satellites have been designed and used for remote sensing imagery that helps in further development of agriculture. India has launched various satellites for that purpose (Table 3.1) that monitors the yield of crop like wheat and paddy. The more details on the functions of this satellites are discussed in section 4.

Table 3.1: Satellite Designed for Benefits of Farmers of India

Sl.No.	*Satellite*	*Launching Date*	*Purpose*
1	Resourcesat-2	20.04.2011	For wasteland inventory
2	Resourcesat-2A	07.12.2016	For measuring land and water resources development
3	RISAT-1	26.04.2012	For paddy and jute monitoring in kharif season

Detection of Plant Disease through Image Processing

Hyper spectral imaging has detected small spots, cankers, discoloration developed on leaf surface due to pathogenic invasion. *Cercospora* leaf shows spots on leaf surface upon fungal infection. The hyperspectral images taken at different time intervals clearly indicates disease progression. Each disease influences the spectral reflectance of plant tissue in a precise way ensuing disease-specific spectral signatures[13].

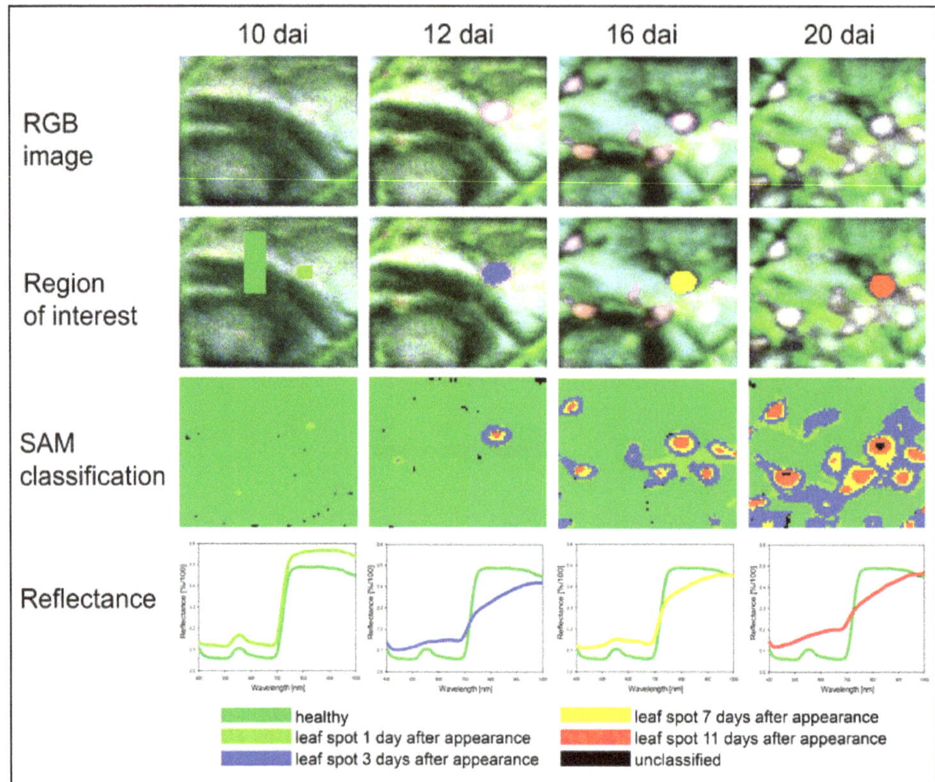

Figure 3.3: Hyper Spectral Imaging of *Cercospora* Leaf Spots Developed Post Fungal Infection.[11]

Hence forth each disease has its unique pattern[13] that can be easily distinguished from others. The software matches these images with the library and provides a meaningful information to farmers.

Pest Management

The other application of these sensors in pest management[14]. Fundamental technologies regarding these data can help determine the possible locations of these infestations. Farmers may then make judgments about a site-specific treatment that can reduce the further progression risk and save money.

Global Positioning System (GPS) and Geographic Information System (GIS) for PA

Precision Agriculture works through doing the right thing at right place and on right time. Integrating high-tech instruments and other data analysis tools the correct set of information can be obtained. In this perspective, GPS becomes part and parcel of precision agriculture[12].Analysis of Remote Sensed images requires real-time information from the field, for different locations and often at various times throughout the crop production season. In conventional practice, these data are recorded on paper and them it converted to digital format for use in remote sensing or GIS. GPS navigated unnamed vehicles are used in PA that provides site-specific farm management[15]. GPS receivers allow the mapping of field boundaries, roads, irrigation systems, and problem areas in crops such as weeds or disease. The precision of GPS allows farmers to create farm maps with precise acreage for field areas[16], road locations and distances between points of interest. It eases in navigation to specific locations in the field.

Variable-rate Technology (VRT)

This technology collects location specific data, in this manner takes the location specific decisions[17]. Multiple variables such as water, fertilizers, soil density are associated with sustainable agriculture development process. The Variable-rate technology recognizes the spatial variability inherent in the agricultural production processes and makes the decision according to the condition of farms at that particular time[18]. As example, soil fertility can vary significantly across a large field therefore applying a single rate of fertilizer will result in areas that are either under- or overfertilized[19]. Variable-rate technology (VRT) optimizes the rate for each location in the field.

The information for VRT can be obtained either from map or sensor. In map-based VRT, the rate of application can be adjusted towards an electronic map, also called a prescription map. From analysing the data obtained from GPS receiver the input rate is optimized[20].

In another method, a device studded sensors are used. Sensor-based VRT requires no map or positioning system. Sensors on the applicator measure soil properties or crop characteristics "on the go." Based on this continuous stream of information, a control system calculates the input needs of the soil or plants and

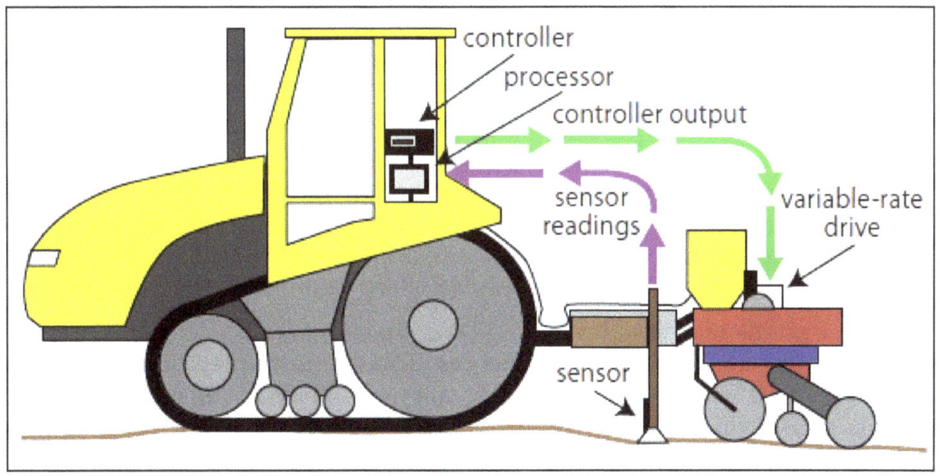

Figure 3.4: The VRT Device[13] that Senses the Soil Parameter and Adjusts the Rate of Seeding Accordingly.

transfers the information to a controller, which delivers the input to the location measured by the sensor.

VRT can offer both economic and environmental benefits when it is used for precise application of pesticides. It can be achieved through using simple light bar guidance systems[21]. This cheap light bar guidance systems offer an easy method to lead equipment across a field to prevent overlapping of pesticides on a particular site.

VRT offers the great promises by minimizing the wastage of nutrients. Nitrogen and phosphate are important plant nutrients that is critical for plant growth. The aim of PA is to apply only the nutrients that benefits the plants, that too in right quantity. The over-application increases the environmental problems like eutrophication. The rate of application can differ with in the field based on soil fertility, types and moisture[22]. There is some type of soils in a field that does not have the potential to validate maximum rates of nutrient application. On the other hand, there might be areas that need to be reduced rates because of sensitivity to the environment.

The other application of VRT in Yield Monitoring. Yield monitors uses GPS, GIS, a computer, and any sensor to quantify the amount of harvested crop[23]. The harvesting instruments are equipped with this yield monitors. The yield monitors can also record the crop moisture, elevation, variety, and a number of other harvest variables.

Advanced Spray Technologies

A "smart sprayer" that applies the herbicide to the target weeds leaving the desired plant aside. It combines GIS, computer software, high voltage light, infrared emitters and silicon photo detectors. This eye-like "vision" technology determines the precise location of individual weeds or patches and then individually-controlled nozzles apply herbicide in small doses only to the weeds[24].

Other Innovation Related to PA

As described on website of PrecisionAg[14]- a global union of people engaged in practicing precision agriculture, a new hand-held device is developed in a year 2017 which samples the DNA from plants. This technology allows the farmer to check the specific genetic traits for plants that aids in selection of compatible plant varieties.

A mobile application named **AGBRIDGE** developed by Scruggs Equipment Co. is a low-cost, universal wireless data transport solution that works with any agriculture controller equipped with USB port. AGBRIDGE is a controlling mobile app that enables the data transport between equipment in the field and the offices of farmers, governments' officers by simply launching the mobile app on any phones[15].

The current technology set up allows the site-specific detection of plant condition and the management practices. The future of precision agriculture techniques aims to apply a plant specific solution[25]. For example if in field one or two plant are having particular set of deficiency. Through this technology particular treatment can be given to that selected plants only. This may minimizes the financial burden on agriculture and cast the way for sustainable development.

Limitation of PA

As discussed in previous sections, the PA has many advantages that helps farmers in decision making. However the continuous technological up-gradation raises many technical problems. The system up-gradation often undermines the historical data records. The farmer has to install different base stations every-time. With updating of the system, there can be a slight shift in geographic coordinates. That subsequently results in discrepancy among the previously recorded data and the new data set of the system,

Furthermore, a sole dependence on sensor based imaging technique for detection of plant disease may sometimes results in delayed detection of disease. As many plant pathogen are cryptic they shows symptoms after very long incubation period.

Precision farming cannot be generalized for every crop. This oversimplification may lead towards the non-accurate decisions. PA adaption needs extensive training for farmers on various technical, economical and analytical issues. Small farmers often avoids the adaptation because of relatively high startup cost. The devices involved in PA needs maintenance and skilled men power for that. That often limits its wide application among the small farm-holders.

Precision Agriculture: Indian Scenario

Precision Agriculture is very famous practice among the developed countries like USA, Canada and Japan. However in developing countries like India where economy dominated by small farm-holders. The major constraints that limits its promotion are:

I. Small holdings
II. Heterogeneity and diversity of cropping systems
III. Dynamic market conditions
IV. Lack of technical expertise knowledge and technology
V. High start-up cost
VI. Lack of awareness

It is observed that the major problem is the size of farms. In India more than 60 per cent of operational holdings have size less than 1ha. Only in few states like Punjab, Rajasthan, Haryana and Gujarat has more than 20 per cent of agricultural lands have operational holding size of more than 4 ha. There is a scope of implementing precision Agriculture for crops like, rice and wheat especially in the states of Punjab and Haryana. A common platform for scientist, government and farmers is needed for adoption of precision agriculture.

Despite of these limitations Indian science has marked his way in precision agriculture through launching the satellites for agriculture applications (Table 3.1). Through these satellites following facilities are available to Indian farmers:

- Crop-production forecasting for 8 major corps like paddy, wheat *etc.*

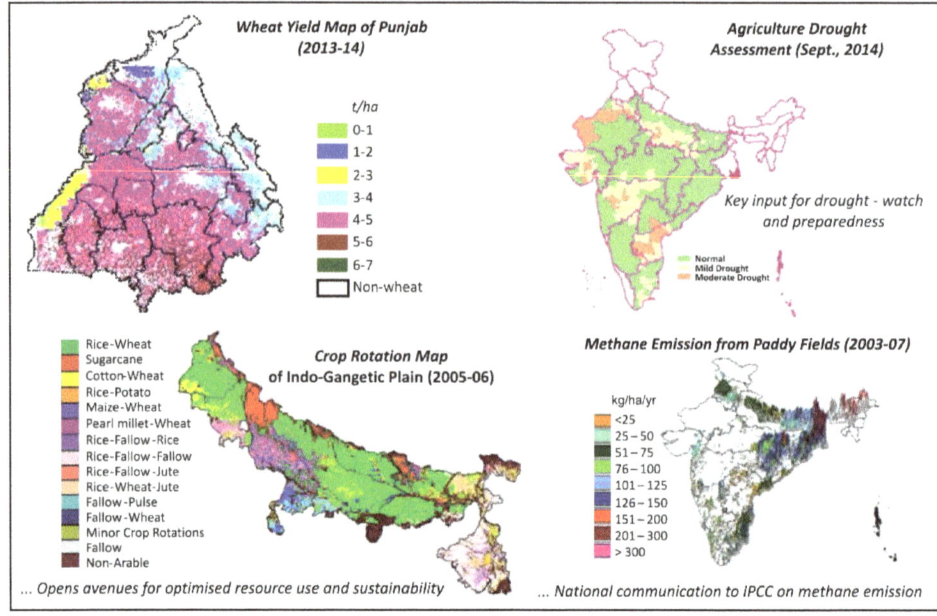

Figure 3.4: Information Obtained through the Remote Sensing Satellites that May Help in the Development of PA in in India (*Source*: website of National Remote sensing Centre, ISRO).

- ✰ An inventory for horticulture crops
- ✰ Drought assessment and monitoring
- ✰ Mapping of agriculture land

The PA requires an evolution in India, particularly for the assessment of water-resources. The guidance and information on weed management and variable rate technology are also not easily available to the Indian farmers limiting the use of PA.

The following strategies may help in the successful adoption of precision agriculture in the country.

I. Formation of team of specialist involving agricultural scientists, engineers, manufacturers and economists to study the overall scope of precision agriculture.

II. Formation of farmer's Union and Co-operative society as many of the precision agriculture tools are costly (GIS, GPS, RS, *etc.*).

III. Government legislation for environment protection that force the farmers for alternative approaches.

IV. Demonstration seminars and subsidise equipment, seed grant for the start up

Conclusions

Farming has evolved through many stages. It began with traditional farming by soil to laboratory flasks and finally progressed to site-specific crop management. More recently there has been growing interest on real-time on-the-go monitoring with ground based sensors. The challenge for the future is to develop precision farming approaches that can provide customized management of farm inputs for individual plants. The technology can designed an ideal farming practice for a farmer through integrating the inputs of weather, history of crops, and water-resources. The plant specific farming, that will be practiced in future may reduce the economic burden and increase the per capita production of crop. Although the recognition and growth of precision agriculture has been rapid since last two decades, some vital strategies are needed to implement this technology for small farm holders. Furthermore this requires continuous research and development of algorithms for the radiometric and geometric correction of remote sensing data and for information extraction. It also needs the easy access to sensing data, a subsequent training and technology transfer program to accelerate the acceptance and implementation of this technology for the agronomy.In this field India is taking baby steps cause of technological limitations; skilled manpower can bridge this technological gap.

References

1. Piperno, D. R. (2011). The origins of plant cultivation and domestication in the New World tropics: patterns, process, and new developments. *Current anthropology, 52*(S4), S453-S470.
2. McBratney A, Whelan B, Ancev T, Bouma J. Future directions of precision agriculture. Precision agriculture. 2005 Feb 1;6(1):7
3. Korte, M., Lee, K. and Fung, C.C. (2012). Sustainability in information systems: Requirements and emerging technologies (pp. 481–485). In: *Proceedings 2012 international conference on innovation, management and technology research (ICIMTR2012)*. IEEE
4. Precision agriculture practices, http://cema-agri.org/ accessed on 25 December, 2017-23.
5. Thrikawala S, Weersink A, Fox G, Kachanoski G. Economic feasibility of variable-rate technology for nitrogen on corn. American Journal of Agricultural Economics. (1999) Nov 1;81(4):914-27.
6. Seelan, S. K., Laguette, S., Casady, G. M., and Seielstad, G. A. (2003). Remote sensing applications for precision agriculture: A learning community approach. Remote Sensing of Environment, 88(1), 157-169.
7. Jackson, R. D. (1984). Remote Sensing of vegetation characteristics for farm management. Proceedings of the Society of Photo-Optical Instrumentation Engineers, 475, 81 – 96.
8. Govender, M., Chetty, K., and Bulcock, H. (2007). A review of hyperspectral remote sensing and its application in vegetation and water resource studies. Water Sa, 33(2), 145-151.

9. Mulla, D. J. (2013). Twenty five years of remote sensing in precision agriculture: Key advances and remaining knowledge gaps. Biosystems engineering, 114(4), 358-371.

10. Christy, C. D. (2008). Real-time measurement of soil attributes using on-the-go near infrared reflectance spectroscopy. Computers and Electronics in Agriculture, 61, 10-19.

11. Mahlein, A. K., Steiner, U., Hillnhütter, C., Dehne, H. W., and Oerke, E. C. (2012). Hyperspectral imaging for small-scale analysis of symptoms caused by different sugar beet diseases. *Plant methods*, *8*(1), 3.

12. Shanwad, U. K., Patil, V. C., Dasog, G. S., Mansur, C. P., and Shashidhar, K. C. (2002, October). Global positioning system (GPS) in precision agriculture. In Proceedings of Asian GPS conference

13. Primicerio, J., Di Gennaro, S. F., Fiorillo, E., Genesio, L., Lugato, E., Matese, A., and Vaccari, F. P. (2012). A flexible unmanned aerial vehicle for precision agriculture. *Precision Agriculture*, *13*(4), 517-523.

14. Grisso, R. D., Alley, M. M., Holshouser, D. L., and Thomason, W. E. (2005). Precision Farming Tools. Soil Electrical Conductivity.

15. PrecionAg, http://www.precisionag.com/regions/asia/2017-the-inflection-year-for-indian-agtech/ assessed on 27 December, 2017.

16. AGBRIDGE https://www.agbridgedata.com/ assessed on 28 December, 2017

17. Bastiaanssen, W. G. M., Molden, D. J., and Makin, I. W. (2000). Remote sensing for irrigated agriculture: examples from research and possible applications. Agricultural Water Management, 46, 137-155.

18. Berni, J. A. J., Zarco-Tejada, P. J., Sua´ rez, L., and Fereres, E. (2009). Thermal and narrowband multispectral remote sensing for vegetation monitoring from an unmanned aerial vehicle. IEEE Transactions on Geoscience and Remote Sensing, 47, 722-738.

19. Holland, K. H., Schepers, J. S., Shanahan, J. F., and Horst, G. L. (2004). Plant canopy sensor with modulated polychromatic light. In D. J. Mulla (Ed.), Proc. 7th intl. conf. precision agriculture. (CDROM). Minneapolis, MN: Univ. Minnesota

20. Link, A., Panitzki, M., and Reusch, S. (2002). Hydro N-sensor: tractormounted remote sensing for variable nitrogen fertilization. In P. C. Robert (Ed.), Precision agriculture [CD-ROM]. Proc. 6th int. conf. on precision agric (pp. 1012e1018). Madison, WI, USA: ASA, CSSA, and SSSA

21. Thorp, K. R., and Tian, L. F. (2004). A review on remote sensing of weeds in agriculture. Precision Agriculture, 5, 477-508.

22. Thomasson, J. A., Sui, R., Cox, M. S., and AleRajehy, A. (2001). Soil reflectance sensing for determining soil properties in precision agriculture. Transactions of the ASAE, 44, 1445-1453.

23. Zhang, N., Wang, M., and Wang, N. (2002). Precision agriculture: a worldwide overview. Computers and Electronics in Agriculture, 36, 113-132

24. Whipker, L. D., and Akridge, J. D. (2006). Precision agricultural services dealership survey results. Staff paper. W. Lafayette, IN, USA: Dept. Agricultural Economics, Purdue University.

25. Yang, C., Everitt, J. H., Bradford, J. M., and Escobar, D. E. (2000). Mapping grain sorghum growth and yield variations using airborne multispectral digital imagery. Transactions of the ASAE, 43, 1927e1938.

Chapter 4

Transgenic Plants and Advanced Technology

Purna Dwivedi

Department of Microbiology, Christ College,
Rajkot, Gujarat-360005
e-mail: purna.dwivedi03@gmail.com

ABSTRACT

The world population is known to be increasing day by day and estimated to achieve 9.2 billion by 2050. To feed such a large mass of people, the established ways of crop production will not be competent enough and thus we naturally would need to combine the time honoured farming methods with advanced plant biotechnology techniques. This need has been well heeded and acknowledged with the implementation of transgenic plants. The transgenic plants, a category in genetically modified organisms, are simply those plants whose DNA is reformed with the insertion of genes introduced from the completely distinct organism. This recombinant technology can lead to express a gene that is not native to the plant or can even be used to modify endogenous genes. The resulting protein encoded by the gene bestows a new characteristic to that plant. The technology is now developed to achieve new measures that can tackle abiotic stresses, drought, extreme temperature or salinity, and biotic stresses, such as insects and pathogens, which would normally prove detrimental to plant growth or survival. Creation of genetically modified crops is an innovative method to improve the nutritional content of the plant, an application that could be of particular use in the developing countries. New-generation GM crops are now also being developed for the production of recombinant medicines and industrial products, such as monoclonal antibodies, vaccines, plastics, and biofuels. The two most commonly employed techniques to achieve genetic modification in plants are, the bacterium *Agrobacterium tumefaciens*, which is naturally able to transfer DNA to plants, and the gene gun', which shoots microscopic particles coated with DNA into the plant cell.

Gene technology had emerged as an additional tool in crop improvement in the late 1980s, and today commercial genetically modified crops are commonly used all around the globe. Genetic engineering of crops has been a controversial subject since 1971 when the first genetically modified organisms were developed. Concern about biosafety has led to Government regulation of transgenic crops in contained and field experiments to assess potential risk before the genetically engineered crops are approved for commercialization. GM crops are tightly regulated by several government bodies all throughout the world. In the following article, topics discussed are the various techniques carried out to produce genetically modified plants, types of outcomes of the genetic modification carried out in them and the reasons for why in the first place they are needed to be genetically modified. It also discusses the pros and cons of the transgenic plants, the statistical data of genetically modified crops and their sales in various countries, the current status of the commercialised transgenic crops and the perspective on their future, debate over the safety issues of their use, the ethnic contradictions and laws in India as well as in other countries to keep every possible threat arising from the transgenic plants in check.

Keywords: *Transgenic plants, Recombinant technology, Commercial transgenic plants, Legal regulations for GMO.*

Introduction

The current rate of food production is in a state to be doubled by the middle of the next century on the existing area of land, practicing sustainable agriculture that conserves natural resources simultaneously. According to the consensus in the global scientific and development community, merely the conventional technology would not be capable of food production to feed a global population is predicted to reach 11 billion by 2050 and the new technologies will be essentiality to intensify the conventional technologies that are currently being used.[1] The transgenic plants have become a driving force of the world's agriculture. It is because of this recombinant technology that the ever growing human population is able to meet its food security and commercial demands. The conventional farming methods alone are incompetent to fulfil the demand so posed. Methodically speaking, transgenic plants are those plants which, by the means of genetic engineering procedures, have been inserted with one or more genes from another species into their genome. The experimental process of introducing a genetic information for the required character in the desired plant have come long way evolving from the techniques include the gene gun method, *Agrobacterium tumefaciens* mediated transformation, to the latest CRISPR-CAS9 technology, adoption various vectors for facilitating gene insertion, implementation of fusion proteins *etc.*

The aim leading to the insertion of a combination of genes in a plant is to maximise its usefulness and benefits. Amongst its many advantages are improving shelf life, higher yield, improved quality, pest resistance, tolerant to heat, cold and drought resistance, against a variety of biotic and abiotic stresses. Transgenic plants can also be produced in such a way that they express foreign proteins with industrial and pharmaceutical value.[2] Transgenic plants containing bacterial enzymes have also been utilized to remove mercury, selenium and polychlorinated biphenyls (PCBs) thus performing the bioremediation of the polluted land.[3] Tobacco and Arabidopsis thaliana are the most genetically modified plants and serve as model organisms for other plant species, due to established transformation methods, easy propagation and well analysed genomes.[4] Among the advantages of GM food is its enhanced ability to withstand prolonged storing phases and long-distance transportation rendering it a longer shelf life. The usage these GM crops, has resulted in better yields and decreased costs. With a promising chance of feeding billions of hungry mouths, the producers of the GM crops have entitled it as a second ¯Green Revolution.[5] The scientific community all over the world supports the option of an equalized and sustainable approach that involves the best of conventional crop technology and high-yielding germplasm, and the best of biotechnology (GM and non-GM traits) to accomplish sustainable intensification of crop productivity on the 1.5 billion hectares of cropland globally. The more than 18 million farmers (up to 90 per cent were small/poor farmers) in up to 30 countries who have planted biotech crops attest to the multiple benefits they derived in the last 20 years as follows:

- ✰ Increased productivity that contributes to global food, feed and fibre security;
- ✰ Self-sufficiency on a nation's arable land;
- ✰ Conserving biodiversity, precluding deforestation and protecting biodiversity sanctuaries;
- ✰ Mitigating challenges associated with climate change; and
- ✰ Improving economic, health and social benefits.[6]

Techniques for Genetic Transformation

The Biolistic Approach

The Gene Gun method, also known as the Micro-Projectile Bombardment or Biolistic method is most commonly used in the species like corn and rice. In this method, DNA is bound to the tiny particles of Gold or Tungsten, which is subsequently shot into plant tissue or single plant cells, under high pressure using gun.[7] These accelerated particles penetrate both into the cell wall and membranes. The DNA separates from the coated metal and integrates itself into the plant genome present in the nucleus. This method has been applied successfully for many crops, especially monocots, like wheat or maize, for which transformation using *A. tumefaciens* has been less successful.[8]

The Agrobacterium Facilitated Approach

The second method, *A. tumefaciens* transformation, has the ability to infect plant cells with a piece of its DNA which further integrates into a plant chromosome, through a tumour inducing plasmid (Ti plasmid). This Ti plasmid is capable of generating many copies of its own bacterial DNA by controlling the plant's cellular machinery. The Ti plasmid contains regions of transfer DNA (t DNA), where a desired gene can be inserted, and be transferred to a plant cell through a process known as the ¯floral dip . In this process, flowering plant is dipped into a solution of Agrobacterium carrying the gene of interest, followed by the transgenic seeds, being collected directly from the plant. *A. tumefaciens* transfer is found to more preferable as it is a natural method as well as capable of transferring large fragments of DNA very efficiently.[7] Drawback of *Agrobacterium* is that this method works especially well for the dicotyledonous plants like potatoes, tomatoes and tobacco plants but on the same sight cannot be applied for monocotyledonous plants. Yet, because it is a natural way of transient transformation, it is the most preferred method.

A significant rise in the number of reports on the successful Agrobacterium-mediated genetic transformation of various plant species, variants and cultivars has been observed during the last two decades. Much of the advancement that have been attained in the protocol establishment for the transformation of new host species depends on a relatively small number of binary vectors and genetically modified Ti-helper plasmids, and on an even smaller number of deactivated Agrobacterium strains and isolates. Thus, progress in the gene transfer of different plant species has been accomplished chiefly, by matching the inoculated plant tissue to the suitable Agrobacterium strain, by genetic modification of Agrobacterium, and by developments in tissue culture and transgene selection techniques.[9]

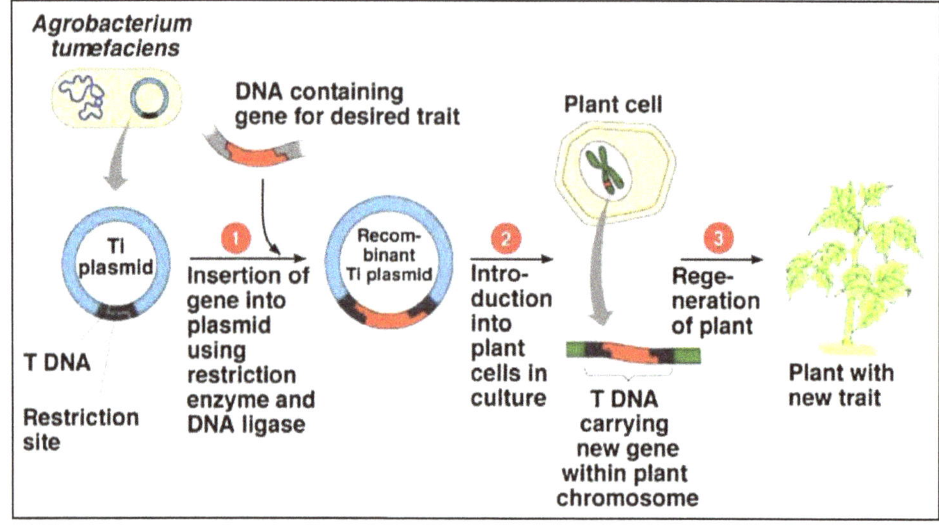

Figure 4.1: Agrobacterium Mediated Transformation.[5]

The Use of Selectable Markers in Transgenic Plants

An appropriate genetic constructs is an important need to be made to facilitate integration and expression of the foreign gene(s) for the successful attainment of effective transfer of genetic material into the desired host. This gives rise to the selection of a selectable marker to allow effective identification of the transformed cells. Selectable markers are preferred, because these under ideal conditions allow establishment and proliferation only of transformed cells which may further regenerate into transgenic plants when transferred to appropriate comprising phytohormones media. A standard genetic construct is made up of a promoter, a transgene and a terminating signal. Mode of introduction of transgenes into plant tissues can be with the help of a separate plasmids or co integrative vectors. A co integrative vector has multiple genes, including selectable markers, all present on the same plasmid.[10] Commonly used promoters for plant transformation include:

Table 4.1: Plant Species and the Mode of Transformation and Filed Trial Conducted on them[10]

Species	Transformation method	Field trials
Banana	Bombardment/*Agrobacterium*	
Barley	Bombardment	Virus resistance
Bean	Bombardment	
Canola	Bombardment/*Agrobacterium*	Herbicide tolerance; pollination control
Cassava	Bombardment/*Agrobacterium*	
Maize	Bombardment/*Agrobacterium*	Insect resistance; herbicide tolerance
Cotton	Bombardment/*Agrobacterium*	Insect resistance; herbicide tolerance
Papaya	Bombardment/*Agrobacterium*	Virus resistance
Peanut	Bombardment/*Agrobacterium*	Virus resistance
Poplar	Bombardment/*Agrobacterium*	Herbicide tolerance
Potato	*Agrobacterium*	Insect resistance; virus resistance; herbicide tolerance
Rice	Bombardment/*Agrobacterium*	Herbicide tolerance
Soybean	Bombardment/*Agrobacterium*	Herbicide tolerance
Squash	Bombardment/*Agrobacterium*	Virus resistance
Sugarbeet	*Agrobacterium*	Herbicide tolerance
Sugarcane	Bombardment	
Sunflower	Bombardment	
Tomato	*Agrobacterium*	Delayed ripening; virus resistance
Wheat	Bombardment	

- ✰ The cauliflower mosaic virus (CaMV) 35S promoter, which is a constitutive promoter, suitable for driving the expression of foreign genes in dicotyledons
- ✰ The maize ubiquitin promoter, also a constitutive promoter, which drives strong
- ✰ Expression of transgenes in monocotyledons.

Organ/tissue-specific promoters are also available to drive expression of transgenes in particular parts of the plant, and specific examples include:

- ✰ The vicilin and phytohemaglutinin promoters, derived from pea and bean, respectively, suitable for seed-specific expression
- ✰ The high molecular weight glutenin promoter from wheat, also suitable for seed-specific expression
- ✰ The s-amylase promoter, for driving expression in the aleuronic layer of cereal grains.

The most common selectable marker genes encode proteins that detoxify metabolic inhibitors such as antibiotics or herbicides. Commonly used selectable markers include:

- ✰ The glucuronidase[11]
- ✰ The luciferase genes[12]
- ✰ The green fluorescent protein from jellyfish[13]

Gateway Vectors

Commonly, the genes to be transferred are cloned between the left and right

T-DNA borders of so-called binary T-DNA vectors that can replicate both in *E. coli* and *Agrobacterium*. The cloning can be time-consuming and laborious because the large size of these vectors. A recent, fast and reliable alternative to the cloning of sequences into large acceptor plasmids, known as the GATEWAY™ conversion technology, is based on the site-specific recombination reaction mediated by λ phage. DNA fragments flanked by recombination sites (att) can be transferred into vectors that contain compatible recombination sites (attB × attP or attL × attR) in a reaction mediated by the GATEWAY™ BP Clonase™ or LR Clonase™ Enzyme Mix (Invitrogen). The entry clones, or the donor plasmids, are constructed by recombination of the DNA fragment of interest with the flanking attB sites into the attP site pDONR201 mediated by the GATEWAY™ BP Clonase™ Enzyme Mix. Subsequently, the fragment in the entry clone can be transferred to any destination vector that contains the attR sites by mixing both plasmids and by using the GATEWAY™ LR Clonase™ Enzyme Mix.[14]

Viral Vectors

Viral vectors have drawn interest because viral infections being rapid and systemic and on the same sight the virus infected cells yield large amounts of virus and viral gene products and this is the reason plant viral vectors have been used to express scFvs (antibody that recognizes the carcinoembryonic antigen (CEA), one of the best characterized tumour-associated antigens) and full-size antibodies.[15] [16] [17] One of the best uses of this is the construction of two tobacco mosaic virus vectors carrying the heavy and light chains of the antibody. Not only the tobacco plants co-infected with the two vectors having the transgenes were expressed, the assembly of the antibody in plant was also confirmed. Transgenic tobacco crop is at the forefront of emerging systems for plant based commercial protein production. Other emerging systems include alternative leafy crops, such as alfalfa, which as a leguminous species requires limited fertilizer input, the use of cereal and legume seed crops for stable antibody accumulation in dry seeds, and the use of fruit and vegetable crops to combine storage with ease of processing and product administration. It is hoped that in future recombinant proteins can be expressed in plants to consistent and high quality levels, which would allow the production of pharmaceutical proteins that can be used regularly in clinical trials.[18]

The Expression of Genome Editing through Fusion Proteins

Use of fluorescent fusion proteins (FP) for expression and tracking has revolutionized our understanding of basic concepts in cell biology. A team led by A Sparks has devised a protocol which strengthens much of the in vivo results that highlights the dynamic nature of the plant secretory pathway. In this protocol the assessment of expression of genes of interest is carried out with the help of transient transformation of tobacco leaf epidermal cells which proved to be a relatively fast technique. Expression of fluorescent proteins (FPs) has been used in many systems to investigate protein interactions, trafficking, turnover, organelle biogenesis, movement and inheritance. In this protocol, FP fusion constructs[19] targeted to various organelles such as the Golgi (sialyl transferase fused to GFP), peroxisomes (PEX10-eYFP) and endoplasmic reticulum (GFP-HDEL) are injected into the leaf lamina of tobacco plants, resulting in transient expression of the fusion protein. Tissue culture of the transiently transformed region allows the generation of plants that stably express the transgene construct. Transient expression of FPs in tobacco epidermal cells is a relatively fast process requiring only 2–4 days from infiltration to expression. A time phase of 2-4 months is required to generate the succeeding generation of stable transgenic plants using a tissue culture approach.[20]

Genome Engineering with Programmable Nucleases

A group of empowering programmable nucleases — including zinc-finger nucleases (ZFNs), transcription activator-like effector nucleases (TALENs) derived from the bacterial clustered regularly interspaced short palindromic repeat (CRISPR)–Cas (CRISPR-associated) system — facilitate targeted genetic alterations in cultured cells, as well as in whole animals and plants. These possess the ability to induce site-specific DNA cleavage in the genome, the repair (through endogenous mechanisms) of which allows high-precision genome editing which makes them of great value in research, medicine and biotechnology. Despite, their differences in several respects, including their composition, targetable sites, specificities and mutation signatures, among other characteristics, knowledge of nuclease-specific features, as well as of their pros and cons, is essential for researchers to choose the most appropriate tool for a range of applications.[21]

Table 4.2: Genome Editing Acronyms, Terms and Definitions[22]

CRISPR	Clustered Regularly-Interspaced Short Paloindromic Repeats	Programable nucleases comprised of bacterially derived endonuclease (Cas9) and a single-guide RNA (sgRNA)
DSB	Double Strand Break	Cleavage in both strands of double-stranded DNA where the two strands have not separated
EMN	Engineered Mega Nuclease	Engineered Mega Nuclease Microbially derived meganucleases that are modified, fused, or rationally designed to cause site-directed Also referred to as LAGLIDADG endonucleases or homing nucleases.
GEEN	Genome Editing with Engineered Nucleases	Genetic engineering where DNA is inserted, replaced, or removed from a genome using SDN.
HDR	Homology-Directed Repair	A mechanism for DSB repair using a DNA sequence homologous to the break site that serves as a template for homologous recombination.
HR	Homologous Recombination	A genetic recombination process where two similar DNA strands exchange nucleotide sequences.
NHEJ	Non Homologous End Joining	A means for repair of DSB without the use of a homologous repair sequence. An error-prone process that often causes small insertions or deletions at the DSB site resulting in mutations.
OMM	Oligonucleotide Mediated Mutagenesis	Site-specific mutation with chemically-synthesized oligonucleotide with homology to the target site (other than for the intended nucleotide modification).
SDN	Site Directed Nuclease	Engineered DNA nucleases that are programmed to specific sites within the genome where they cleave a DNA chain by separating nucleotides.

TALEN	Transcriptional Activator-Like Effector Nuclease	Programmable nucleases comprised of the DNA binding domain of Xanthomonas-derived TAL effectors fused with FokI restriction endonuclease.
ZFN	Zinc Finger Nuclease	Programable nucleases comprised of the DNA binding domain of a zinc-finger protein and the DNA-cleaving nuclease domain of the *Fok*I restriction endonuclease.

The Zinc Finger Nucleases (ZFNs)

Zinc finger nucleases (ZFNs) are chimeric proteins composed of a synthetic zinc-finger-based DNA-binding domain and a DNA cleavage domain. ZFNs can play a helpful role in gene editing as it can be designed to cleave almost any long stretch of double-stranded DNA by modification of the zinc finger DNA binding domain[23 24]. ZFNs form dimers from monomers composed of a non-specific DNA cleavage domain of *Fok* I endonuclease fused to a zinc finger array engineered to bind a target DNA sequence. The DNA-binding domain of a ZFN is typically composed of three-to-four zinc-finger arrays (Figure 4.2A). The amino acids at positions –1, +2, +3, and +6 relative to the start of the zinc finger α-helix, which contribute to site-specific binding to the target DNA, can be changed and customized to fit specific target sequences. The other amino acids form the consensus backbone to generate ZFNs with different sequence specificities. The *Fok* I nuclease undergone dimerization can cleave DNA and with the help of two ZFNs with their C-terminal regions bound to opposite DNA strands of the cleavage site. The ZFN monomer can cut the target site the two palindromic ZF binding sites. To generate ZF arrays that recognize specific DNA sequences, the modular assembly method described

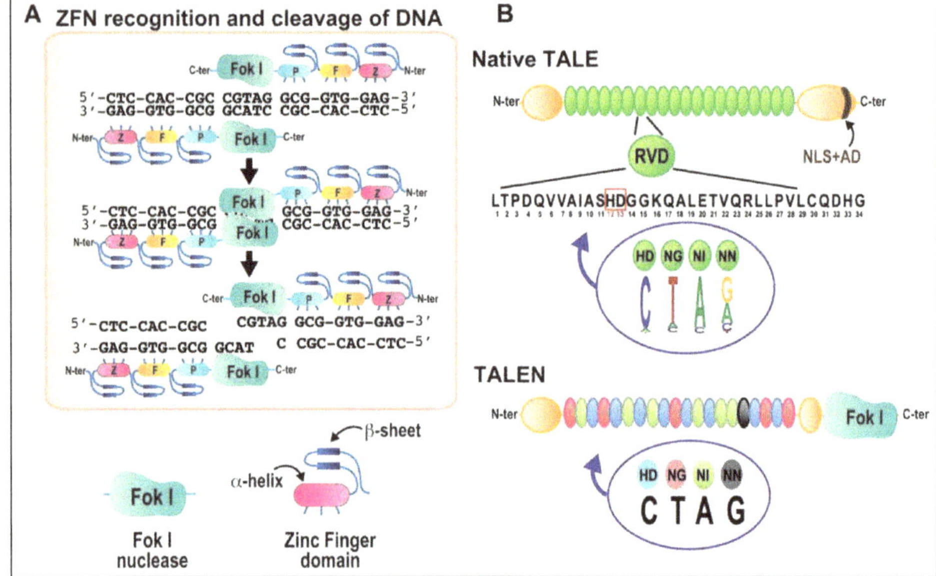

Figure 4.2: Mechanisms of Target Recognition by (A) ZFN and (B) TALEN.

above is initially established, and individual zinc fingers with known specificities for triplet sequences are combined to cover the required sequence.[25-27]

ZFN has been reported as a useful genome editing technique to create target-specific mutations in Arabidopsis using a heat shock promoter (HSP)[28]. A maize line containing a herbicide-resistant marker and a synthetic ZFN target site was produced by using the ZFN target site and the corresponding ZFNs, where the site-specific additional herbicide-resistant marker gene (second trait) flanked with a new ZFN target site was integrated. Therefore, this system allows multiple trait stacking at a specific locus.[29]

Transcription Activator like Effector Nucleases (TALENs)

Transcription activator-like effector nucleases (TALEN) is a recently developed platform for genome editing using engineered nucleases (GEEN). TALE proteins are DNA binding domains derived from various plant bacterial pathogens of the genus *Xanthomonas*, which secrete TALEs into the host plant cell during infection following which TALE moves to the nucleus, where it recognizes and binds to a specific DNA sequence in the promoter region of a specific gene in the host genome[30]. TALEN is composed of a DNA binding domain and an endonuclease *Fok* I domain. Like ZFN, TALEN dimerizes when two monomers recognize individual DNA target sites (Figure 4.2B).

Application TALEN in Plants

TALEN technology has been used in dicot species such as tobacco and Arabidopsis and in monocot species such as rice, *Brachypodium*, barley and maize [31 32 33 34].

- TALEN-mediated genome editing in plants was first reported in rice, where the rice disease susceptibility gene and the sucrose efflux transporter gene *OsSWEET14* (Os11N3) promoter region was disrupted through NHEJ, which resulted in plants that were resistant to *Xanthomonas oryzae* [35].
- In a study conducted, the phytic acid biosynthesis pathway was targeted in maize, which produced independent transformants at four targeted loci with NHEJ-based disruptions in approximately 39.1 per cent of the transformants [32]. These reports show that TALEN-mediated genome editing technology can precisely modify predetermined loci in crop plants leading to improved varieties that are more environmentally friendly and disease or stress resistant.
- Recently, Gurushidze *et al.* (2014)[36] developed gene knockout systems using TALENs to disrupt genes in barley embryonic pollen cultures consisting primarily of haploid cells. These results outcomes have high applicability for the detailed study of gene function and molecular breeding in various crop species.

The CRISPR-CAS9 Technology

A rapidly emerging and escalating gene transfer technology CRISPR/Cas9 is among the latest favourite site specific gene editing tool due to its flexibility, high efficiency, and simplicity which enables this system to be utilized for many applications, including target site mutation, deletion, gene depression and activation. CRISPR-Cas9 is a rapidly developing technology used to produce gene-specific modifications in both mammalian and plant systems and has played a huge part in the increase in genome editing studies in recent years. Although most CRISPR induced modifications created in plants that are reported till date have been small insertions or deletions however, there a few large target gene deletions which have been affirmed, especially for Indica rice. [37]

CRISPR, or Clustered Regularly Interspaced Short Palindromic Repeats, is an integral part of a bacterial defence system. The CRISPR molecule is made up of short palindromic DNA sequences that are repeated along the molecule and are regularly-spaced. These palindromic DNA sequences have foreign DNA sequences from organisms that have previously attacked the bacteria named as the ¯spacers . The CRISPR molecule is inclusive of CRISPR-associated genes, or CAS genes which encrypt proteins helicases and nucleases, respectively.[38] The CRISPR immune system protects the bacteria from repeated virus attacks through three steps:

1. Adaptation – When DNA from a virus invades the bacteria, the viral DNA is processed into short segments and is made into a new spacer between the repeats. These will serve as genetic memory of previous infections.
2. Production of CRISPR RNA – The CRISPR sequence undergoes transcription, including spacers and CAS genes, creating a single-stranded RNA. The resulting single-stranded RNA is called CRISPR RNA, which contains copies of the invading viral DNA sequence in its spacers.
3. Targeting – The CRISPR RNAs will identify viral DNA and guide the CRISPR-associated proteins towards them. The protein then cleaves and destroys the targeted viral material. [39]

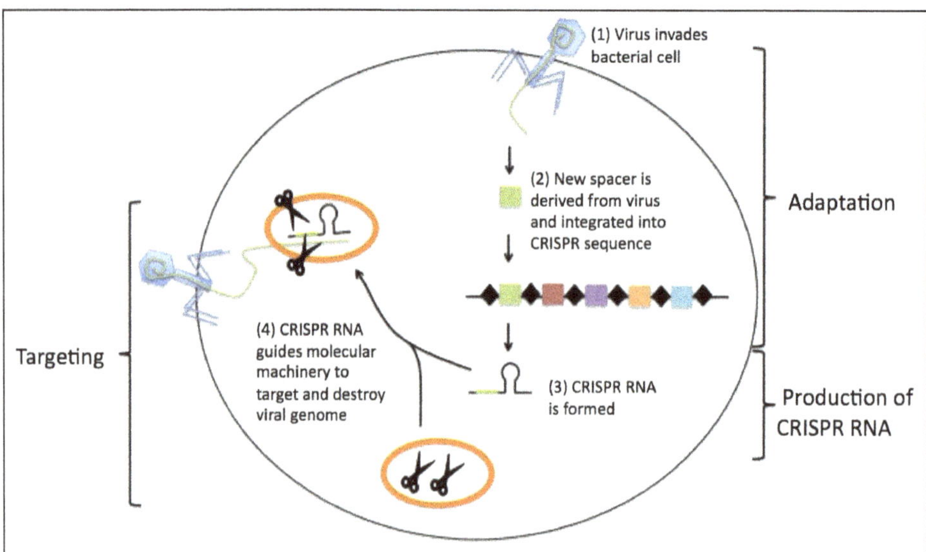

Figure 4.3: The Steps of CRISPR-Mediated Immunity.[24]

The characteristic of CRISPR-Cas9 system to identify a specific DNA sequence is very well utilized by the scientists and applied in the process of development of improvement of crops. Based on their specific gene of interest instead of viral DNA as spacers, scientists design their own sequences. If it is a known gene sequence, it can be easily used in CRISPR where it will then act just like a spacer for the system and guide the Cas9 protein to a DNA matching sequence.

The following is what CRISPR-Cas9 permits researchers to perform:

- ✰ Gene Knock-Out
- ✰ DNA-Free Gene Editing
- ✰ Gene Insertions or ¯Knock-ins
- ✰ Transient Gene Silencing[40]

Applications CRISPR - Cas9

The CRISPR - Cas9 system is found to be broad spectrum technique which can be applied to nearly every organism. Early studies using CRISPR - Cas9 for gene editing have focused on crops important for agriculture. Its various benefits comprising of improved traits, such as yield, plant architecture, plant aesthetics, and disease tolerance of the crops.

- ✰ The team of Ying Wang from Syngenta Biotechnology China designed several CRISPR sgRNAs (signal guide RNAs) and successfully deleted fragments of the dense and erect panicle1 (*DEP1*) gene in the Indica rice line IR58025B. The mutant plant so produced showed improvements in yield-related traits, such as dense and erect panicles and reduced plant height. [37]
- ✰ A team of researchers from the Chinese Academy of Agricultural Sciences led by Yupeng Cai also used the CRISPR-Cas9 system to induce mutations on *GmFT2a*, an integrator in the photoperiod flowering pathway of soybean. The developed soybean plants showed late flowering, resulting in increased vegetative size. The mutation was also found to be stably inherited in the following generation.[41]
- ✰ A team of Beijing Key Laboratory of Vegetable Germplasm Improvement, led by Shouwei Tian targeted *ClPDS*, the phytoene desaturase in watermelon, using CRISPR-Cas9 to achieve the albino phenotype. All genome-edited watermelons harbored mutations in *ClPDS* and showed full or mosaic albino phenotype.[42]
- ✰ Cold Spring Harbor Laboratory, together with various research institutions, also used CRISPR-Cas9 to generate mutations in the flowering suppressor SELF-PRUNING5G (SP5G) in tomato to manipulate photoperiod response. The mutations brought about by CRISPR-Cas9 caused rapid flowering and enhanced the compact growth habit of field tomatoes, resulting in a quick burst of flower production and early yield.[43]

While still in a young and in rapidly evolving stage, CRISPR has already proved its worth in the increase in genome modification studies in recent years. The system holds wide applications in plant and animal improvement, as well as in the medical field. As a relatively young technique, various discoveries and innovations for its efficient use in wider applications are in the offing.

Stress Tolerance by Transgenic Plants

A method invented by a team at Virginia Tech Intellectual Properties, Inc. reports a surprising discovery that genetically engineered plant to contain and express traits for increasing the growth rate, biomass or stress tolerance of a plant by genetically modifying the plant to contain and overexpress a functional gene product of an ascorbic acid synthesis-cell wall synthesis network. Examples of the functional gene products include myo-inositol oxygenase, glucuronic acid reductase, L-gulono-1, 4-oxidase, glucuronate kinase *etc.* Some examples include Arabidopsis, lettuce, tobacco, soybeans, potato, tomato, canola, rice, corn, and wheat and hybrid poplar. The transgenic plants that are genetically engineered to over-express at least one gene of the ascorbic acid synthesis-cell wall synthesis network, as suggested by the experiential results of strong interconnection of the AsA biosynthetic pathway and the non-cellulosic cell wall biogenesis pathway together, have a more robust growth of the aboveground and belowground biomass of the plant. This also results in increased tolerance to stress, as intermediates of the ascorbic acid route are diverted to pathways that promote biomass growth and tolerance to stress. In some cases, an increased level of vitamin C of the plant was also observed as a result of genetic modification step so carried out. In other cases, no such increase in the level of vitamin C of the plant was detected. The consequences of increased growth rate are advantageous as it unlocks the opportunity for harvesting mature crops even in areas with short growing seasons. The amplification in aboveground biomass would progress in greater quantities of produce per plant, while parallel increases in belowground biomass result in sequestration of larger quantities of carbon, helping to alleviate the problem of greenhouse gas build up. Similarly, a successful cultivation crops or other plants of interest under high soil salinity conditions can be achieved as a result of increases in stress tolerance of plants that were not previously possible.[44]

Global Statistics

Transgenic crops have delivered substantial agronomic, environmental, economic, health and social benefits to farmers, and increasingly to the consumers in the last 20 years of commercialization of biotech crops. The substantial multiple benefits of the transgenic crops has been very well heeded by both large and small farmers in industrial and developing countries and has resulted into their rapid adoption. In 20 years, an accumulated 2 billion hectares of biotech crops have been grown commercially comprised of 1.0 billion hectares of biotech soybean, 0.6 billion hectares of biotech maize, 0.3 billion hectares of biotech cotton, and 0.1 billion hectares of biotech canola (Table 4.3, Figures 4.4 and 4.5). Biotech products derived from this 2 billion hectares significantly contribute food and shelter to the current 7.4 billion people. As far as the economic benefits are concerned, US$ 81.7 billion was generated in industrial countries and US$86.1 billion in developing countries out of the US$ 167.8 billion additional gain in farmer income generated by transgenic in the 20 years of commercialization (1996 to 2015).[6]

Table 4.3: Global Area of Biotech Crops, 2015 and 2016 by Crop (Million Hectares)[6]

Crops	*2015*	*Per cent*	*2016*	*Per cent*	*+/–*	*Per cent*
Soybean	92.1	51	91.4	50	-0.7	-1.0
Maize	53.6	30	60.6	33	+7.0	+13.0
Cotton	24.0	13	22.3	12	-1.7	-7.0
Canola	8.5	5	8.6	5	+0.1	+1.0
Alfalfa	1.0	<1	1.2	<1	+0.2	+20.0
Sugar beet	0.5	<1	0.5	<1	0	0
Papaya	<1	<1	<1	<1	<1	<1
Others	<1	<1	<1	<1	<1	<1
Total	**179.7**	**100**	**185.1**	**100**	**+5.4**	**+3.0**

In 2016, four biotech crops (soybean, maize, cotton and canola) comprised the most extent of hectares (Table 4.3). The adoption trend provided in Figure 4.4 shows the plateauing optimal rate for biotech soybean, an increase in biotech maize, and marginal increases in canola, while cotton still has a downward trend due to global low price (Figures 4.4 and 4.5).

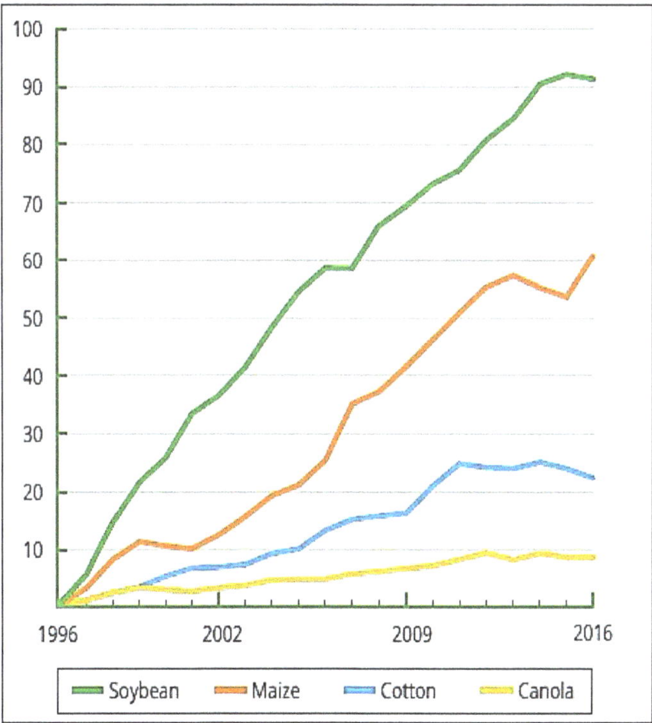

Figure 4.4: Global Area of Biotech Crops, 1996 to 2016 by Crop (Million Hectares).[6]

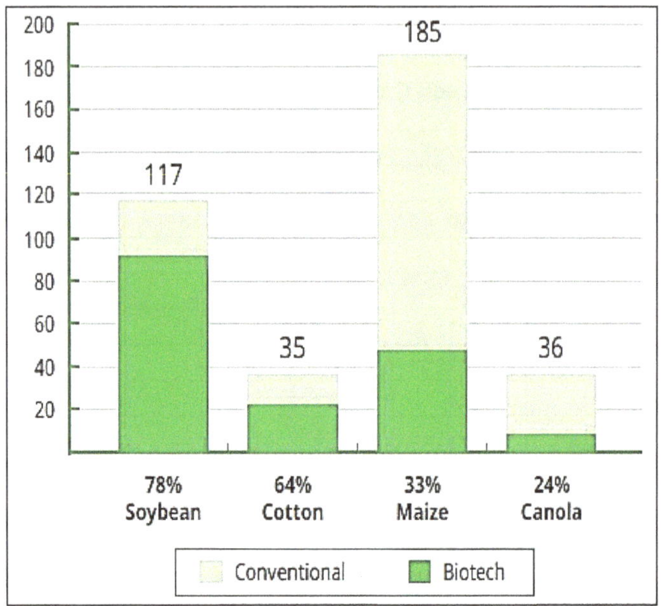

Figure 4.5: Global Adoption Rates (per cent) for Principal Biotech Crops, 2016 (Million Hectares).[6]

Regulatory System for Transgenic Plants in Selected Countries

All around the world, there are regulatory bodies comprising scientific as well as non-scientific societies which have been set up by the governments to primarily approve, disapprove and keep a check on the utilisation of the transgenic plants. The plant phenotype occurring as the result of a given biotechnology process should be the emphasis of safety determinations and this scientific position is very well supported by the regulators assessing the transgenic plants worldwide.

- The regulatory point of view of Canada for evaluating transgenic plant holding a novel trait for environmental release is strongly based upon its phenotype. [45]
- The regulatory paradigm followed in the United States under the coordinated framework distributes the authority among the US Food and Drug Administration (FDA), Environmental Protection Agency (EPA) and Department of Agriculture (USDA). The USDA serves as the lead US regulator under the coordinated framework and draws its authority to regulate transgenic crops to the extent that the derived plant may behave as a plant pest or harmful weed. Animal and Plant Health Inspection Service (APHIS) is responsible for regulating the introduction (importation, interstate movement and field release) of transgenic organisms that may pose a plant pest risk. EPA-Environmental Protection Agency evaluates potential environmental impacts, and aimed to regulate the pesticidal property rather than the crop. A probable human health risk posed by

Table 4.4: Status of Biosafety Research Trials of Biotech Crops in India, 2016 (*Source*: MOEF and CC, 2016; Analyzed by ISAAA, 2016)[6]

Crop	*Gene(s)/Event*	*Developer*	*Status*
Chickpea	cry7Ac, cry1Aabc/IPCa2 and MP9	ICAR-Indian Institute of Pulses Research, Kanpur	BRL-I
Cotton	GHB 614 (Glytol)	Bayer Biosciences Pvt. Ltd., Hyderabad	BRL-II
Cotton	WideStrike	Dow Agro Science Pvt. Ltd	Hybrid Seeds Production
Maize	NK603	Monsanto	BRL-II
Maize	cry7F, cry1Ab and cp4EPSPS genes/TC1507 x MON 810 x NK 603 (DAs-01570-1 x MON-00810-6 x MoN-00003-6	Pioneer Hi-Breed Private Limited, Hyderabad	BRL-I
Maize	TC1507 x MON810	Pioneer Hi-Breed Private Limited, Hyderabad	BRL-I
Mustard	Bar, barnase and barstar/events bn 3.6 and modbs 2.99	Delhi University	Environmental Release
Pigeonpea	cry1Ac, cry1Aabc/IOCc2 and SS5	ICAR-Indian Institute of Pulses Research, Kanpur	Event Selection
Rice	Abiotic stress tolerance namely drought and salinity and nutrition stress	Bioseed Research India pvt. Ltd., Hyderabad	Event selection
Rice	cry2Aa2a	RasiSeeds Research Farm, Telangana	Event selection
Sugarcane	DREB	Sugarcane Research Institute, U.P Council of Sugarcane Research (UPCSUR), Shahjahanpur	Event Selection

the transgenic plant is analysed by Food and Drug Administration, FDA, if the plant is intended for human consumption, especially as it relates to allergens, anti-nutrients and toxins. [47]

☆ The European Union, EU, legislation describes GM crops as an organism whose genetic material has been altered in a way that it differs from the natural mating/recombination. The recombinant nucleic acid techniques are explicitly subject to regulation and mutagenesis is explicitly excluded.[46] The EU precautionary approach and its unique application to the defined process of genetic modification is often reflected in emerging regulatory networks elsewhere in the world where new biosafety laws are being adopted and implemented [47 48]

Regulatory System in India

The two main agencies responsible that for implementation of the rules notified for the procedures for manufacture, import, use, research and release of genetically modified organisms (GMOs) as well as products made by the use of such organisms under the Environmental Protection Act 1986 (EPA) are the Ministry of Environment and Forests (MoEF) and the Department of Biotechnology (DBT), Government of India, which have further six defined competent authorities as per the rules for handling of various aspects of the rules:

1. Recombinant DNA Advisory Committee (RDAC)
2. Review Committee on Genetic Manipulation (RCGM)
3. Genetic Engineering Approval Committee (GEAC)
4. Institutional Biosafety Committees (IBSC)
5. State Biosafety Coordination Committees (SBCC)
6. District Level Committees (DLC).

Out of these, the three agencies that are involved in approval of new transgenic crops are:

1. IBSC set-up at each institution for monitoring institute level research in genetically modified organisms.
2. RCGM functioning in the DBT to monitor ongoing research activities in GMOs and small scale field trials.
3. GEAC functioning in the MoEF to authorize large-scale trials and environmental release of GMOs. [49]

Conclusions

Pros and Cons

A major promoting fact backing the growing of transgenic plants is that only it has proved to be catching the pace of the growing population by fulfilling its food demands. After decades of dramatic increases in food production, due to the green revolution, the rate of growth has again observed to decline hinting that the conventional methods of food production needs to be substituted. The increase in the food production due to ¯green revolution methods such as high-yielding hybrid seeds and intensive use of fertilizers, irrigation and chemical pesticides has rendered severe environmental damage. The use transgenic crops allow farmers to spend less money while producing more food that too utilizing fewer pesticides and herbicides further reducing their exposure to dangerous pesticides. Insect resistant GM crops, such as those containing the bacterial Bt gene (which makes the plant itself toxic to key pests), allow farmers to dramatically reduce their use of spray insecticides. Next-generation seeds may allow farmers to maintain high yields while using less water and chemical fertilizer. Implementation of transgenic plant would necessitate less tilling to remove weeds, thereby protecting the soil, foods with better texture, flavour and nutritional value are produced with a longer shelf life for easier shipping. If it's allowed to flourish, GM technology will eventually provide widespread benefits for virtually all the people, as well as the global environment.

On the other hand, the demerits of the transgenic plants are that they have been blamed to create ¯super weeds that have evolved a resistance to glyphosate, a common herbicide in GMO food production. The insect-resistant crops may harm species that are not their target, such as monarch butterflies. Further, the insects that GM crops are designed to kill could evolve and develop resistance to those crops, resulting in a super pest, ultimately requiring farmers to use more aggressive control measures, such as increased use of chemical sprays. Cross-pollination can cover quite large distances, where new genes can be included in the offspring of traditional plants or crops resulting in difficulty in distinguishing between crop fields of organic and transgenic plants. Another drawback of transgenic plants is that the genetic modification carried out in them often adds or mixes proteins that were not indigenous to the original plant, which might cause new allergic reactions in human body.

Future Prospects

Current molecular biology allows targeted gene mutations to be achieved effectively by GEEN. In gene modification, these targetable nucleases have the potential to become alternatives to standard breeding methods to identify novel traits in economically important plants and animals. Currently, the promising nuclease system CRISPR/Cas9 is becoming more widely used because it is easy to set up, and it is easy to design targets and constructs. An important issue in plant genome editing is how to deliver and express the engineered nucleases in plant cells, because not all useful plant species have established regeneration and transgenic methods. The selection of appropriate plant tissues, and the optimization of methods for transformation and culture are major issues that remain to be resolved to provide opportunities to generate novel, useful crops. Thus, efficient systems to deliver genome editing tools into plant cells must be developed. As new plant breeding techniques develop, these efforts, together with a deeper understanding of the structure and function of whole genomes, will enable the development of future technologies in breeding new and important traits in plants. [27]

Public Understanding of Genome Editing

Many new breeding techniques have been evolved since the advent of the genetically modified plant by the plant research and development community that represent options for increased innovation and which may find greater public and regulatory acceptance over the use of transgenic approaches. Yet, to achieve the general public's view of foods derived from products of modern biotechnology to be completely acceptable is perhaps the greatest hurdle faced for definition and implementation of regulatory processes that remain constant with scientific perceptive of new plant breeding technologies including genome editing.

In the given situation conveying concepts of modern biotechnology to the general public, there is considerable potential that the public may not immediately embrace genome editing and, therefore, may outpace the ability of scientists to communicate the opportunities afforded by genome editing for crop improvement.[50]

References

1. James C, Krattiger AF. (1996) Global review of the field testing and commercialization of transgenic plants: 1986 to 1995. ISAAA Briefs.

2. Herbers K, Sonnewald U. (1999) Production of new/modified proteins in transgenic plants. Current opinion in Biotechnology; 10(2):163-8.
3. Meagher RB. (2000) Phytoremediation of toxic elemental and organic pollutants. Current opinion in plant biology; 3(2):153-62.
4. Koornneef M, Meinke D. (2010) The development of Arabidopsis as a model plant. The Plant Journal; 61(6):909-21.
5. Rani SJ, Usha R. (2013) Transgenic plants: Types, benefits, public concerns and future. Journal of Pharmacy Research; 6(8):879-83.
6. James C. ISAAA briefs. (2012) Global status of commercialized biotech/GM Crops.
7. HS Chawla. (2002) Introduction to plant biotechnology. Science Publishers.
8. Shrawat A, Lorz H. (2006) Agrobacterium-mediated transformation of cereals: a promising approach crossing barriers. Plant Biotechnol J; 4(6):575e603
9. Tzfira T, Citovsky V. (2006) Agrobacterium-mediated genetic transformation of plants: biology and biotechnology. Current opinion in biotechnology;17(2):147-54.
10. Christou P. Transformation technology. (1996) Trends in Plant Science; 1(12):423-31.
11. Jefferson RA, Kavanagh TA, Bevan MW. (1987) GUS fusions: beta-glucuronidase as a sensitive and versatile gene fusion marker in higher plants. The EMBO journal; 6(13):3901.
12. Ow DW, De Wet Jr, Helinski Dr, Howell SH, Wood KV, Deluca M. (1986) Transient and stable expression of the firefly luciferase gene in plant cells and transgenic plants. Science; 234(4778):856-9.
13. Chalfie M, Tu Y, Euskirchen G, Ward WW, Prasher DC. (1994) Green fluorescent protein as a marker for gene expression. Science:802-5.
14. Karimi M, Inzé D, Depicker A. (2002) GATEWAY™ vectors for Agrobacterium-mediated plant transformation. Trends in plant science; 7(5):193-5.
15. Verch T, Yusibov V, Koprowski H. (1998) Expression and assembly of a full-length monoclonal antibody in plants using a plant virus vector. Journal of immunological methods; 220(1):69-75.
16. Hendy S, Chen ZC, Barker H, Santa Cruz S, Chapman S, Torrance L, Cockburn W, Whitelam GC. (1999) Rapid production of single-chain Fv fragments in plants using a potato virus X episomal vector. Journal of immunological methods; 231(1):137-46.
17. McCormick AA, Kumagai MH, Hanley K, Turpen TH, Hakim I, Grill LK, Tusé D, Levy S, Levy R. (1999) Rapid production of specific vaccines for lymphoma by expression of the tumor-derived single-chain Fv epitopes in tobacco plants. Proceedings of the National Academy of Sciences; 96(2):703-8.
18. Schillberg S, Twyman RM, Fischer R. (2005) Opportunities for recombinant antigen and antibody expression in transgenic plants—technology assessment. Vaccine; 23(15):1764-9.

19. Runions J, Hawes C, Kurup S. (2007) Fluorescent protein fusions for protein localization in plants. Protein Targeting Protocols: 239-56.

20. Sparkes IA, Runions J, Kearns A, Hawes C. (2006) Rapid, transient expression of fluorescent fusion proteins in tobacco plants and generation of stably transformed plants. Nature protocols; 1(4):2019-25.

21. Kim H, Kim JS. (2014) A guide to genome engineering with programmable nucleases. Nature Reviews Genetics; 15(5):321-34.

22. Wolt JD, Wang K, Yang B. (2016) The Regulatory Status of Genome-edited Crops. Plant biotechnology journal; 14(2):510-8.

23. Durai S, Mani M, Kandavelou K, Wu J, Porteus MH, Chandrasegaran S. (2005) Zinc finger nucleases: custom-designed molecular scissors for genome engineering of plant and mammalian cells. Nucleic acids research; 33(18):5978-90.

24. Camenisch TD, Brilliant MH, Segal DJ. (2008) Critical parameters for genome editing using zinc finger nucleases. Mini reviews in medicinal chemistry; 8(7):669-76.

25. Bae KH, Do Kwon Y, Shin HC, Hwang MS, Ryu EH, Park KS, Yang HY, Lee DK, Lee Y, Park J, Sun Kwon H. (2003) Human zinc fingers as building blocks in the construction of artificial transcription factors. Nature biotechnology; 21(3).

26. Segal DJ, Beerli RR, Blancafort P, Dreier B, Effertz K, Huber A, Koksch B, Lund CV, Magnenat L, Valente D, Barbas CF. (2003) Evaluation of a modular strategy for the construction of novel polydactyl zinc finger DNA-binding proteins. Biochemistry; 42(7):2137-48.

27. Osakabe Y, Osakabe K. (2014) Genome editing with engineered nucleases in plants. Plant and Cell Physiology; 56(3):389-400.

28. Lloyd A, Plaisier CL, Carroll D, Drews GN. (2005) Targeted mutagenesis using zinc-finger nucleases in Arabidopsis. Proceedings of the National Academy of Sciences of the United States of America; 102(6):2232-7.

29. Ainley WM, Sastry-Dent L, Welter ME, Murray MG, Zeitler B, Amora R, Corbin DR, Miles RR, Arnold NL, Strange TL, Simpson MA. (2013) Trait stacking via targeted genome editing. Plant biotechnology journal; 11(9):1126-34

30. Boch J, Scholze H, Schornack S, Landgraf A, Hahn S, Kay S, Lahaye T, Nickstadt A, Bonas U. (2009) Breaking the code of DNA binding specificity of TAL-type III effectors. Science; 326(5959):1509-12.

31. Christian M, Qi Y, Zhang Y, Voytas DF. (2013) Targeted mutagenesis of Arabidopsis thaliana using engineered TAL effector nucleases. G3: Genes, Genomes, Genetics; 3(10):1697-705.

32. Liang Z, Zhang K, Chen K, Gao C. (2014) Targeted mutagenesis in Zea mays using TALENs and the CRISPR/Cas system. Journal of Genetics and Genomics; 41(2):63-8.

33. Shan Q, Wang Y, Chen K, Liang Z, Li J, Zhang Y, Zhang K, Liu J, Voytas DF, Zheng X, Zhang Y. (2013) Rapid and efficient gene modification in rice and Brachypodium using TALENs. Molecular plant; 6(4):1365-8.

34. Wendt T, Holm PB, Starker CG, Christian M, Voytas DF, Brinch-Pedersen H, Holme IB. (2013) TAL effector nucleases induce mutations at a pre-selected location in the genome of primary barley transformants. Plant molecular biology; 83(3):279-85.

35. Li T, Liu B, Spalding MH, Weeks DP, Yang B. (2012) High-efficiency TALEN-based gene editing produces disease-resistant rice. Nature biotechnology; 30(5):390-2.

36. Gurushidze M, Hensel G, Hiekel S, Schedel S, Valkov V, Kumlehn J. (2014) True-breeding targeted gene knock-out in barley using designer TALE-nuclease in haploid cells. PLoS One; 9(3):e92046.

37. Wang Y, Geng L, Yuan M, Wei J, Jin C, Li M, Yu K, Zhang Y, Jin H, Wang E, Chai Z. (2017) Deletion of a target gene in Indica rice via CRISPR/Cas9. Plant Cell Reports: 1-1.

38. Barrangou R, Fremaux C, Deveau H, Richards M, Boyaval P, Moineau S, Romero DA, Horvath P. (2007). CRISPR provides acquired resistance against viruses in prokaryotes. Science; 315(5819):1709-12.

39. Harvard University. (2015). CRISPR: A game-changing genetic engineering technique. http://sitn.hms.harvard.edu/flash/2014/crispr-a-game-changing-genetic-engineering-technique/.

40. Cong L, Ran FA, Cox D, Lin S, Barretto R, Habib N, Hsu PD, Wu X, Jiang W, Marraffini LA, Zhang F. (2013) Multiplex genome engineering using CRISPR/Cas systems. Science; 339(6121):819-23.

41. Cai Y, Chen L, Liu X, Guo C, Sun S, Wu C, Jiang B, Han T, Hou W. (2017) CRISPR/Cas9-mediated targeted mutagenesis of GmFT2a delays flowering time in soybean. Plant Biotechnology Journal.

42. Tian S, Jiang L, Gao Q, Zhang J, Zong M, Zhang H, Ren Y, Guo S, Gong G, Liu F, Xu Y. (2017) Efficient CRISPR/Cas9-based gene knockout in watermelon. Plant cell reports; 36(3):399-406.

43. Soyk S, Müller NA, Park SJ, Schmalenbach I, Jiang K, Hayama R, Zhang L, Van Eck J, Jiménez-Gómez JM, Lippman ZB. (2017) Variation in the flowering gene SELF PRUNING 5G promotes day-neutrality and early yield in tomato. Nature genetics;49(1):162-8.

44. Nessler CL, Lorence A, Chevone B, Mendes P, inventors; Virginia Tech Intellectual Properties, Inc., assignee. Stress tolerant transgenic plants over-expressing ascorbic acid and cell wall synthesis genes. United States patent US 9,000,267. 2015 Apr 7.

45. Smyth S, McHughen A. (2008) Regulating innovative crop technologies in Canada: the case of regulating genetically modified crops. Plant biotechnology journal; 6(3):213-25.

46. Parliament, E. (2001) Directive 2001/18/EC of the European Parliament and of the Council of 12 March 2001 on the deliberate release into the environment of genetically modified organisms and repealing Council Directive 90/220/EEC. *Off. J. Eur. Comm. L*, **106**, 1–38.
47. Okeno JA, Wolt JD, Misra MK, Rodriguez L. (2013) Africa's inevitable walk to genetically modified (GM) crops: opportunities and challenges for commercialization. New biotechnology; 30(2):124-30.
48. Gupta K, Karihaloo JL, Khetarpal RK.(2008) Biosafety regulations of Asia-Pacific countries. Book:96p.
49. Ahuja V, Jotwani G (2010) The Regulation of Genetically Modified Organisms in India; krishikosh.egranth.ac.in
50. Paarlberg R. A dubious success: the NGO campaign against GMOs. (2014) GM crops and food;5(3):223-8.

Chapter 5

Policy Networks and Agriculture Innovation: A Study of System of Rice Intensification in Bihar, India

Vikas Kumar

Formerly Project Assistant at Gujarat National Law University, Gandhinagar Gujarat and also done Ph.D. from Central University of Gujarat.
e-mail: vikaskumarcug@gmail.com

ABSTRACT

This paper emphasizes the critical role of policy networks for the implementation of agricultural innovation in terms of System of Rice Intensification. Further, it covers the agricultural policy since last one decade and figure out the changes in policy to promote the system of rice intensification technique. Besides, it also looks the development of agricultural supports and their mission or objectives. These policy analyses with the different time frame. It is well known that, agriculture is the backbone of Bihar economy and have a vital source of income for the rural society. Therefore, proper policy for agriculture sector is essential to improve livelihoods and welfare of the masses. It is essential to have a more inclusive and rational approach which deals both the demand and supply side issues, captures the complex relationships among the actors, and comprises agricultural policies with other policies for development of economy.

Keywords: *Policy networks, Agriculture policy, Rice, System of rice intensification, Bihar.*

Introduction

The state of Bihar has considered to be undergoing for a second Green Revolution in the country. According to National Farmers Commission have focused the need for enhanced development of agriculture in the state for securing food security of the country and Late Dr. Abdul Kalam, former President of India has been described Agriculture as Core Competence of Bihar. Though, the limitation of green revolution did not success in the state because high yielding varieties of rice and wheat are responsive to high fertilizer doses mainly under irrigated ecology. Therefore, the larger parts of Bihar are now facing a crisis of sustainability and it is hence, Bihar is conducting Rainbow Revolution in the country that would be achieved through sustainable farming technologies for instance, System of Rice Intensification (SRI). The relevance of agriculture to Bihar's economy is reflected in varying degrees at grass root level. According to Fourth Annual Employment and Unemployment survey[1] (2015), the contribution of the service sector is 60 per cent, followed by 23 per cent by agriculture and 17 per cent by manufacturing in Bihar's economy. The 56 per cent of the state population is employed in the agriculture sector, followed by the services (36 per cent) and manufacturing (8 per cent) sectors.

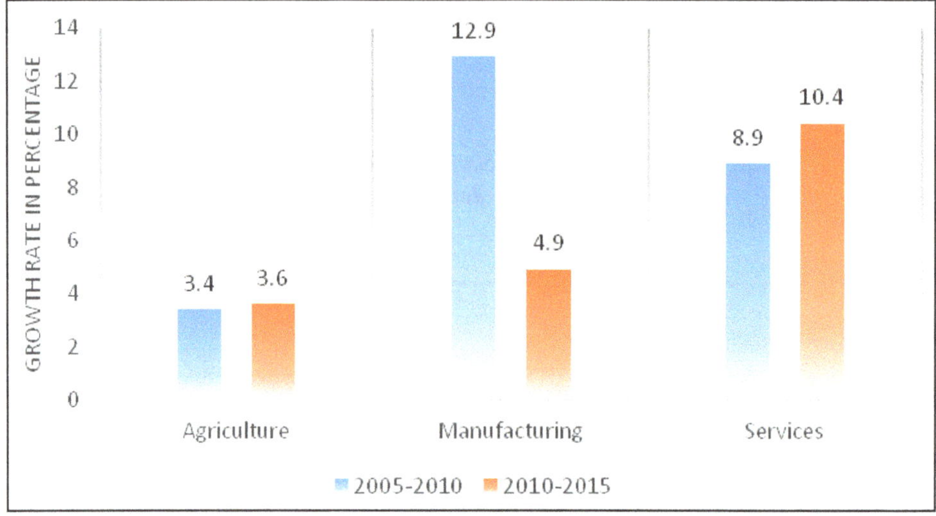

Figure 5.1: Growth Rate of Sectors in Bihar (*Source*: Central Statistics Office).

At an overall level, agricultural growth remained slow (below 4 per cent) in the state and the growth rate of agriculture has been just 0.2 per cent increased from 2005-10 to 2010-15. Apart from that, agricultural growth remained confined to a few well-endowed pockets which have created regional disparities. However, the data and figure represents that the growth of agriculture in Bihar has performed poorly, declining in the early 1990s by 2 per cent per annum and growing by less than 1 per cent per annum since 1994-95 but later on it has performed better 3.6 per cent in the year of 2010-15.

Further, taking this as an account, the contribution of agriculture plays vital role in the state economy as 77 per cent of the workforce is in agriculture and generating nearly 25 per cent of the State Domestic Product. However, the area under cultivation is gradually shrinking and natural hazards such as drought and floods also play a

1 http://labourbureaunew.gov.in/UserContent/Annual_Emp_Ump_July15.pdf?pr_id=ixSYU0Ryea0 per cent 3D.

role to affect production. The hurdles of agriculture in Bihar can be solved through enhanced cropping intensity, change in cropping pattern, improvement in seeds of high yielding varieties, cultivation practices, *etc.* The Government is planning to re-orient agriculture through diversification policy and other measures. The major objective of the policy is to enhance productivity of food grains, and so as to fulfill food security mission and create new markets at competitive prices. Hence, based on the argument the objectives of the paper is to:

1. To overview the concept of Policy Networks.
2. How the actors of Policy Networks support in the Agriculture Innovation especially in the context of System of Rice Indemnification (SRI).

Hence, based on the above introduction the, the chapter has been categorized into six different sections including introduction. The second section discusses about the conceptual framework of policy networks, it deals with the basic definitions of policy, programs and projects. Similarly, third section focused on the actors of policy networks in agriculture specific to the system of Rice Intensification. Fourth, the section discusses about the Policies for overall growth of Agriculture in Bihar and more focused on the system of rice intensification. The Fifth section demonstrates about the Agriculture Road Map of Bihar and their achievement in the context of System of Rice Intensification. Last but not the least conclude the arguments.

Policy Networks: A Conceptual Framework

In the period of 1970, the term Policy Network first time used in political science. Broadly, it sets of actors who engage in the making policy whether they are inside or outside the government and simply it can be also said the relationship between these actors. Although, there are various political scientists defined the term their own way (Thatcher, 1998). In addition, the Policy networks defined or conceptualized in two ways first, it is sets of political actors who involved in resource exchange and second, who involved in the process specially rules and norms.

Further, Lubell and Fulton (2007) the idea of Policy Networks has been developed through traditional research which can be divided into three parts: (1) the classical diffusion of innovation model and its posterity, (2) theories of social capital, and (3) theories of cultural evolution. Though, the notion of policy networks has significant implications for institutional and government decision making as well (Berry and Berry, 1992). The aim of the argument is to deliver a theoretical basis for main objective: Rice Cultivators to policy networks is one of the most significant catalysts for the adoption of system of rice intensification. Although, this paper with policy networks and diffusion of technology. This study helps to classify the most pertinent theoretical perspectives for understanding the role of policy networks to implement the technique and how public organization influence networks strength.

Policy Networks in Diffusion of Innovation in Terms of SRI

The diffusion of innovation models stresses the significance of policy networks as part of the procedure by which an innovation is imparted through specific channels after some time among the individuals from a social system (Rogers

1962). Basically, the information spread through policy networks, each actor of the innovation system estimates the costs and benefits of a particular innovation and adopts that innovation if beneûts outweigh costs. In the context of system of rice intensification, policy networks comprise farmers, government agencies, and other local organizations as members of the agricultural system. These networks spread information about the existence and effectiveness of different types of policy, program and the technique. Norman Uphoff (2007) one the main author who helps to promote SRI and he states that, SRI is more technique rather than technology and it is the set of elements and visions changes towards cultivation of rice successfully. He also argued that, the practices of SRI are to be adapted by farmers and there is always scope for the further innovation. Similarly, according to Bray (1986) pointed that SRI is based on more farmer skills and field level rather than external inputs. The flexibility of principles can be applied by farmers in any situation.

Although, there is mixture kind of views occurred from the researchers regarding SRI. The phenomena of SRI have been taken seriously not only because of scientific argument, it's also because of the involvement of other actors (such as farmers, NGOs, research institutions and extension organizations) which reflects the value of the system and have their own experience. Therefore, it is a natural bottom-up innovation process and farmers and other government and non-government agencies engaged to diffuse at local, regional and national levels. The SRI is stimulated through different types of material and resources, including legitimacy and access to the media and governance structures.

Bill Gates, visited a village in Bihar where SRI has been implemented by NGO with support from India's rural development bank, NABARD[2]. The author tries to relate the interaction between local and global dynamics in the governance of technological innovation in agriculture. Though, the debate is going that whether SRI should be implemented or not or in simply it can be said that how farming should be done. But it is not simple as look like Glover (2011) raise the question that, it is a not matter of how farming should be while it is a question about agricultural science should be done, by whom and with what aims. Basu and Leeuwise (2012) on playing the role of networks in the adaptation of SRI and the study suggested that there is a mixed culture of networks which played a significant role in the spreading of SRI. For instance, local newspaper plays an important role to advertise SRI for adoption. It also support in agriculture innovation system to have contributed to awareness and get opinions from the experts. Authors more focused on theoretical consideration of innovation rather than on farm level study and suggested that, SRI was adopted by higher level organizations and institutions.

However, about SRI two things could be drawn in the policy framework: first how these types of innovation and discovery processes could be promoted and facilitated, secondly, how different level of stakeholders (international institution of agricultural and civil society) joins together to drive scientific knowledge into farmers practice. There is required, a new institutional arrangements and

---

2 http://www.pradan.net/index.php?option=com_content and task=view and id=159 and Itemed=106.

collaboration between actors and networks such as scientific researchers and the potential users and beneficiaries of agricultural research.

Networks of Actors in Policy to Support SRI

The actors in the innovation system of SRI have used their networks to perform better and access knowledge. The networks of actors may depend on the region and specific objectives, but actors in the networks are associated to other actors through many networks and group, formally and informally. Though, actors play different role in these networks for instance, farmers play as role of end users and as an informer. Therefore, the diffusion of SRI has been spread pre-existing networks and research stations exist. Nevertheless, in SRI new networks are formed during the process and diffusion. Farmers in Patna district gained vital skills for SRI farming by participating in a wide network of actors. These skills are preparation of nursery, planting, weeding and harvesting, *etc.* Most of the skills came to farmers through ATMA training or workshop, field staff and private organization. The innovation system needs a participation and involving of actors through networks, farmers and other actors for instance research institute and ATMA. The question raised by farmer and providing solutions by KVK enhanced the knowledge of agriculture. Hence, in this process multiple sources of knowledge and variations of communication and adaptation patterns are used for farming[3].

The Figure 5.2 represents to the networks and their relation of actors. The relation and networks have been shown with colors and arrows. The dash arrow denotes to indirect links and week networks between two actors and Simple line arrow represents to the direct links and strong networks with actors. It can be observed from the national organizations have strong relationships with most of the actors and it works as a network to facilitate SRI technique. Similarly, sources of technical assistance have also a strong relationship with other actors to promote SRI. This is so, because technical assistance provides technology to farmers to enhance agriculture growth. These technologies are in the form of product and process, for instance, Hybrid seeds, planting technique of Paddy cultivation. There is also a strong relation between policy maker and national organization and other actors because policy maker support financially to the organization. Hence, all the networks linked to other networks directly or indirectly. The reason of networks may be differ from each other and specific. For instance, Farmers are directly linked with SRI for their increase income and similarly, Ministry of Agriculture, GoI and Department of Agriculture GoB directly linked with SRI because to fulfill NFSM, NRDM, BRLDP *etc.*

Policies for Overall Growth of Agriculture in Bihar

In 2006 the new agricultural policy was prepared by the State government, to build upon the natural advantages that the State has in agriculture. Bihar has a good fertile land, endowed water resources and beneficial climatic conditions

---

3 The information is based on field visit and Interaction with farmers and resource person. It may be vary from place to place.

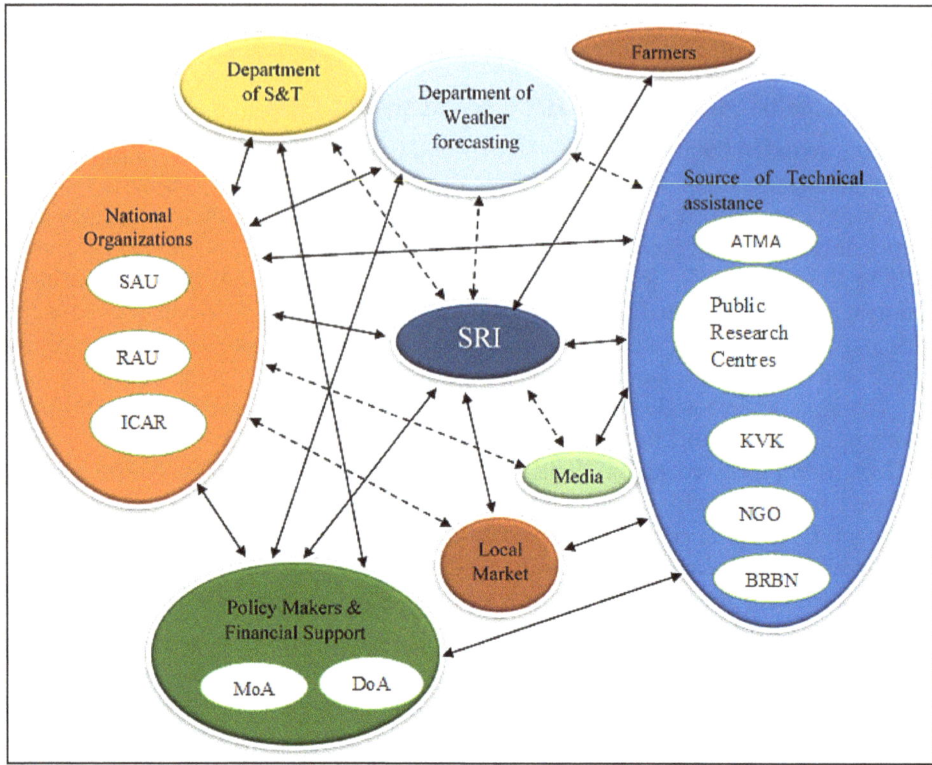

Figure 5.2: Actors of Policy Networks to Promote SRI Innovation (*Source*: Prepared by Author, 2017).

that mean it is having tremendous potential to the agriculture sector. In-spite of well available resources in the state, the productivity of crops of Bihar compares poorly with other states. Hence, at the principal of the new agricultural policy for Bihar is the focus on increasing productivity of crops which is low comparison of the national average. Therefore, the major initiatives have been taken by the State government in last one decade[4]:

- Food security, Increase in farmer's income, Increase in crop productivity and Environmental conservation has been fixed as the four targets of the new agricultural policy regime.
- ATMAs have been constituted in 23 districts of the State which did not have its ATMA coverage under the centrally sponsored programme. Thus, all the districts of the State now have ATMA coverage.
- A megaproject for establishment of soil testing laboratories in all 534 blocks of the State has been sanctioned, to take a soil testing facilities right to the door of the farmers.

4 http://bameti.org/pdf/state_profile.pdf accessed on 15th October 2016.

- ☆ 31 new seed testing laboratories are to be established in the State to give each district its own seed testing laboratory.
- ☆ The Chief Minister Horticulture Mission has been started in 19 districts of the State which were not covered under National Horticulture Mission, thereby universalizing the programme in the State.
- ☆ Micro-nutrient testing laboratories have been established in 3 districts of the State.
- ☆ Research and Educational infrastructure of Rajendra Agricultural University, which happens to be the only agricultural university of the State, has been strengthened.
- ☆ Agricultural Produce Marketing Board has been abolished
- ☆ Bihar State Seed Corporation has been revived, and seed production has been started on 45 state agricultural farms which were lying inoperative.
- ☆ Agricultural Produce Marketing Board has been abolished.
- ☆ Farmers' Commission has been established.
- ☆ Land Reform Commission has been established

Though, it is also realized that in the light of geophysical characteristics, there should be a distinct development strategy for flood-prone and draught-prone areas of Bihar. Therefore, specific strategies are devised and deployed for Paddy crop.

Strategy for Rice Cultivation

Rice is cultivated in all districts of Bihar. Out of 38 districts, 25 districts are characterized as a low productivity group which accounts for 63 per cent of 36.57 lakh hectares of total area under rice in the state. Further, one district, namely, Rohtas is under high productivity group, *i.e.* yield more than 2,500 kg/ha. Triennium average productivity of a high productivity group comprising of one district was 2,597 kg/ha as against the State's, average productivity of 1,530 kg/ha[5]. The major constraints in production are flash floods and submergence, drought in uplands, zinc deficiency and bacterial blight. According to the GoI, (2008)[6] the appropriate technological interventions and strategies are:

- ☆ Propagation of system of rice intensification (SRI) Technology.
- ☆ Cultivation of short duration and drought tolerant varieties Vandana, Tulasi, Rajashree.
- ☆ Cultivation of varieties like ARRH 2, DRRH 2 in normal situation and Rajendra Mahsuri, Rajendra Sweta and Swarna in flood prone and submergence areas.
- ☆ Cultivation of bacterial blight resistant varieties such as Ajaya, IR 64.

---

5 http://drdpat.bih.nic.in/ accessed on 15th October 2016

7 Government of India, 2008. Chapter 10 Developmental Strategies, Policies and Institutional Directions. Bihar's Agriculture Development: Opportunities & Challenges-A Report of the Special Task Force On Bihar available on http://bihar's per cent 20agriculture per cent 20development.pdf.

- ✰ Application of zinc sulphate in zinc-deficient areas.
- ✰ Propagation of hybrid varieties.
- ✰ Propagation of Boro rice in the non rainy season as the productivity is very high due to the absence of disease, pests and weeds, but it requires committed irrigation. Further, it should also be supported by the Strong seed programme and fine/scented variety for raising income.
- ✰ Propagation of Replacement of long duration varieties with short and medium duration varieties.

Programs and Project Initiatives for Agriculture Development

Besides, there are 14 major development programs which are handled and monitored by Department of Agriculture, Government of Bihar. Out of 14, 5 state sponsored, 4 centre sponsored and 4 Mission Mode projects[7]. However, the National Food Security Mission (NFSM) and Rastriya Krishi Vikas Yojana (RKVY) are main programs which linked to Rice cultivation.

National Food Security Mission (NFSM)

NFSM was launched in Bihar in the year of 2007-08. The main objectives of this program are to increase productivities of rice, wheat and pulses along with to maintain or increase the fertility of soil. Though, this program has some positive effects in rural area by allocating seeds and fertilizers but, huge number of farmers do not have access NFSM, especially remote villages and poor farmers. Further, fund allocation of this program is carried out by Department of Agriculture. In the year of 2009-10 86 per cent of the fund is allocated but gradually, it reduced to 59 per cent in 2010-11 and 35 per cent in 201112. The fund allocation reduced because due to another state program being implemented such as National Rural Livelihood Mission and Agriculture Mechanization *etc.* Also, the seeds of paddy distributed by State Government did not come into practice by the majority of farmers because farmers did not have knowledge about the seeds or their less confidence in new technology[8].

Rastriya Krishi Vikas Yojna (RKVY)

This project was launched in the year of 2007-08 with an objective to increase investment in agriculture and their allied sectors. It also helps to reduce the yield gap and introduce the agriculture and allied sectors in an integrated manner. In this project, mechanization is the major element which accounts for 85 per cent of the total outlay of the project but, only one third outlay of agriculture mechanization could be utilized in 2010-11 and performance remained commendable in 2011-12. The mechanization specially, laser leveler and Rota vector could not be implemented satisfactorily due to the small size of land holding in Bihar[9].

---

7 http://www.bihartimes.in/articles/RKP/agriculturetransformation.html accessed on 15th October 2016.

8 *ibid.*

9 http://www.bihartimes.in/articles/RKP/agriculturetransformation.html accessed on 15th October 2016.

However, all these projects did not affect more on farmers because of their small size of land holdings, low socio-economic status and poor access to officials of the agriculture department. Furthermore, there are various new innovative programs have been introduced by State Government such as Mukhayamantri Teevra Beej Vistar Yojana, Beej Gram Yojana *etc.* These programs have mentioned in the Bihar Agriculture Road Map. Two agriculture, road map is prepared for five year plans. First Agriculture Road Map was prepared for the year of 2007 to 2012 which is completed now and second road map is prepared for the year of 2012 to 2017. The details of both agriculture, road maps are discussed in the next section.

Agriculture Road Map-I: SRI Achievements

In the year of 2008, first time agriculture road map was prepared ended on 31st March 2012. The map was used as a medium to popularize quality seeds, new farm implements, the use of green manure, vermin compost and latest technologies to enhance productivity. In order to achieve major objectives of increasing the farm income, while assuring food and nutritional security and enhancing agricultural growth with justice, a series of programs are planned. These programs cover all aspects of agriculture, from inputs to marketing of final products. They fall into four major groups:

1. Inputs, access, supply and quality.
2. Transfer of technology and extension.
3. Income generation schemes.
4. Marketing.

During the ending year of road map 2011-12 farmers have made new records in Rice and Potato productivity. In this road map two ambitious programs initiated: 1) Chief Minister's crash seed program, and 2), seed village scheme. However, in the year of 2010 more than 7000 farmers were engaged as Kisan salahkar at Panchayat level. After forming of these infrastructures, many ambitious productivity enhancement programs were implemented. The first program was the SRI method of Rice and Wheat cultivation in which more than 10 per cent of the farming community of Bihar benefitted and SRI rice cultivation was practiced in 3.5 lakh hectares and SRI wheat in 2.40 lakh hectares. Second program was for the cultivation of hybrid rice, which covered an area of more than 4.0 lakh hectares. Besides this, the Government has also taken initiatives towards organic farming program which aims at reaching green manure, vermin compost and bio fertilizer to every farmer in five years. In the year of 2011, a new method was adopted to distribute subsidy. An input distribution cum training camp was organised at the block level for timely supply of inputs and cash subsidy distribution.

Furthermore, this map also focused on irrigation because irrigation and waterlogging are two major constraints for agriculture development. Therefore, the water resources sector was included and they were assigned the responsibility to increase the irrigation intensity from present levels of 82 per cent to 159 per cent in 2017 and 209 per cent in 2022. It happened mainly from 14.64 lakh private tubewells. Though, tubewell irrigation is dependent on the use of diesel, therefore the cost of irrigation is increasing with ever increasing cost of diesel and now it is beyond the capacity of even medium and big farmers use diesel for applying adequate irrigation. However, the progress of SRI and rice cultivation farming is discussed below:

Progress of SRI

SRI campaign was launched in the year of 2011 by Chief Minister of the State. This technique is, ideally, suitable for the small and marginal farmers. The progress of this scheme is given in Table 5.1

Table 5.1: Progress of SRI in Bihar

Sl.No.	*Item*	*Target*	*Achievement*
1	Demonstration (Ha.)	70400	70386
2	Demonstration (No. of Farmers)	176000	180000
3	Financial (Rs. In lakh)	5280	5278.92
4	No. of Conoweeders	118945	74497
5	Total coverage including demo. (Ha.)	350000	334542

Source: Agriculture Road Map-II GoB (2016).

The table represents progress of SRI technique till the year of 2011-12. It can be observed from table that, 96 per cent of the target area has been achieved, but number of conoweeders did not have up to level. The reason for failure lie in weeder machine is not working properly. Hence, farmers does not satisfy with machine and therefore, farmers do weeding manually.

Hybrid Rice

Under the program for promotion of hybrid rice varieties was implemented during kharif season. In the year of 2011-12 hybrid rice area has doubled in comparison to the previous year coverage. The details of the scheme are given in Table 5.2.

Table 5.2: Progress of Hybrid Rice

Sl.No.	*Item*	*Target*	*Achievement*
1	Demonstration (Ha.)	200000	199463
2	Demonstration (No. of Farmers)	500000	550000
3	Financial (Rs. In Lakh)	6000	5983.28
4	Total coverage including demo. (Ha)	400000	405371
5	Seed sale on subsidy (Q)	30000	29919
	Seed sale without subsidy (Q)	30000	31198

Source: Road Map-II, GoB (2016).

Promotion of Dhaincha

A program for the cultivation of Dhaincha as green manure crop was implemented for maintaining the soil fertility. This will add 200 quintal per hectare green matter into the soil, which will enhance the microbial population in the soil. This will have the additional advantage of nitrogen fixation. The details of the scheme are as below:

Table 5.3: Promotion of Dhaincha

Sl.No.	*Item*	*Target*	*Achievement*
1	Demonstration (Ha.)	370024	370024
2	Demonstration (No. of farmers)	925000	925000
3	Seed distribution (quintals)	99776	99775

Source: Agriculture Road Map-II, GoB (2016).

Expenditure Outlay Plan to Implement Programs and Projects

By launching of Agriculture Road Map in 2008, the state took a major step forward in the holistic development of agriculture in the state, plan outlay for agriculture increased forty times from Rs. 20.43 crore in 2005-06 to 797.86 crore during 2011-12. The detail of outlay plan is given in Figure 5.3.

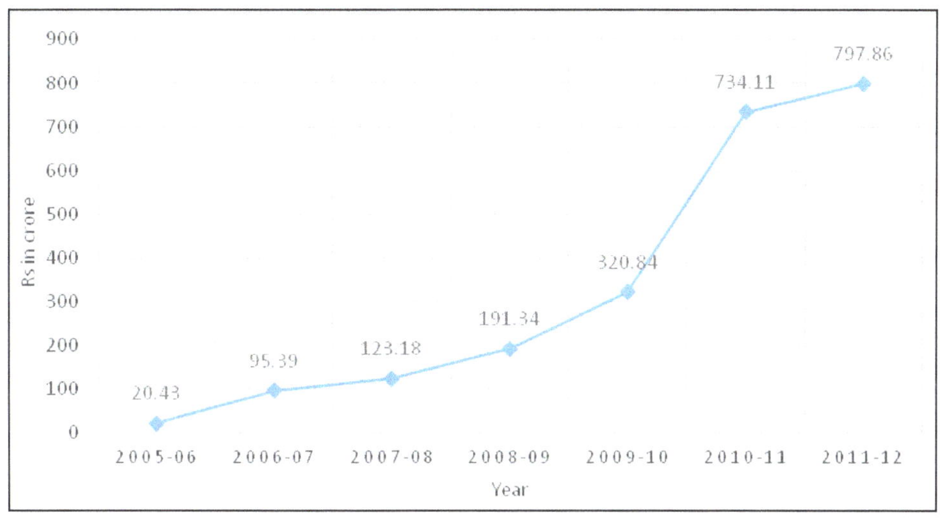

Figure 5.3: Expenditure on Implement Programs and Projects (*Source*: Agriculture Road Map-II, GoB (2016).

The Figure 5.3 shows agriculture road map has led to forty fold increase in the plan outlay of the agriculture department in past five years. However, Agriculture production and productivity enhancement programs will be implemented with support from State and Central Government. The program initiated during first road map has continued to be further strengthened in second agriculture road map. It is broader based than the first Road Map.

Agriculture Road Map-II

After, to get the feedback from the first agriculture road map, the second map has been prepared in the year of 2012 and the programs is set for the 2012-2017. The major goal of Agriculture Road Map-II is[10]:

- Increase in farmers' income
- Food Security
- To create gainful employment and to check migration
- To ensure equitable farm agriculture growth with focus on gender and human aspects
- Conservation and sustainable use of natural resources
- One product from Bihar in every Indian's plate

The vision of this map is to increase crop productivity in qualitative as there is limited scope for an increase in area. Current fallow and other fallow land will be brought under cultivation with appropriate interventions. Hence the strategy for Paddy cultivation are following:

- Increase in farmers' income and reduction in cost of cultivation through adoption of modern agriculture techniques and management method: The cost of the quality of agricultural produce will be reduced by encouraging use of Zero tillage, compost and green manure. Farmers' income will increase with the adoption of techniques *viz.* SRI of Rice and Wheat cultivation.
- Sustainable Agriculture Production compatible with the changing climatic conditions through adoption of appropriate crop, enterprise mix, recycling of organic waste other appropriate methods. Organic waste will be used for vermin composting to enrich the soil fertility. Crop straw will be harvested with appropriate technique and utilized for fodder purposes.
- To establish agriculture as a prestigious profession to attract educated youth towards agriculture and to reward for great contributions: The work of the agriculture scientists, extension workers and farmers would be recognized and rewarded.

However, besides these, an integrated seed plan is prepared for next five years. This is based on crop wise, agro climatic zone wise and variety wise. In this plan, government collaborates with the private sector to produce and supply of quality seed including hybrid varieties. This plan assigned specific roles to ICAR institutions, Agriculture Universities, KVKs, and Government Farms, National and State Seed Corporations and Private seed companies. This plan includes Breeder, Foundation and Certified seed. It also includes Production, Processing and Storage of inbred lines and hybrid varieties.

---

10 Agriculture Road Map-II, Government of Bihar, 2016. Available on http://www.Krishiroadmapeng.pdf. Access on 16th October 2016.

Further, the ICAR institutions and agriculture universities would be responsible for the purity and production of Breeder seed developed in the public sector. Further, multiplication of Breeder seed to Foundation seed will take place in government seed multiplication farms. Certified seed will be produced by the registered seed growers of seed corporations and in the seed villages. Strict quality control will be strictly observed at every step of Seed Production, Processing and Storage. Private sector seed companies are playing an important role, particularly in hybrid seeds. As the private hybrid varieties are not certified, the quality of private hybrid varieties is not subject to the mandatory testing under seeds Act[11]. In order to take maximum benefit from the private sector varieties is allowed only after it has been tested for suitability in the agro climatic situation of the state. Such testing is done by the agricultural universities/KVKs/ICAR institutions. Hence, to achieve the targets for the seed replacement rate, the requirement for Breeder, Foundation and Certified seed is assessed as given Table 5.4.

Table 5.4: The Requirement of Paddy Seed Year-wise (Unit in quintals)

Year/Type		*2012-13*	*2013-14*	*2014-15*	*2015-16*	*2016-17*
High Yielding Varieties	Certified Seed	297000	309750	348000	342000	336000
	Foundation Seed	3713	3872	4350	4275	4200
	Breeder Seed	46	48	54	53	53
Hybrid	Hybrid Seed	75000	82500	90000	97500	105000

Source: Agriculture Road Map-II, GoB (2016).

Though, to meet the seed requirement for achieving the targets of SRR, the on-going schemes are to be continued with suitable modifications. Mukhyamantri Tibra Beej Vistar Yojna and Seed Village program has been merged into one integrated program. Though, the cost of the seed is higher farmers are tempted to sow the home kept seed. It affects productivity. Therefore, subsidy is provided to the farmers so that farmers can adopt new seeds. However, the provision for seed subsidy under central schemes is there, but State government is also providing additional subsidy from its own resources. Currently, subsidy is provided at a rate of Rs. 7 per Kg for Paddy. Moreover, seed subsidy has been administered through government seed companies. The subsidy amount is released by the seed companies at the source so that the farmers get the seed at subsidized rates. It has brought transparency and need to be continued for benefitting the farmers. The physical and financial target for the Paddy seed subsidy program is shown in Table 5.5

However, the productivity milestone set for the road map could not be achieved. The productivity levels recorded in demonstration plots are much higher than the productivity levels reported. It has opened the discussion for the veracity of the

11 Certification Agency notified under Section 8 of the Seeds Act, 1966. Eligibility Requirements for Certification of Crop Varieties of those Seed of only those varieties which are notified under Section 5 of the Seeds Act, 1966 shall be eligible for certification.

productivity data. Pilot testing of remote sensing technology for the assessment of the crop area and production has started which can be utilized after it is validated. The extension services have to play a major role to implement this program and policy. The most challenging job is extension services in agriculture because it involves bringing in behavioural change in farmers.

Table 5.5: The Physical and Financial Target for Paddy Seed Subsidy Program (Physical unit in quintal and financial unit in Rs. Lakh)

Year	*2012-13*	*2013-14*	*2014-15*	*2015-16*	*2016-17*
High Yielding Varieties					
Physical	297000	309750	348000	342000	336000
Financial	2079	2168	2436	2394	2352
Hybrid					
Physical	75000	82500	90000	97500	105000
Financial	81	100	100	200	300

Source: Agriculture Road Map-II, GoB(2016).

Agricultural Extension for SRI and Overall Paddy Cultivation

The main object of the extension services is to be converted knowledge into skills to help farmers increase their income. The present extension system has reconstructed to make it capable of dissemination of agricultural technology to farmers with transparency and need based priorities. A system has developed for technology development and extension continuum. The District Agriculture officer is the main principal officer who also responsible for the development of agriculture at the district level and leads role in ATMA governing council and other committees at the district level for effective coordination. ATMA and BAMETI has been strengthened. The Block Agriculture officer is engaged in distributing assistance to farmers for the ambitious scheme like SRI. As para extension worker Kisan Salahkar is an integral part of the extension service. For an effective extension service, the extension workers would need to go to villages and up to the farmers in the field. The physical and financial extension program for Paddy is shown in the Table 5.6.

Table 5.6: The Physical and Financial Extension Program for Paddy Cultivation (Physical in ha. and Financial in Lakh)

Demonstration		*2012-13*	*2013-14*	*2014-15*	*2015-16*	*2016-17*	*Total*
SRI	Physical	1.4	1.6	1.8	1.8	1.8	8.4
	Finance	10500	12000	13500	13500	13500	63000
Hybrid Rice	Physical	2	2	2	2	2	10
	Finance	6000	6000	6000	6000	6000	30000
Boro Paddy	Physical	0.10	0.2	0.4	0.5	0.5	1.7
	Finance	750	1500	3000	3750	3750	12750

Source: Agriculture Road Map-II, GoB (2016).

The Table 5.6 represents the physical and financial extension program and it can be observed that, since last two-three years financial flow is constant and demonstration area is same. However, the innovation in agriculture policies or program need attention at the national level as well as state level for enhancing the agricultural production and productivity. On the other hand, it is also important to promote and adopt SRI practices in enhancing sustainable agriculture and now time has come to build confidence of small and marginal farmers in Bihar through right policies by ensuring easy credit availability, remunerative prices for agricultural products, supply of drought resistant varieties and short-duration high yielding varieties, establishment of self-help groups and encouraging direct marketing and selling of agriculture products by the farmers.

Conclusion

The State government declared 2011 as the SRI year by calling 'SRI Kranti (or revolution)' in first agriculture road map (GoB, 2016). Later, SRI came to be known as the System of Root Intensification, applying to many crops beyond rice and it has been taken up in this form by the ATMA and other government agencies. In-spite of all these policies and programs the situation of farmers are not better, especially in the case of small and marginal farmers. Thus, it is the innovation in agriculture need to focus on the boosting of rural infrastructure, the advancement of agri-business and subsidiary farm enterprises and creation of more employment to avoid migration from rural areas to urban areas. The fragile climate and rise in temperature is an inevitable process in Bihar. There is a need to focus on development of drought resistant, less water intensive and short duration crop in drought prone district of the state. SRI is the cost-effective, innovative farming techniques which Bihar farmers can adapt.

Though, there are many policy challenges for Bihar agriculture. The main challenges are food security and promotion of rural non-farm sector in order to generate income and sustain livelihoods of farmers. Hence, the major concern areas are credit and infrastructure, market, diversification, institutions, education/skill deficit. The marginal and small farmers can get benefit if programs and policy run and implement properly. To this point, there is need to monitor these program at field level and group approach is needed for inputs and marketing. Besides this, environmental concerns have to be addressed in order to have sustainable agricultural growth.

References

Berry, F.S. and Berry, W.D. 1992. Tax innovation in the states Capitalizing on political opportunity. *American Journal of Political Science* 36:715–42.

Bray, F. 1986. The Rice Economies: Technology and Development in Asian Societies. Basil Blackwell.

Glover, D. 2011. Science, practice and the System of Rice Intensification in Indian agriculture. *Food Policy*, 36(6), 749–755. doi:10.1016/j.foodpol.2011.07.008

Government of Bihar 2016. Department of Agriculture http://krishi.bih.nic.in/

Lubell and Fulton Local Policy Networks and Agricultural Watershed. *Journal of Public Administration Research and Theory*, Management doi:10.1093/jopart/mum031

Rogers, E. M. 1962. *Diffusion of Innovations*. Glencoe: Free Press. p. 11.

Thatcher, M. 1998. The development of policy network analyses. *Journal of Theoretical Politics* 10(4): 389–416

Uphoff, N. 2007. Agroecological alternatives: Capitalizing on genetic potentials. *Journal of Development Studies*. 43:1, 218-236.

Chapter 6

Role of Transcriptomics, Proteomics, and Metabolomics in Linking Genome and Phenome; Importance of Understanding the Phenotypes for Expiating the Outcome of Genomic Technologies-Knockout Mutant Studies and High Throughput Phenotyping

Abhinandan S. Patil[1], *Viralkumar B. Mandaliya*[2], *Kirankumar G. Patel*[3] *and S.A. Patil*[4]

[1]*Plant Sciences Institute, Agricultural Research Organization, Rishon Lezion-7528809, Israel*
[2]*Gujarat National Law University, Gandhinagar-382426, Gujarat, India*
[3]*P. D. Patel Institutes of Applied Sciences, Charotar University of Science and Technology, Anand-388421, Gujarat, India*
[4]*Deptt. of Zoology, Smt. Kasturbai Walchand College, Sangli-416416, Maharashtra, India*
**e-mail: agrilstar25@gmail.com*

ABSTRACT

Three omics are derived from the field of biochemistry and involves the analysis of small-molecule metabolites and polymers such as nucleic acid, protein, starch. Although this field is relatively new, there have been significant recent advances and there is scope for many direct applications in plant biotechnology. Metabolomics might be considered to be the key to integrated systems biology because it is frequently a direct gauge of the desired phenotype, measuring quantitative and qualitative traits such as starches in cereal grains or oils in oilseeds. This chapter discusses importance of understating the phenotypes for expiating the outcome of genomic technologies like knockout mutant studies and high throughput phenotyping. Application of transcriptomics, proteomics, and metabolomics, gene knockout techniques, and high-throughput techniques are a handful to plant and animal biologist for exploiting them in the well-being of human beings.

Keywords: *transcriptomics, proteomics, metabolomics, knockout mutant*

Introduction

Since the first observation by Gregor Mendel that phenotypic traits of pea plants are faithful manifestations of their genetic inheritance, altered phenotypes, which are readily observed, described, and quantified, have been central to the discovery of gene functions and molecular relationships among genes in the field of genetics. The lack of high-throughput technologies to access well-networked and integrated phenotypes from heterogeneous sources and across multiple scales of biological conditions has prevented the effective use of phenotypic information. As a result, development of phenotypic databases dramatically lags behind the rapid advance in genomic databases.

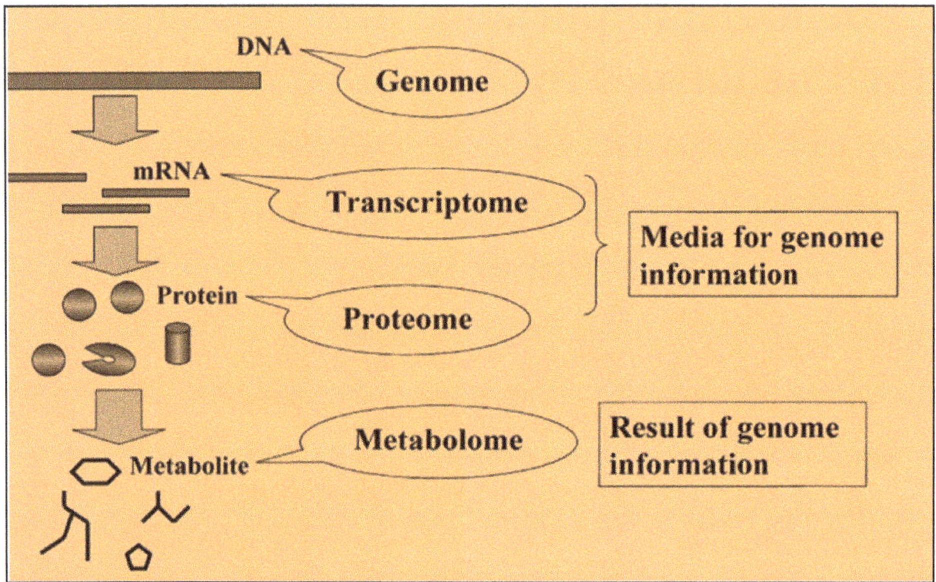

Figure 6.1: Genome to Omics.

Definition of 3-omics

Transcriptomics

The genome is made up of DNA, a long, winding molecule that contains the instructions needed to build and maintain cells. For these instructions to be carried out, DNA must be transcribed into corresponding molecules of ribonucleic acid (RNA), referred to as transcripts. A transcriptomics is a study and collection of all the transcripts present in a given cell.

Role of Transcriptomics

The application of microarrays and sequence-based methods to expression profiling has added an extra dimension to current genomic data and has founded several statistics-based disciplines within bioinformatics. Owing to their extended linear dynamics, sequence-based methods have the potential to determine more accurately quantitative levels of gene expression. Furthermore, they do not require prior sequence information and so have the advantage of being able to identify novel genes or to assess gene expression in uncharacterized plants. With the scaling-up of EST sequencing projects, it is becoming possible to mine these datasets to estimate expression information, although this remains more a byproduct of EST sequencing than a true transcriptomic tool. The predominant methods for sequence-based expression analysis are a serial analysis of gene expression (SAGE) and massively parallel signature sequencing (MPSS).

Proteomics

Science focused on determining the structures and functions of all the proteins produced by living organisms.

Role of Proteomics

- ☆ **Definition**-Proteomics refers to the analysis of protein profiles. The amino acid sequence of a protein determines the protein's three-dimensional structure and function (Banks *et al., 2000*).
- ☆ *One of the goals of* functional genomics and its approaches is to understand what the function of each of the genes and their protein products are (Tytus *et al., 2006*).
- ☆ Systemic deletion approaches can demonstrate gene function by demonstrating functional deficiencies in an organism when the gene is removed (Banks *et al., 2000*).
- ☆ *It is worth noting that function* is a protean concept. DNA and RNA fulfill the tasks of storage, transfer, and processing of genetic information contained in the genome of living organisms (Tytus *et al., 2006*).
- ☆ *Proteins form* complex cellular machinery for the realization of this genetic program resulting in the phenotype independency and in response to changing environment conditions (Nakanishi *et al., 2001*).

Challenges in the Utilization of Proteomics

1. Certain disadvantages are limiting the use of proteomics.
2. Proteins are dynamic and interacting molecules, and their changeability can make proteomic snapshots difficult. There is the need for a more sensitive analytical system and the absence of an effective method for large-scale data comparison (Pandey and Mann, 2000).
3. Very closely related proteins may not guarantee a functional relationship (Dumwell *et al., 2001*).
4. The false positive rate of motif assignment is high due to the high probability of matching short motifs in unrelated proteins by chance (Rossignol, 2001).
5. Proteins possess different levels of energy, for instance, hydrogen bonds, hydrophobic effects, Van der-Waal forces and electrostatic forces thus difficult to deal with proteins.

6. Within the proteome, the many observed layers of complexity begin with an RNA processing mechanism called alternative splicing in which a single gene can produce multiple versions of a protein (Rossignol, 2001).

Metabolomics

As the systematic survey of all metabolites present in a plant tissue, cell and cellular compartment under defined condition.

Role of Metabolomics

Like proteomics, metabolomics was derived from the field of biochemistry and involves the analysis (usually high throughput or broad scale) of small-molecule metabolites and polymers such as starch. The foundations of metabolomics are descriptions of biological pathways and current metabolomics databases, such as Kyoto Encyclopedia of Genes and Genomes, are frequently based on well-characterized biochemical pathways. On a more applied level, the bioinformatics of metabolomics involves the identification and characterization of a broad range of metabolites through reference to quantitative biochemical analysis.

Although this field is relatively new, there have been significant recent advances and there is scope for many direct applications in plant biotechnology. Metabolomics might be considered to be the key to integrated systems biology because it is frequently a direct gauge of the desired phenotype, measuring quantitative and qualitative traits such as starches in cereal grains or oils in oilseeds. Moreover, metabolomes can be correlated with genetics through proteomes, transcriptomes, and genomes and therefore bypass the more traditional quantitative trait locus approach applied to molecular crop breeding.

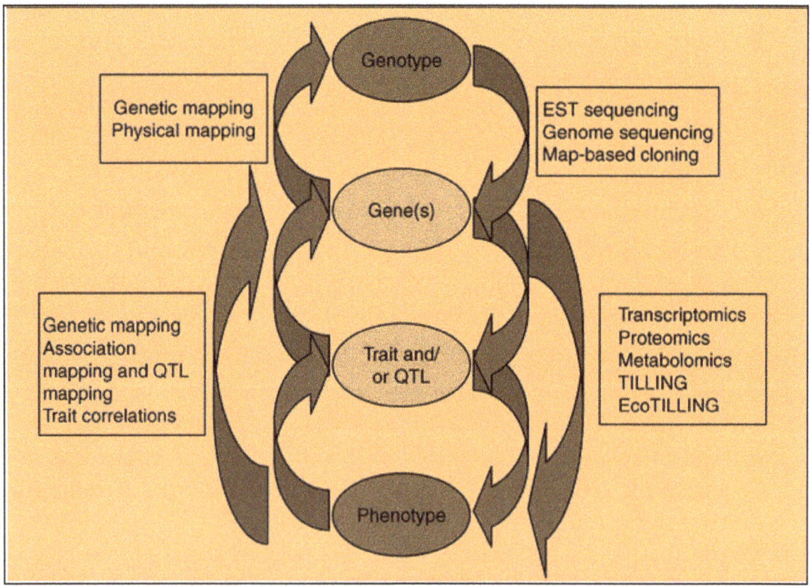

Figure 6.2: Genomics-based Approaches for Enhancing the Prediction of the Phenotype from a Genotype.

The better prediction of the phenotype that a particular genotype will produce is a primary goal of genomics-based breeding. The figure indicates how the various tools and techniques available today can be used to enhance our understanding of the various components between the genotype and the phenotype. On the left side are those strategies essentially based on classical genetics approaches (often enhanced by modern molecular tools), which can resolve the complexity of a phenotype, trait or QTL at a finer level in the genome. The right side indicates the application of modern genomics approaches to move from a genotype to phenotype. For example, genome and EST sequencing in combination with gene prediction algorithms and map-based cloning lead to the discovery of essentially the full set of genes in a genome. These genes can then be used in transcript profiling (transcriptomics), protein profiling (proteomics) and metabolite profiling (metabolomics) experiments to better understand their role in a trait or phenotype. TILLING and Eco-TILLING identify allelic variants of a gene, producing useful germplasm for discovery and confirmation of the role(s) of the particular gene(s) in a final phenotype. These can also be used as sources of superior haplotypes for use in direct enhancement of the phenotype. Traditionally, we have relied on classical genetic approaches such as trait correlation analyses and QTL mapping to dissect a complex phenotype into simpler trait components and/or QTL. QTL mapping has been enhanced in resolution with the availability of high-density molecular marker maps. Association mapping can also be applied to these high-density maps to directly identify the gene(s) associated with a particular phenotype and/or trait, without the need for segregating genetic populations. Genetic and physical mapping, using both cytogenetic and large-insert libraries such as bacterial artificial chromosome (BAC) and yeast artificial chromosome (YAC) based approaches, of the genes underlying QTLs provide detailed information regarding the organization of the genes in the genome as well as a basis for understanding the epistatic interactions or epigenetic phenomenon in the genome so that appropriate crop improvement strategies can be devised.

Importance of Understating the Phenotypes for Expiating the Outcome of Genomic Technologies

Knockout Mutant Studies

If the injected or transfected DNA contains a sequence homologous to a sequence in the mouse genome, it will sometimes be inserted into that sequence by homologous recombination.

Definition

The insertion of this foreign DNA into a gene will disrupt or "knock out" the function of the gene just like the insertions of the transposable genetic element.

Indeed, this approach has been used to generate knout mutation in 100 of mouse gene.

Importance of Knockout Studies

1. To study a range of process in mammals including, development, physiology, neurobiology, and immunology.

2. It has provided model systems for studies of numerous inherited human disorders from sickle cell anemia to heart disease to many types of cancer.
3. Knockouts are primarily used to understand the role of a specific gene or DNA region by comparing the knockout organism to a wild-type with a similar genetic background.
4. Knockouts organisms are also used as screening tools in the development of drugs, to target specific biological processes or deficiencies by using a specific knockout or to understand the mechanism of action of a drug by using a library of knockout organisms spanning the entire genome, such as in *Saccharomyces cerevisiae*.

Procedure of Knockout Mutation in Mouse

See Figures 6.3 and 6.4.

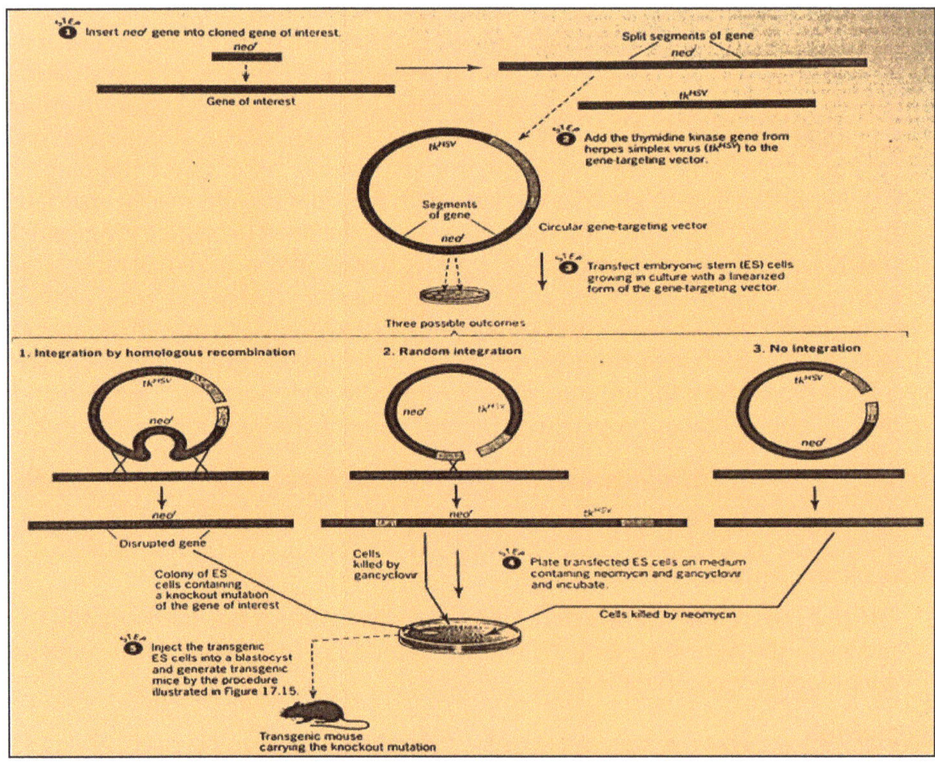

Figure 6.3: Generation of Knockout Mutations in Mice by Homologous Recombination.

High Throughput Phenotyping

Lower-cost, automated and semi-automated methods for data acquisition and analysis are now being developed, enabled by inexpensive cameras and computers with open-source software. Most recent applications have been in crops and model

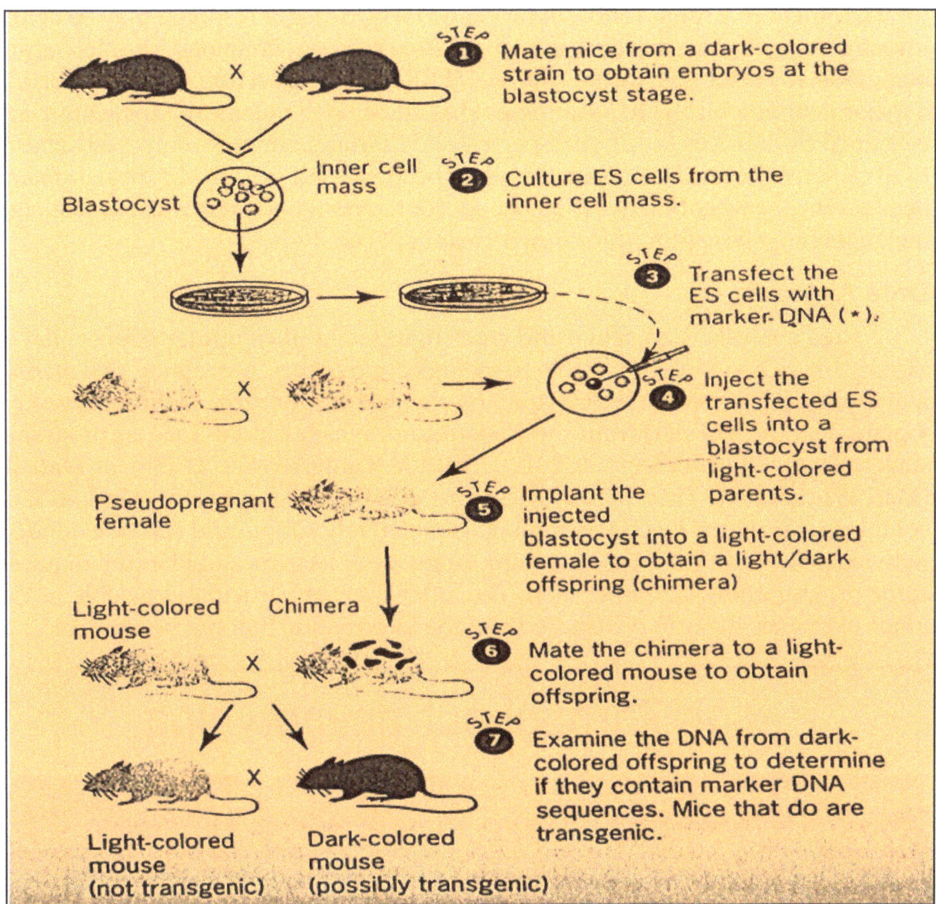

Figure 6.4: Scheme for Production of Transgenic Mice by Embryonic Stem (ES) Cell Technology.

organisms, but the tools can be extended to systematics and ecology, fields that often require huge amounts of specimen data. In this essay, we describe a few available tools to encourage readers to consider ways to increase the throughput of their own research. Further, terminology high-throughput phenotyping could apply to any morphological, physiological, or biochemical phenotype, here we focus on morphology or other phenotypes (*e.g.*, drought response) that can be captured using images. "High throughput" was defined by Fahlgren *et al.* (2015) as "hundreds of plants per day", but for many projects, even tens of plants per day would be a massive leap forward.

Data Recording

The appropriate method of image acquisition is determined first by the biological question and scale (macroscopic or microscopic) and second by the budget. Different camera types can provide different information (Fahlgren *et al.*, 2015). For example, shape and size of a herbarium specimen can be captured with a digital camera recording visible light. Conversely, drought response may be better investigated with near-infrared imaging. State-of-the-art imaging technologies are being assessed in the field by the ARPA-E TERRA-REF project (http://terraref.org/), a major goal of which is to determine what additional biological information can be gained from pricey (*e.g.*, hyperspectral and thermal) cameras compared to basic RGB cameras. Regardless of camera type, speed, or scale of data, the measurement needs to fit the scientific question. In addition, enough experimental and image metadata must be captured for downstream data analysis.

Data Analysis

Image analysis is an active and challenging field of computer science that is rapidly providing tools applicable to biological problems. A common first step in manipulating a photograph is extracting the relevant portion of the image (*e.g.*, a plant, leaf, or spikelet) from the background, which can be done in programs such as ImageJ (Schneider *et al.*, 2012), PlantCV (Fahlgren *et al.*, 2015b), or MatLab (MathWorks). The first two of these are open source, whereas MatLab is a commercial product. Basic use of ImageJ is relatively simple and can be extended with macros. MatLab is a programming language of its own, and PlantCV requires some programming skill in Python. The latter two are particularly flexible in the kinds of images that can be handled and the information that can be extracted.

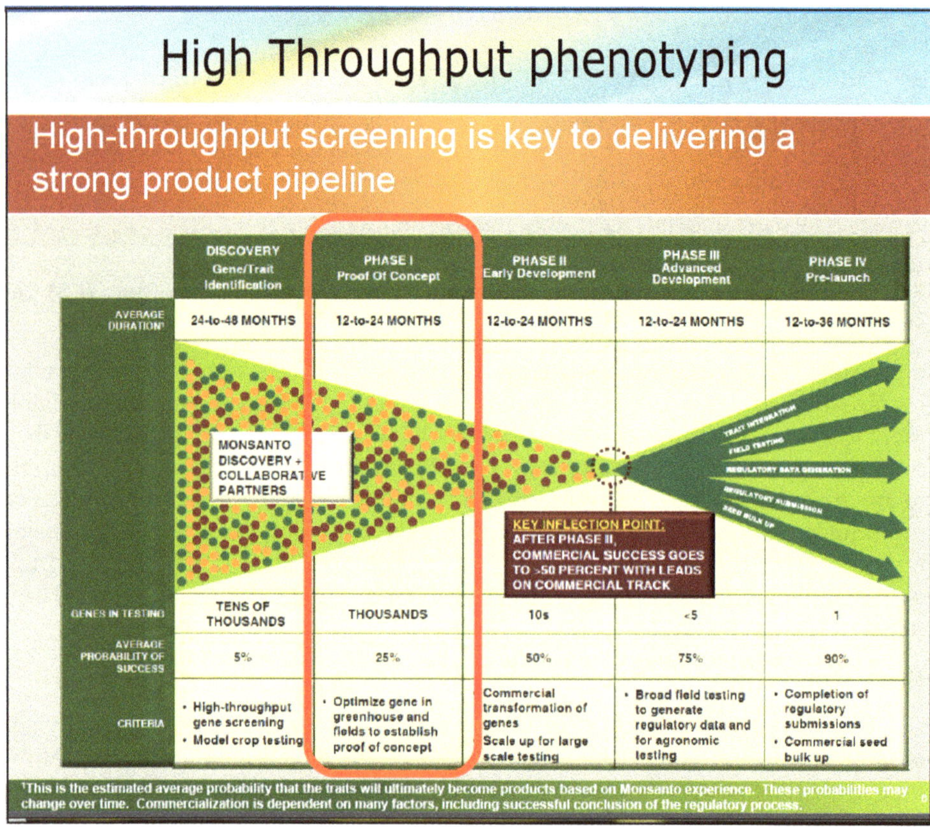

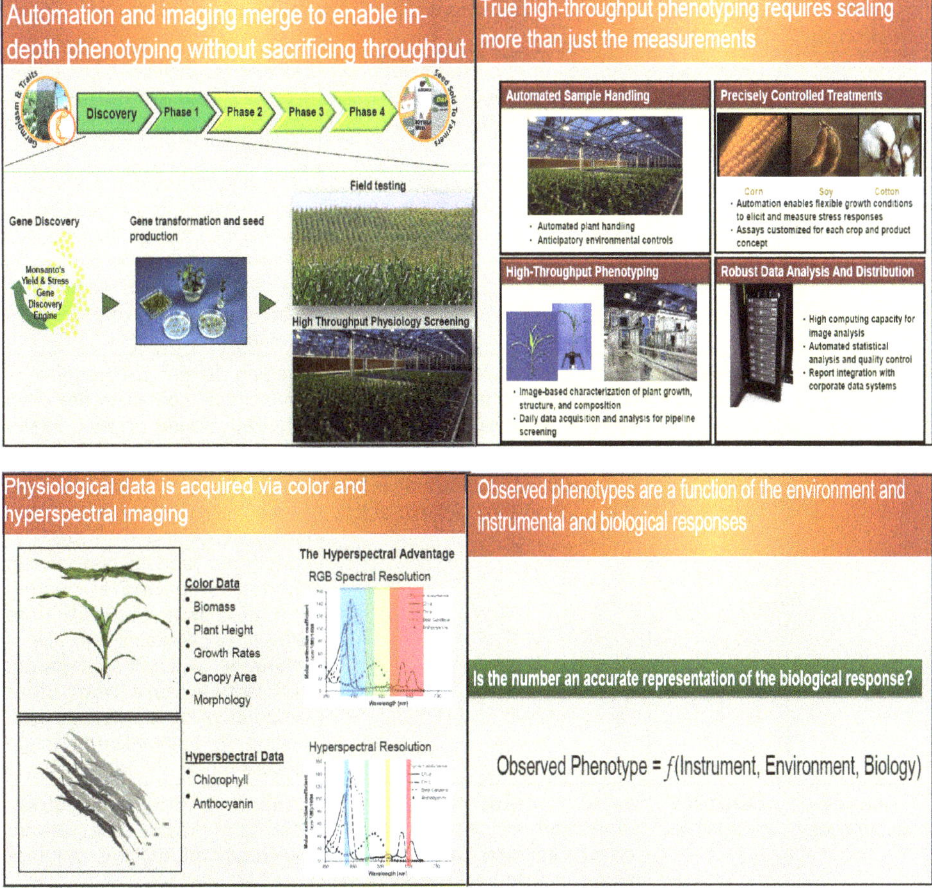

Table 6.1: The Advantages and Limitations of Imaging Techniques for Plant Phenotyping under different Growing Environments

Imaging Techniques	*Growing Environment*	*Applications*	*Limitations*
Visible imaging	Controlled environment	Growth dynamics, Shoot biomass, Yield traits, Panicle traits, Root architecture, Imbibition and germination rates, leaf morphology, seedling vigor, coleoptile length and biomass at anthesis, seed morphology, root architecture	Only provides plant physiological information
	Field	Imaging canopy cover and canopy color; color information can be used for green indices; the use of 3D stereo construction from multiple cameras or viewpoints allows the estimation of canopy architecture parameters	No spectral calibration; Only relative measurement; shadows and sunlight can result in under or overexposure and limit automatically processing image

Imaging Techniques	*Growing Environment*	*Applications*	*Limitations*
Fluorescence imaging	Controlled environment	Photosynthetic status, indirect measurement of biotic or abiotic	Difficult to analysis complicated whole-shoot of non-rosette species; pre-acclimation conditions required
	Field	Photosynthetic status, indirect measurement of biotic or abiotic stress	Difficult to measure at the canopy scale, because of the small signal to noise ratio, though laser-induced fluorescence transients can extend the range available, while solar-induced fluorescence can be used remotely
Thermal imaging	Controlled environment	Surface temperature; stomatal conductance water stress induced by biotic or abiotic factors	Imaging sensor calibration and atmospheric correction are often required; sound physics-based results interpretation needed
	Field	Stomatal conductance; water stress induced by biotic or abiotic factors	Imaging sensor calibration and atmospheric correction are often required; Changes in ambient conditions lead to changes in canopy temperature, making a comparison through time difficult, necessitating the use of reference. Difficult to separate soil temperature from plant temperature in sparse canopies, limiting the automation of image processing.
Imaging spectroscopy	Controlled environment	water content composition parameters for seeds; leaf area index; Leaf and canopy health status; panicle health status; leaf growth; Coverage density	Sensor calibration required; cost, large image data sets for hyperspectral imaging, complex data interpretation
	Field	Biochemical composition of the leaf or canopy; pigment concentration; water content; indirect measurement of biotic or abiotic stress; canopy architecture, LAI or NDVI	Sensor calibration required; changes in ambient light conditions influence signal and need frequent white reference calibration; canopy structure and camera geometries or sun angle influence signal. Data management is challenging
LIDAR	Controlled environment	Canopy height and canopy architecture; estimation of LAI; volume and biomass; reflectance from the laser can be used for retrieving spectral information	Specific illumination required for some laser scanning instruments
	Field	Canopy height and canopy architecture; estimation of LAI; volume and biomass; reflectance from the laser can be used for retrieving spectral information	Integration or synchronization with GPS and encoder position systems is required for georeferencing

Table 6.2: Relative Advantages and Disadvantages of Typical Phenotyping Platforms

Phenotype Platform Type	*Advantages*	*Disadvantages*
Controlled environment based	Automatically continuous operation; good repeatability	Generally expensive; can only monitor a very limited number of plots
Ground-based	Very flexible deployment; good capacity for GPS/GIS tagging; very good spatial resolution	Generally take a long time to cover a field, so subject to varying environmental conditions
Aerial based	Can cover the whole experiment in a very short time, getting a snapshot of all of the plots without changes in environmental conditions	Limitations on the weight of the payload; spatial resolution depends on speed and altitude

Conclusions

Application of transcriptomics, proteomics, and metabolomics, gene knockout techniques, and high-throughput techniques are a handful to plant and animal biologist for exploiting them in the well-being of human beings.

References

1. Genetics, Simmons and snustads, international student version.
2. Website: Monsanto company
3. Shu, Q.Y., Lagoda, P.J.L. Mutation techniques for gene discovery and crop improvement. Mol Plant Breed. **5**, 193-195 (2007).
4. Waugh, R., Leader, D.J., McCallum, N., Caldwell, D. harvesting the potential of induced biological diversity. Trends in Plant Sci. **11**, 71-79 (2006).
5. Puchta H. The repair of double-strand breaks in plants: mechanisms and consequences for genome evolution. J Exp Bot. **56**, 1–14 (2005).
6. Till B.J., Cooper J., Tai T.T., Caldwell D., Greene E.A., Henikoff S., Comai L. Discovery of chemically induced mutations in rice by TILLING. BMC Plant Biol. **7**, 19 (2007).
7. David Edwards, Plant bioinformatics: from genome to phenome.

Chapter 7

Seed Patenting: Approach of US, Europe and India

Rujitha Shenoy

Assistant Professor, Inter University Centre for IPR Studies, CUSAT, Cochin

e-mail: rujithashenoy@gmail.com

ABSTRACT

Plant and seed patent became a matter of discretion either to protect by way of patents or sui generis system or both after signing of TRIPS Agreement for the member countries. After compliance with TRIPS countries followed different strategies to protect their social and economic interests. Patenting seeds have raised havoc among the farmers in the light of decision of united states supreme court in Monsanto v bowman. The basic rule of patent exhaustion/first sale doctrine as interpreted by the court in case of self-replicating technologies will be examined. The paper examines the conflict between the rights of patent holders right to manufacture as well as first sale doctrine for sold goods creating certain limitation on the rights of the patent holder. In this context the paper explores the different strategies adopted by the countries to protect the interest of farmers. In the light of this issues it examines the provisions in the Indian legislature to protect the interest of the farmers and the seed policy of India is in tune with protecting the interest of the farmers. As the Indian patent Act make it clear that seeds and plants or parts thereof cannot be patented the paper also explores the battle over Bt cotton. This provision is a result of India opting to provide sui genesis legislation that provides intellectual property protection for plant varieties including transgenic varieties under a separate and specialized law known as the Protection of Plant Varieties and Farmers' Rights (PPVFR) Act, 2001. In this context examines the patent granted by Indian patent office to Monsanto for genetically modified plants, seeds and clams for gene.

Introduction

Agriculture is the backbone of the Indian economy. It has made a significant contribution for the economic development of Industrialized country. It plays a key role in developing and under developing country. In India 28 per cent of the income comes from agriculture.[1] Nearly two-thirds of its population depends directly on agriculture. Agriculture provides direct employment to 70 per cent of working people in the country. It is the main stay of India's economy.

Apart from those who are directly involved in the agrarian sector, a large number of the population is also engaged in agro-based activities. Agriculture meets the foods requirements of large population of India. It ensures food security for the country. Substantial increase in the production of food grain like-rice, wheat *etc.* and non-food grains like-tea, coffee, spices, fruits and vegetables, sugar, cotton *etc.* has made India self-sufficient.[2] This shows the very need of protection of farming community to sustain agriculture. In the context of globalization, where country is having obligations of WTO requirements there is a need to examine the existing legal regime after the TRIPS compliance adopted by India for the protection of farmers and to ensure food security.

India's Protection of Plant Varieties and Farmers' Rights Act

The international obligations relating to protecting plant breeder's rights based on TRIPS obligation under the requirements under Article 27.3 of the TRIPS agreement made India to enact Plant variety and farmers rights protection Act by way of a model of effective sui generis systemasrequiredunderTRIPS.

India's Protection of Plant Varieties and Farmers' Rights Act of 2001 is the most far-reaching legislation with regard to establishing rights for farmers to save, use, exchange and sell farm-saved seed. The Act represents a sui generis attempt to balance the rights of farmers and breeders, considering the huge farming population in the country. The attempt is to analyse the positive elements and negative elements aspect of this legislation and how far the farmers rights have protected and ensure food security.

The intellectual creation of plant breeders as well as farmers in developing new varieties will definitely fall under the umbrella of Intellectual property. India has taken care to protect the efforts of farmers also by recognizing their rights and giving protection. The positive elements of the act is the unique provision which confers three concurrent rights - to breeders, to farmers and to researchers.[3] When it comes to Farmers' Rights, the Act recognizes the farmer as cultivator, conserver and breeder. The Act establishes nine rights for farmers, of which the most important in this regard are the right to seed and the right to compensation for crop failure[4]:

The provisions on the right to seed specify that farmers are entitled to save, use, sow, re-sow, exchange, share and sell farm produce, including seeds of varieties protected by plant breeders' rights. They are, however, not allowed to sell seeds

1 https://ippmedia.com/en/features/importance-agricultural-sector-country per cent E2 per cent 80 per cent 99s-economic-development.

2 http://www.publishyourarticles.net/knowledge-hub/essay/essay-on-the-importance-of-agriculture-in-the-indian-economy/3300/.

3 S.30 and s.39,42THE PROTECTION OF PLANT VARIETIES AND FARMERS' RIGHTS ACT, 2001.

4 S.39(2) of PPVPFACT 2001.

of protected varieties as branded packages. All the same, this stands as the most liberal legislation to date in this sphere, allowing farmers all the customary rights they previously enjoyed.

The Act seeks to protect farmers from exaggerated claims by seed companies regarding the performance of their registered varieties. The breeder is obliged to disclose to farmers the performance of the variety under given conditions. If the material fails to perform according to this information, farmers may claim compensation from the breeding company through the Authority set up to administer the Act.

Not only does the 2001 Act protect the rights of farmers to save, use, exchange and sell farm-saved seed, it also seeks to ensure that these seeds are of good quality, or at least that farmers are adequately informed about the quality of seed they buy[5]. In addition, safeguards are provided against innocent infringement by farmers. Farmers who unknowingly violate the rights of a breeder are not to be punished if they can prove that they were not aware of the existence of such a breeder's right[6].

The research exception provision promotes research while preventing the premature exploitation of protected varieties in the name of research is positive one. The provision of compulsory licensing is also a positive element of this act by providing to invoke this provision at any time, after the expiry of three years from the date of issue of a certificate of registration of a variety,[7] any person interested may make an application to the Authority alleging that the reasonable requirements of the public for seed or other propagating material of the variety have not been satisfied or that the seed or other propagating material of the variety is not available to the public at a reasonable price and pray for the grant of a compulsory license to undertake production, distribution and sale of the seed or other propagating material of that variety.[8]

Another aspect is the exemption from fees for farmer or group of farmers or village community shall not be liable to pay any fees in any proceeding before the Authority or Registrar or the Tribunal or the High Court under this Act.[9]

Another provision is regarding benefit sharing provisions such that a proportion of the benefit will accure to a breeder of such variety or such proportion of the benefit accruing to the breeder from an agent or a licensee of such variety, as the case may be, for which a claimant shall be entitled as determined by the Authority if new variety is developed from the existing variety.

The disclosure requirement is another aspect where every application for registration must include a denomination of the variety and describe (1) the geographical origin of the material, and (2) all information regarding the contribution

---

5 Sec.39 PPVPFR Act 2001.

6 Sec42 PPVPFR Act 2001.

7 Sec47 PPVPFR Act 2001.

8 SEC.49 PPVPFR Act 2001.

9 S.44 PPVPFR Act 2001.

of the farmer, community, or organization in the development of the variety.[10] Further, the application must state that all genetic or parental material used to develop the variety has been lawfully acquired. Moreover, section 40 requires the breeder to disclose information "regarding the use of genetic material conserved by any tribal or rural families in the breeding or development of such [new] variety. Exceptions to registration of variety which says variety becomes un registerable if it is likely to deceive the public, hurt the religious sentiments of any class or section of Indians, or cause confusion regarding the variety's identity, or is not different from every denomination which designates a variety of the same botanical species or of a closely related species registered under the Act.[11]

The major advantage is by recognizing the extant variety so as to protect traditional knowledge and indigenous rights which includes matters known and existing in the public domain. At the same time recognizing the right of the state over it by granting the rights to determine their production, sale, marketability, distribution, importation or exportation of extant variety. In essence, an extant variety encompasses a farmers' variety, or a variety about which there is common knowledge, or a variety in the public domain, as well as any variety included under section 5 of the Seeds Act. The registration of extant variety makes it protected.[12]

The negative aspect of the act is with respect to the extant registration is two it is imposing a term of protection for extant varieties which creates an impression that matters in the public domain are not available in perpetuity.[13] Secondly, allowing any third party to register an extant variety could presumably lead to more extant variety to come in to public domain. Plants that are not commercially usable or being used may never be registered, leaving the registry incomplete at the same time helps to appropriate by anybody after the term of protection. The term common knowledge has been left broadly undefined may affect the actual intent of the act. The term common knowledge has been left broadly undefined may create confusion and,fixing criteria for registration of farmers variety may not be attractive. The compensation or the benefit shared actually flows to them through the gene fund lacks clarity. The lack of clarity of on extant variety and farmers variety is causing problems there by blocking the benefits to flow to farmers. The disclosure requirement verification is required. The protection for local communities is inadequate because the breeder is not required to show prior informed consent from the community from which he obtained the traditional knowledge.

Ensuring Farmers' Rights to save, use, exchange and sell seed in this way must be seen as a success with regard to this component of Farmers' Rights, as these rights are basically fully ensured through the Act.[14] Whether the provision on compensation

---

10 S.17 PPVPFR Act 2001.

11 Sec.40 PPVPFR Act 2001.

12 S.15 PPVPFR Act 2001.

13 Srividhya Raghavan, Jamie Mayer O' Shields, "Has India Addressed it' s Farmers' Woes? A Story of Plant Protection Issues", 20 Geo. Int'l Envtl. L. Rev. 97 Fall, 2007.

in case of crop failure can be implemented in practice is another question, as there have been no cases so far.[15] On the whole, India's Protection of Plant Varieties and Farmers' Rights Act is the most advanced in terms of Farmers' Rights to save use, exchange and sell seed to date. It applies to all farmers in India, and to all crop species. So far, twelve crop species have been brought under the scope of the Act, and more species will follow. The practice of saving, using, exchanging and selling seeds may well exist elsewhere, but India is the only country so far where a law has been passed establishing and securing Farmers' Rights to this extent.

Seed Patenting in United States

The history of seed development in Unites states reflects the extreme propertisation of seeds and genetic resources deviating from its earlier trend of seed development, distribution, and ownership in the hands of public sector and augmented by hundreds of small, often family-run, seed breeder businesses, which acted mainly as distributors of publicly developed seed varieties.[16] This contrasts sharply with the situation today in which the top ten companies control 65 per cent of proprietary, or intellectual property (IP)-protected, seed.[17]

The initiatives of patent office, the Secretary of the Treasury, U.S. Department of Agriculture (USDA) were to gather seeds and seed data from their all around the globe and to collect and distribute seeds to farmers across the country. Thus creating a vibrant agricultural germplasm base.[18]

Simultaneous to liberal seed programmes government enacted legislations which provided publicly funded resources for institutions of higher learning devoted to agriculture, referred to as land grant universities, and also for experimental and research services for rural communities.[19] These resulted in sweeping of potentional profits of seed compant. They decided to shift away from government programmes and become private entities. The growth of seed company resulted in giant multi national company holding seed monopolies and later witnessed the lobbying of the seed companies for the strong IPR regime, The success of the seed companies

---

14 Srividhya Raghavan, Jamie Mayer O' Shields, "Has India Addressed it' s Farmers' Woes? A Story of Plant Protection Issues", 20 Geo. Int'l Envtl. L. Rev. 97 Fall, 2007.

15

16

17 Kristina Hubbard, Farmer to Farmer Campaign on Genetic Eng'g, Nat'l Family Farm Coal., Out of Hand: Farmers Face the Consequences of a Consolidated Seed Industry p4 (2009), available at http://farmertofarmercampaign.com/Out per cent 20of per cent 20Hand.FullReport.pdf.

18 The vibrant seed trade between early European settlers and Native Americans established an important agricultural germplasm base that is still evident today in American farming. During the colonial era, the landed gentry formed "agricultural societies" that saved, cultivated, and exchanged seeds, though these were not widely distributed to the general populace. U.S. farmers saved seeds and developed steady genetic improvement; in fact, some of the most well-known seed varieties such as Red Fyfe wheat, Grimm alfalfa, and Rough Purple Chili potato are the result of farmer breeding and cultivation.

19

and the breeders resulted in legislations for the protection of seeds, plants and plant varieties. These include: The Plant Patent Act (PPA) of 1930 which allowed asexually reproduced plants, excluding tuber-propagated plants, to receive patent protection,[20] The Plant Variety Protection Act (PVPA) 1970 gave plant breeders 25 years exclusive IPR via a Certificate for a newly developed plant variety, including sexually reproduced plants and tuber-propagated plant varieties.[21] However, the PVPA granted exemptions to allow researchers and farmers to save seed. 1980: The Bayh-Dole Act allowed public institutions to obtain patents on publicly funded research. The judicial trend from 1980's starting from *Diamond v. Chakrabarty granted patents for genetically modified bacteria* and spurred the initiation of public-private partnerships, where industry funds public research to advance their own goals and often appropriates the resulting technology. Thus was followed by granting patents for transgenic plants in The *Ex parte Hibberd* case[22] where patents were granted for sexually-reproduced plants and thus expanded the scope of subject matter to plants, seeds. Again in *J.E.M. Agricultural Supply v. Pioneer Hi-Bred*[23] upheld granting of plant utility patents in the U.S other than in plant patent act. The Genetic Engineering Technology revolutionized the agriculture. The genetically engineered crops were granted patents after the JEM case*d* decision. In the years following the case, the Patent and Trademark Office (PTO) received over 1,800 applications for plant patents.[24]

International Patent Regime

On an international level, the World Trade Organization's Trade-Related Aspects of Intellectual Property Rights (TRIPS) Treaty, the United Nations,' World Intellectual Property Organization (WIPO), and the International Union for the Protection of New Varieties of Plants (UPOV) have encouraged and projected the American IPR paradigm around the world.[25] The interpretational technique of courts helped the multination to gain patents for GE crops and the misleading definition of invention further spurred patenting by claims for isolated part of nature, through a trivial modification of existing thing in nature by technology.

---

20 http://www.etcgroup.org/sites/www.etcgroup.org/files/publication/472/01/raficom46usplantpatentact.pdf.

21 http://www.greenhousegrower.com/varieties/plant-patent-law-protecting-the-variety-pipeline/.

22 227 USPQ 443 (PTO Bd. Pat. App. and Int. 1985).

23 [1] J.E.M. Ag Supply, Inc. v. Pioneer Hi-Bred International, Inc., 122 S. Ct. 593, 596 (2001).

24 James, Clive (1996). "Global Review of the Field Testing and Commercialization of Transgenic Plants: 1986 to 1995". The International Service for the Acquisition of Agri-biotech Applications. Retrieved 11 September 2012.

25 More than 90 percent of U.S. soybean acreage and 80 percent of corn acreage is planted with Monsanto's patented traits.At present, four agrichemical companies own a full 43 percent of the world's commercial seed supply. The number of small, independent seed companies has rapidly declined: Ten multinational corporations hold approximately two-thirds – 65 percent – of global commercial seed for major crops.

GE seed patents are now a central mechanism by which to gain control and ownership of genetic material of seeds writ large. IPR rules, particularly following the 1985 *Diamond v. Chakrabarty* decision, have expedited the adoption of GE seeds and simultaneously, GE seed technology broadens the scope of seed patenting. These schemes codify a weak and misleading definition of "invention," allowing companies to "isolate" a part of nature, or slightly modify an existing process or "product," and then patent it, as if it were novel. Yet the purported innovation is based on centuries of collective community knowledge and traditional seed breeding Monsanto controls 60 per cent of the global corn and soybean seed markets.[26] The number of indepemdent domestic Industries fall down from 300 to less than 100 because of monopoly held by few multinational seed companies.[27]

Monsanto v Bowman[28]: A "patent" Example

This case is highly important it shows the devastating effects of patents on farmers right to sell, resow and save seeds. Monsanto invented and patented Roundup Ready soybean seeds, which contain a genetic alteration that allows them to survive exposure to the herbicide glyphosate. Monsanto sold the patented seeds stating that it can be used once and can be used for consumption or for selling but not for re planting. Bowman purchased soybeans intended for consumption; planted them; treated the plants with glyphosate, killing all plants without the Roundup Ready trait; harvested the resulting soybeans that contained that trait; and saved some of these harvested seeds containing trait to use in next season for planting.[29] Monsanto sued Bowman for infringement as he was cultivating using Monsanto's seeds. The district court rejected Bowman's defense of exhaustion. The Federal Circuit affirmed district court's decision.The Supreme Court held that patent exhaustion does not permit a farmer to reproduce patented seeds through planting and harvesting without permission.[30] By planting and harvesting patented seeds, Bowman made additional copies of Monsanto's patented invention, which means "making" of the patented product there by patent infringement. In such a case of replicating technologies falls outside the protections of patent exhaustion otherwise it may result in patentees rights futile. Under the doctrine of patent exhaustion, the authorized sale of a patented article gives the purchaser, or any subsequent owner, a right to use or resell that article. Such a sale, however, does not allow the purchaser to make new copies of the patented invention.[31]

The impact of this decision is that farmers have to approach Monsanto again and again for planting the seeds paying prices on each purchase making the life

---

26 Hubbard, Farmer to Farmer Campaign on Genetic Eng'g, Nat'l Family Farm Coal., Out of Hand: Farmers Face the Consequences of a Consolidated Seed Industry p4 (2009).

27 I. Matthew Wilde, "Independent seed companies a dying breed," WCF Courier, August 22, 2012, http://wcfcourier.com/business/local/article_7cef1ffc-b0bb-56a8-8d83-faf894bf76ad.html.

28 Monsanto v Bowman 11-796, 569 U.S. (2013).

29 Ibid p .1.

30 Ibid p. 4-10.

31 Id p. 3.

of farmers miserable. The implication of this decision reflects the negative side of patenting seeds which thwarts the food security of a nation.

Seed Patents in Europe

In case of biotechnology inventions it is governed by European Biotechnology Directive The exclusion from patentable subject matter is given under art.4, art.5[32] and art. 6[33] Article 4 says

1. "The following shall not be patentable:
   (a) Plant and animal varieties;
   (b) essentially biological processes for the production of plants or animals.
2. Inventions which concern plants or animals shall be patentable if the technical feasibility of the invention is not confined to a particular plant or animal variety.
3. Paragraph 1(b) shall be without prejudice to the patentability of inventions which concern a microbiological or other technical process or a product obtained by means of such a process."

Here it can be seen that plants and animal varieties are excluded. But the plant which are produced by conventional techniques like crossing and non conventional methods like genetic engineering can be patentable, Based on this European Patent Office (EPO) has granted over 120 patents on conventionally bred (non-GMO) plants and animals.[34]. No patents on seeds" NGOs and many farmers' organizations and breeders have taken position to ban these patents as these patents restrict access to seeds for breeding, Recently, European Parliament and the European Commission also requested that granting of patents on plants and animals **means of an "essentially biological processes"**be restricted to the sole field of genetic engineering.[35] The NGO's have raised concern on the interpretation "essentially biological process" as the ban effectively only concerns plants and animals that

---

32 Article 5-1. The human body, at the various stages of its formation and development, and the simple discovery of one of its elements, including the sequence or partial sequence of a gene, cannot constitute patentable inventions.2. An element isolated from the human body or otherwise produced by means of a technical process, including the sequence or partial sequence of a gene, may constitute a patentable invention, even if the structure of that element is identical to that of a natural element.3. The industrial application of a sequence or a partial sequence of a gene must be disclosed in the patent application.

33. 1. Inventions shall be considered unpatentable where their commercial exploitation would be contrary to *ordre public* or morality; however, exploitation shall not be deemed to be so contrary merely because it is prohibited by law or regulation. 2. On the basis of paragraph 1, the following, in particular, shall be considered unpatentable: (a) processes for cloning human beings; (b) processes for modifying the germ line genetic identity of human beings; (c) uses of human embryos for industrial or commercial purposes; (d) processes for modifying the genetic identity of animals which are likely to cause them suffering without any substantial medical benefit to man or animal, and also animals resulting from such processes.

34 https://www.gmo-free-regions.org/gmo-free-regions/european-union/gmo-news-related-to-the-european-union.html?tx_sosnews_list per cent 5Bpage per cent 5D=77 and cHash=06aa4042c39be06bff4401fbab214784.

are the result of crossing and selection.[36] The concerns raised are on the narrow interpretation so the legal definition of "essentially biological" breeding should include all methods and biological materials used in conventional plant breeding.For example, it has to be made clear that plant characteristics derived from conventional breeding and plant varieties are not within the scope of patents granted on methods of genetic engineering.[37]

Indian Patent Act: Seed Patents

In India agriculture was based on free exchange of Knowledge and seeds, So as to ensure food security methods of agriculture and plants were excluded from patentability in the Indian Patent Act 1970 to ensure that the seed, the first link in the food chain, was held as a common property resource in the public domain.[38] In this manner, it guaranteed farmers the inalienable right to save, exchange and improve upon the seed was not violated. To comply with TRIPS Agreement two amendments have been made in the 1970 Patent Act. The 2002 and 2005 Amendment made changes in the definition of what is NOT an invention. Though care has been taken to prevent patenting of plants and seeds and living organisms, the lack of clarity in the provisions and the confusing biotechnology guidelines opened up the flood gates of patent application for genetically modified plants animals and seeds. The analysis oft the provisions are as follows:

S. 3 (c): "the mere discovery of a scientific principle or the formulation of an abstract theory or ***discovery of any living thing*** or ***non-living substance occurring in nature*** – not an invention.

This section makes it clear that discovery of plants or living organisms are not patentable. So isolation of a cell leading to plant can be called as mere discovery. But the word "mere" gives the impression that you can patented an isolated tissue leading to a plant.

S.3(h) a method of agriculture or horticulture;

This section makes it clear that nobody can patent method of agriculture as it should be freely available for the farming community and no monopoly over it

According to Section 3(i) of the Indian Patent Act, the following is not an invention:

"Any process for the medical, surgical, creative, prophylactic or other treatment of human beings or any process for a similar treatment of animals or plants or render them free of disease or to increase their economic value or that of their products."

---

35 https://www.publiceye.ch/en/media/press-release/patents_on_seeds_europe_misses_the_boat/

36 http://www.ifoam-eu.org/en/news/2016/11/04/no-patents-seeds-press-release-eu-commission-says-plants-and-animals-derived.

37 No Patents On Seeds Press Release: Eu Commission Says Plants And Animals Derived From Conventional Breeding Should Be Regarded As Non-Patentable, http://www.ifoam-eu.org/en/news/2016/11/04/no-patents-seeds-press-release-eu-commission-says-plants-and-animals-derived.

38 https://www.grain.org/es/article/entries/2166-india-seed-act-patent-act-sowing-the-seeds-of-dictatorship.

In the 2005 Amendment however, the mention of "plants" have been deleted from this section. This deletion implies that a method or process modification of a plant can now be counted as an invention and therefore can be patented. Thus the method of producing Bt cotton by introducing genes of a bacterium thurengerisis in cotton to produce toxins to kill the bollworm can now be covered by the exclusive rights associated with patents. In other words, Monsanto can now patent methods of treatment of plant which gives economic benefit of Bt cotton in India.

(j) plants and animals in whole or any part thereof other than microorganisms but including seeds, varieties and species and essentially biological processes for production or propagation of plants and animals;

The 2005Amendment has also added a new section (3j). This section says plants and animals as well as seeds and plant variety not patentable. So the plant can be either genetically modified or genetically modified seed or genetically engineered animals not patentable. But the Biotechnology guidelines which deviated from legislative intent and followed the path of United States and Europe made the Indian examiners to grant patents on it. Thus allowed patents for methods as well as for the plant's production or propagation of genetically engineered plants to count as an invention. Since plants produced through the use of new biotechnologies are not technically considered "essentially biological," which is the jurisprudence of Europe and United States also borrowed by Indian examiners and granted patents on genetically modified seeds. Thus section 3(j) has found another way to create room for multinational seed corporations like Monsanto.

Biotechnology Patent Examination Guidelines, 2013

It lists out **ten claims** as the claims that usually forms part of biotechnology patent applications Gene sequences, host cells, **plant** and animal **tissue culture.** Extensively used these claims in the illustrations to explain how to analyse biotechnology patent claims and grant patents. It's clear that these claims are treated as permissible claims by the Patent Office. But the guidelines goes without saying isolated biological materials are non-patentable subject matter. It gives the impression that gene patents can be allowed. So that a plant/seed having particular characteristic due to particular gene which is patented will give monopoly over that plant/seed. This the way out found by the multinational seed companies to enforce their property rights.

In the Guidelines for Processing of Patent Applications Relating to Traditional Knowledge and Biological Material" also it goes without saying isolated biological materials not patentable subject matter. The claims relating to extracts/alkaloids and/or isolation of active ingredients of plants, which are naturally/inherently present in plants. Instead it goes for defining when it is novel/having inventive step when use of such plants is pre-known as part of teachings of TK.

Granted Indian Patent Analysis

Many patents has been granted for transgenic plants as well as seeds. Some times in guise of method included claims of seeds too, The table given below shows few patents granted on transgenic plants and seeds

Patent no, 228182 Patent application no 2554/CHENP/2005	Monsanto Technology LLC.	DNA constructs and methods to enhance the production of commercially viable transgenic plants
528/DELNP/2007 A Patent no	Monsanto Technology	MAIZE SEED WITH SYNERGISTICALLY ENHANCED LYSINE CONTENT
1409/KOLNP/2003 Patent no	Monsanto Technology	TRANSGENIC HIGH TRYPTOPHAN PLANTS
5701/DELNP/2007	Monsanto Technology	TRANSGENIC PLANTS WITH ENHANCED AGRONOMIC TRAITS
2939/DELNP/2006	Monsanto Technology	HIGH LYSINE MAIZE COMPOSITIONS AND METHODS FOR DETECTION THEREOF
3227/DELNP/2007	Monsanto Technology	HIGH YIELDING SOYBEAN PLANTS WITH LOW INOLENIC ACID
573/KOL/2007	Uttar Banga Krishi Vishwavidyalaya	PUFFED RICE WITH VITAMIB-B
7136/DELNP/2008	Monsanto Technology	"Nucleic Acid Constructs And Methods For Producing Altered Seed Oil Compositions"
3278/DELNP/2008	Monsanto Technology	"A DNA CONSTRUCT FOR INCREASED LYSINE IN SEED"
71/MUM/2008	Monsanto Technology	A PROCESS FOR ISOLATION OF SEED MUCILAGE FROM THE SEED OF OCIMUM,
17/08/2007	Monsanto Technology	TRANSGENIC PLANTS WITH ENHANCED AGRONOMIC TRAITS"

Cases Study: 1

For example in the granted patents on MAIZE SEED WITH SYNERGISTICALLY ENHANCED LYSINE CONTENT[39] the claims of the invention are as follows:

The invention also provides a method for providing maize seed with synergistically increased lysine content, including:

(a) Providing a transgemc maize plant häving in its genome transgenic DNA including sequence for zein reduction and sequence for lysine biosynthesis,

(b) Expressing the transgenic DNA in seed of the transgenic maize plant, the expressing resulting in a synergistically increased lysine content of the seed, and

(c) Harvesting the seed with synergistically increased lysine content.

Embodiments of the method of the invention include providing a transgenic maize

The claims clearly mentions the isolated gene. Maize seed with lysine content, maize plant as well as harvesting the maize seed. All these claims attract sec 3(h) (i) (j) which makes it non patentable subject matter.

---

39 Patent no. 528/DELNP/2007 A.

Case Study 2

The invention TRANSGENIC PLANTS WITH ENHANCED AGRONOMIC TRAITS" describes its invention as:

Disclosed herein are inventions in the field of plant genetics and developmental biology. More specifically, the inventions provide plant cells with recombinant DNA for providing an enhanced trait in a transgenic plant, plants comprising such cells, seed and pollen derived from such plants, methods of making and using such cells, plants, seeds and pollen. In particular, the recombinant DNA of the inventions express transcription factors with homeobox domains. This shows how patents are granted in India for a non patentable subject matter.[40]

Case Study 3

In the invention titled "PUFFED RICE WITH VITAMIB-B[41]". The claims are

1. Vitamin enriched puffed rice comprising 0.1 to 0.6 per cent riboflavin based on total weight of rice incorporated into puffed rice by soaking parboiled rice in solution of riboflavin.
2. Vitamin enriched puffed rice as claimed in claim 1 wherein the amount of riboflavin is 1 to 7mg, preferably 5 mg per kg rice.

Here the claims are directly for the rice itself which was not the intent of sec 3 of the patent Act.

The above patent analysis shows how patents are granted for the non-patentable subject matter.

7288/DELNP/2009	CORN PLANTS AND SEEDS ENHANCED FOR ASPARAGINE AND PROTEIN
6560/CHENP/2008 A	CORN PLANT AND SEED CORRESPONDING TO TRANSGENIC EVENT MON89034 AND METHODS FOR DETECTION AND USE THEREOF

In the above given table the claims for transgenic seed been removed and then only granted patents due to objection/opposition both are patents of Monsanto.

Monsanto v Nuziveedu – On Going Patent Litigation

Monsanto is holding a patent on a nucleic acid sequence which will show herbicide resistance if inserted in a cotton plant. The Plaintiff sells 50 gms of transgenic seeds to the defendants for Rs. 50,00,000/- under a sub-license agreement. The sub-license agreement required the defendant to pay "trait value" for the sale of every 450 gms of the hybrid seed developed using the transgenic seed.[42] Farmers' now have to pay 'trait value' to Monsanto and R and D cost for the hybrid seed to the seed company, In 2015 the Govt. of India started regulating the price of cotton seeds by the "Cotton Seeds Price (Control) Order, 2015"[43]

---

40 17/08/2007.

41 573/KOL/2007.

The Order fixed the maximum sale value and in doing so also fixed the "trait value". Since the trait value fixed by the Govt. was less than the sub-license amount Nuziveedu requested Monsanto to revise the sub-license which was rejected by the latter. When they could not reach a consensus on the issue Monsanto terminated the license and alleged that the further sales by Nuziveedu is infringement.Nuziveedu challenged the patent of Monsanto in the counter claim stating that there can be no patent for plants and seeds containing "nucleic acid sequence". Therefore once the "nucleic acid sequence" is implanted into the donor seeds no further claim can be made with the seeds, The defendants contended that the plaintiffs can only claim 'benefit sharing' under the PVFRA for the use of its patented trait by the defendant in their plant variety. Here the court held that since the application of patent revocation is pending and use of trait by defendant's amount to infringement there should pay trait value decided by government order.

Here the interesting thing is that in United States the use of seeds after sale is not allowed and they have to get from Monsanto again. The US court held that patent exhaustion won't remain. But in Indian Contest even though we are having Plant varies protection and farmers right act, which gives right to save and sell the seeds. This provision been incorporated to avoid US type situation in Bowman case. Then also for the second sale of seeds Monsanto is charging trait value. This shows equivalent to again buying from the Monsanto. The defendant's contention of benefit sharing mechanism to applied if such varieties is registered under the Act by Monsanto. At the same time Monsanto stood for patent rights on gene constructs. This shows there is no demarcation between patent rights and plant variety protection rights. So there is a need for having clear demarcation whether rights over both can be claimed or how legislation differs from each other in terms of rights

Conclusion

Seed is pivotal for a farmer is concerned so monopoly over seeds will deter the sustenance of a agriculture of a country itself. The TRIPS flexibilities while utilized by the developing countries should protect their agriculture from the hands of multinational, So a clear demarcation of rights under plant variety as well as subject matter of patents to be made clear and avoid over lapping of legislation which will defeat the intend of the legislations. Otherwise it will drastically affect the farmers as well as the agriculture thereby food security.

---

42 Monsanto Technology Llc And Ors. vs Nuziveedu Seeds Limited and Ors,Del HC,2017. P.30.

43 https://nsai.co.in/newsletter/182-dec-15-cotton-seeds-pricecontrol-order-2015.

Chapter 8

Scientometric Analysis on Cloning from 2004-17

Rahil Mathakia and Viralkumar B. Mandaliya

Gujarat National Law University, Gandhinagar-382426, Gujarat, India
e-mail: viral_mandaliya@yahoo.com

ABSTRACT

The present study was emphasized on the Scientometric study on cloning. The Indian Citation Index database (www.indiancitationindex.com) was employed to know the publication status on "Cloning" from various countries in Indian journals. Total publication records observed was 798 from 2004-17, and the highest number of record count was observed in the year 2014. The top contributing author was Rai A from ICAR - Indian Veterinary Research Institute (ICAR-IVRI). An Indian Journal of Biotechnology journal was found as top journal for the publication on "Cloning".

Keywords: *Bibliometric, Genetic engineering, ICI database, Indian Citation Index, r-DNA technology.*

Introduction

Bibliometrics is an indicative measure for the output of research in a form of published literature. Bibliometric analysis is generally used by the researchers to understand the trends and growth of literature in given field. Simply, it enables the user to explore (i) research trends both within a country and globally, (ii) the patterns of collaboration among countries, institutions and individual researchers, (iii) trends of a country's share in the global activities in particular field, (iv) growth of the literature in specific field, (iv) the top and leading authors and institutions in the field, and (v) the leading publication in the field.

The historical observation regarding bibliometric has shown that Pritchard (1969)[1] was the pioneering person to define it in his own words during his research article "Statistical Bibliography or Bibliometrics?" He had remarked that term statistical bibliography is clumsy, not very descriptive, and can be confused with statistics itself or bibliographies on statistics, hence he had suggested that the word "Bibliometrics, *i.e.* the application of mathematics and statistical methods to books and other media of communication" be substituted for "statistical bibliography". In the 1960s, term 'scientometrics' was become popular in Science after its first time usage by Vassily V. Nalimov[2]. The Scientometrics is based on indexed database to do statistical analysis of scientific publication based on various parameters.

Cloning in general term referred as copying. Cloning is a process of making a copy. The product developed in this cloning process referred as clone. The material to be cloned *i.e.* copied, could be DNA fragment, gene fragment, whole unicellular cell, or whole organism. The first cloned mammal known in history was a sheep named Dolly[3]. This sheep was died in 2003, and currently on display at the National Museums of Scotland, Edinburgh.

Scientometric analyses of Cloning from the Indian National Perspective

The present study is aimed to Scientometric analysis on publications on "Cloning". Hadagali GS and Hiremath RS (2014) from Karnatak University, Dharwad had made Scientometric analysis on Cloning research from the year 1999-2010 using web of science[4]. Kelageri PC (2016) from University of Agricultural Sciences, Dharwad (Karnataka) also worked on the same line had done Scientometric analysis from the year 2004-09 using ISI web of knowledge[5].

India has developed Indian Citation Index (ICI) database[6] to conduct such Scientometric analysis[7]. ICI database is covering the data from year 2014-17 from top Indian scholarly journals. ICI enable a researcher to determine the status[8]

---

1 Pritchard, A (1969). Statistical bibliography or bibliometrics? Journal of Documentation, 24, 1348-349.

2 Hood, W.W. and Wilson, C.S. The Literature of Bibliometrics, Scientometrics, and Informetrics. Scientometrics (2001) 52: 291. https://doi.org/10.1023/A:1017919924342.

3 Campbell *et al.*, Sheep cloned by nuclear transfer from a cultured cell line. Nature. 1996:380 (6569): 64–66.

4 Hadagali GS and Hiremath RS (2014). Scientometric Analysis of Literature on Cloning, 1999-2010. Journal of Advances in Library and Information Science 3(3): 210-221.

5 Kelageri PC (2016). Cloning research: a scientometric study. International Journal of Library Science and Information Management 2(3): 70-78.

6 Parameshwar S, Goutami, and Patil DB (2016), Publication trends in library and information science: A bibliometric analysis of library herald. Library Herald, 54 (3), 316-330, DOI: 10.5958/0976-2469.2016.00023.3

7 Chand P (2011), Indian Citation Index (ICI): A dream of Indian research community comes true. Library Herald, 49(1), 34-47.

8 Ram S, Kataria S, and Ahmad S (2014), an assessment of the visibility of Indian Journals in Social Science Citation Index – Journal Citation Report. Journal of Information Management, 1(1), 1-16.

of research and development from every States/Union territories of India[9]. The current data status of ICI as per their release note on 30th Nov 2017 is the current Index paper title count stands at 613 thousand, their paper wise reference count is at 11.62 million, and it were indexed from 1,031 total journals from India[10]. The present Scientometric analysis on Cloning was performed using ICI database from the year 2004-17.

Material and Method

The complimentary access was provided by IndianCitationIndex.com to access the database. Indian Citation Index database (www.indiancitationindex.com) was searched on 6th December 2017 for the analysis on the sector "Cloning" from the year 2004-17. The internet facility was provided by Information and Communication Technology (ICT) Division, Gujarat National Law University, Gandhinagar.

Results

An Analysis of Total Publication on "Cloning"

ICI database was searched on 6th December 2017 to analyze the total record counts on the sector "Cloning" from year 2004-17. The total record count observed was 798 articles which includes the contribution from various countries in Indian journals. Then specific search was made in context to country India, and the total record counts observed was 555 articles. Table 8.1 has shown total record counts from ICI database from various countries in ICI indexed Indian journals on 6th December 2017. The highest number of record count observed in the year 2014 (Figure 8.1).

Table 8.1: Total Record Counts Observed on "Cloning" from Indian Citation Index, Year 2004-17

Year	*Record Counts*	*Year*	*Record Counts*
2004	43	2011	56
2005	42	2012	63
2006	38	2013	75
2007	48	2014	92
2008	62	2015	85
2009	50	2016	77
2010	46	2017	21

An Analysis of International Contribution on "Cloning"

Here, top countries have been identified from ICI database which shown the contribution on Cloning in Indian Journal (Figure 8.2). The contribution recorded as

9 Parameshwar S (2017). Publication Trends in Library and Information Science: A Bibliometric Analysis of Pearl: Journal of Library and Information Science. Pearl: A Journal of Library and Information Science, 11(2): 134-142.

10 Indian Citation Index, http://www.indiancitationindex.com.

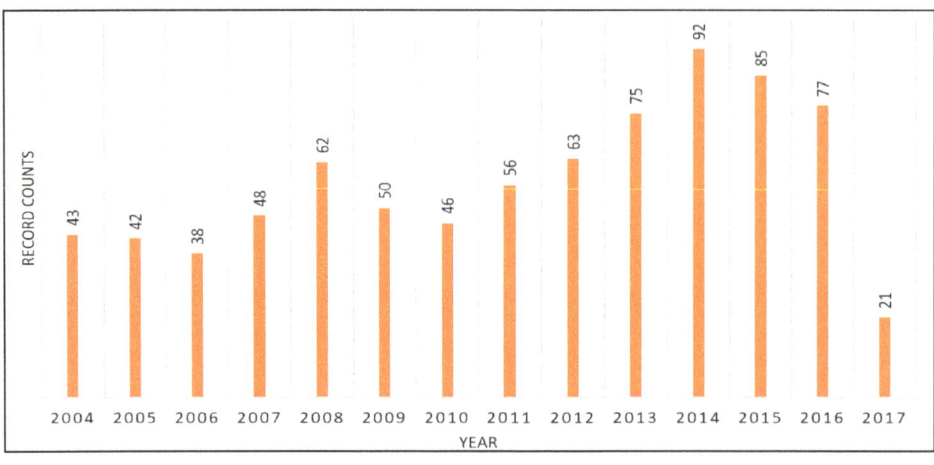

Figure 8.1: The Total Record Counts Year-wise Presented for Publication on "Cloning" from Year 2004-17.

total 235 articles which includes collaborative as well as independent contribution from foreign countries. The highest number of record is observed from China which is 133 articles (56 per cent) on Cloning (Figure 8.2).

Table 8.2: International Contribution of Foreign Countries in the Sector of "Cloning" (2004-17) in Indian Journal

Sl.No.	*Countries*	*Record Counts*	*Percent (per cent) Proposition*
1	China	133	56.60 per cent
2	Iran	26	11.06 per cent
3	United States of America	21	8.94 per cent
4	Japan	16	6.81 per cent
5	South Korea	9	3.83 per cent
6	Egypt	9	3.83 per cent
7	Indonesia	7	2.98 per cent
8	Thailand	5	2.13 per cent
9	Australia	5	2.13 per cent
10	Russia	4	1.70 per cent

An Analysis of Contribution from States/Union Territories of India on "Cloning"

The contribution of articles from the Indian territorial perspective were analyzed. The contribution was gathered from 36 state/union territories (UTs) across the nation. Among total of 36 State/UTs, Uttar Pradesh, Delhi, and Tamil Nadu were the top most State/UTs (Table 8.3) for contribution on "Cloning" and it was counted as one half among all States/UTs (Figure 8.3).

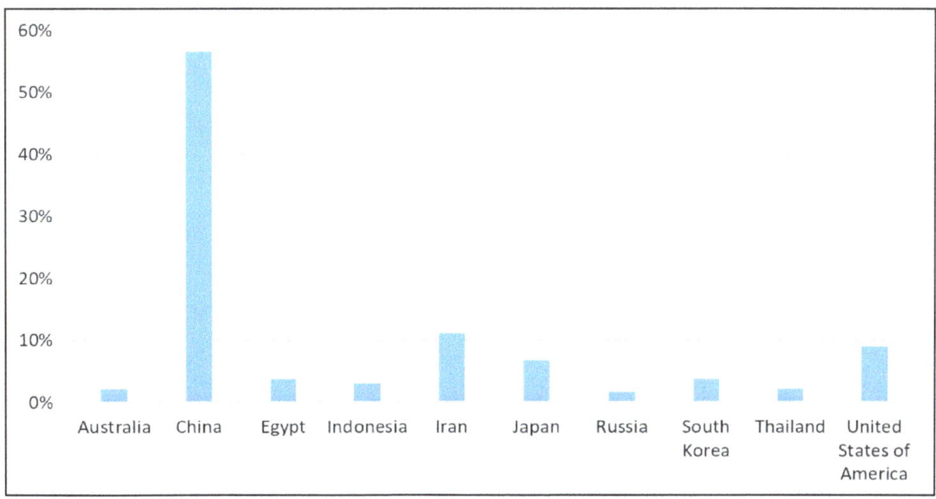

Figure 8.2: International Contribution of Various Countries on "Cloning" (2004-17) in Indian Journal.

Table 8.3: Contribution from States/UTs of India on "Cloning" (2004-17)

Sl.No.	*States*	*Counts*
1	Uttar Pradesh	145
2	Delhi	87
3	Tamil Nadu	66
4	Karnataka	54
5	Punjab	43
6	Uttarakhand	41
7	Maharashtra	33
8	Kerala	31
9	Haryana	30
10	Rajasthan	29

An Analysis of Top Authors in the Sector of "Cloning"

Top authors who contributed on "Cloning" were identified in this study (Table 8.4). Top author is who contribute the numbers of article in one topic in his/her career. The top author contributor was Rai A (Figure 8.4) from ICAR - Indian Veterinary Research Institute (ICAR-IVRI) whose top cited articles "Cloning of canine parvovirus *VP2* gene and its use as DNA vaccine in dogs" was cited 4 times by various authors.

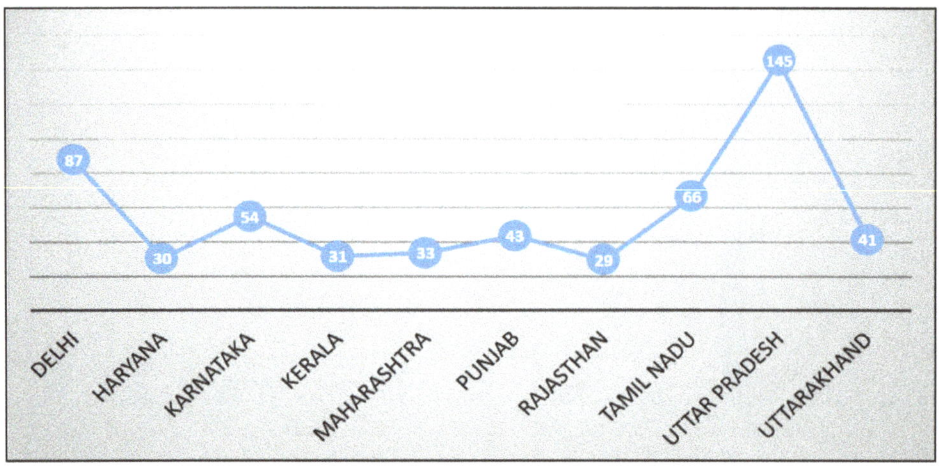

Figure 8.3: Coverage of States/UTs in Number of Publication on the Sector "Cloning" (2004-17) Observed from Indian Citation Index.

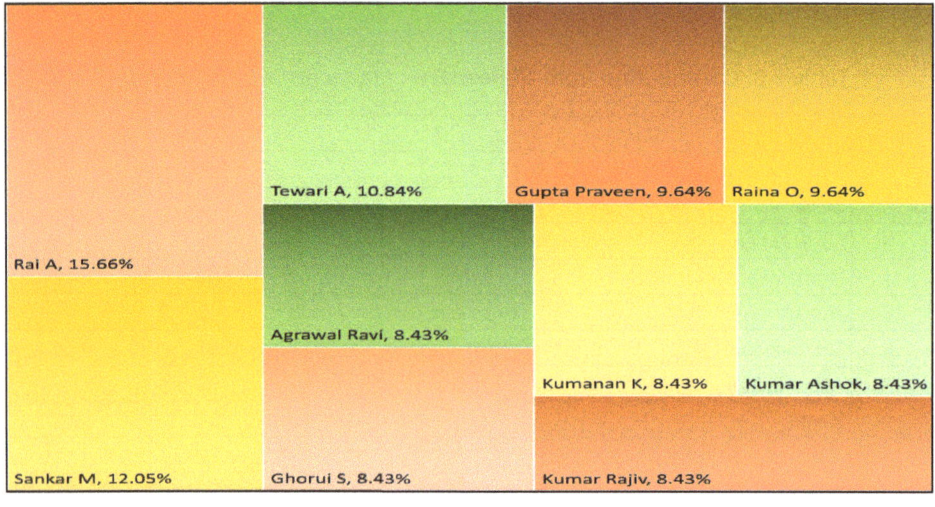

Figure 8.4: Top Authors on the Sector "Cloning" identified from Indian Citation Index (2004-17).

An Analysis of Top Authors from UP in the Sector of "Cloning"

The highest number of contribution was recorded from Uttar Pradesh (Table 8.4). An additional search was made with the curiosity to know about the top most authors from Uttar Pradesh in comparison with top authors across the nation identified and listed in Author-wise analysis (Table 8.5). Here, Rai A is first top most author from Uttar Pradesh (Figure 8.5) and the same has been listed as third top most author across the nation (Figure 8.4).

Table 8.4: Top Authors Observed on the Topic "Cloning" from Indian Citation Index (2004-17)

Sl.No.	*Authors*	*Record Counts*	*Percent (per cent) Proposition*	*Top Cited Article*	*Time Cited*	*Affiliation*	*State*
1	Rai A	13	15.66 per cent	Cloning of canine parvovirus *VP2* gene and its use as DNA vaccine in dogs	4	ICAR - Indian Veterinary Research Institute (ICAR-IVRI)	Uttar Pradesh
2	Sankar M	10	12.05 per cent	Intraspecific and gender variation in *hmcp4* gene of cysteine proteinase in *Haemonchus contortus*	1	ICAR - Indian Veterinary Research Institute (ICAR-IVRI)	Uttar Pradesh
3	Tewari A	9	10.84 per cent	Isolation and characterization of paraflagellar rod protein gene (*Pfr1*) in *Trypanosoma evansi* and its conservation among other kinetoplastid parasites	1	ICAR - Indian Veterinary Research Institute (ICAR-IVRI)	Uttar Pradesh
4	Gupta Praveen	8	9.64 per cent	Cloning and expression of fusion gene of Newcastle disease virus in a eukaryotic expression system	3	ICAR - Indian Veterinary Research Institute (ICAR-IVRI)	Uttar Pradesh
5	Raina O	8	9.64 per cent	Molecular cloning, comparative sequence analysis and prokaryotic expression of GRA5 protein of *Toxoplasma gondii*	1	ICAR - Indian Veterinary Research Institute (ICAR-IVRI)	Uttar Pradesh
6	Agrawal Ravi	7	8.43 per cent	Molecular and immunological characterization of heat shock protein 70 (*HSP70*) gene from buffalo	1	ICAR - Indian Veterinary Research Institute (ICAR-IVRI)	Uttar Pradesh
7	Ghorui S	7	8.43 per cent	Cloning and sequence analysis of dippa-tubulin gene of *Trypanosoma evansi* isolates from Indian dromedaries (*Camelus dromedarius*)	0	ICAR - National Research Centre on Camel (ICAR-NRCC)	Rajasthan
8	Kumanan K	7	8.43 per cent	Cloning and expression of fusion (F) protein gene of newcastle disease virus (NDV)	1	Tamil Nadu Veterinary and Animal Sciences University (TNVASU)	Tamil Nadu
9	Kumar Ashok	7	8.43 per cent	Characterization of goat lingual antimicrobial peptide cDNA	1	ICAR - Indian Veterinary Research Institute (ICAR-IVRI),	Uttar Pradesh
10	Kumar Rajiv	7	8.43 per cent	Cloning and expression of chicken granulocyte-macrophage colony stimulating factor (*GMCSF*) gene	2	ICAR - Indian Institute of Horticultural Research (ICAR-IIHR)	Karnataka

Table 8.5: Top Authors from UP on the Sector "Cloning" (2004-17) identified from Indian Citation Index

Sl.No.	*Authors*	*Percent (per cent) Proposition*
1	Rai A	16.05 per cent
2	Sankar M	13.58 per cent
3	Tewari A K	11.11 per cent
4	Raina O K	9.88 per cent
5	Gupta Praveen K	9.88 per cent
6	Saravanan B C	8.64 per cent
7	Singh Harkirat	8.64 per cent
8	Kumar Ashok	7.41 per cent
9	Kumar Rajiv	7.41 per cent
10	Chaturvedi Uttara	7.41 per cent

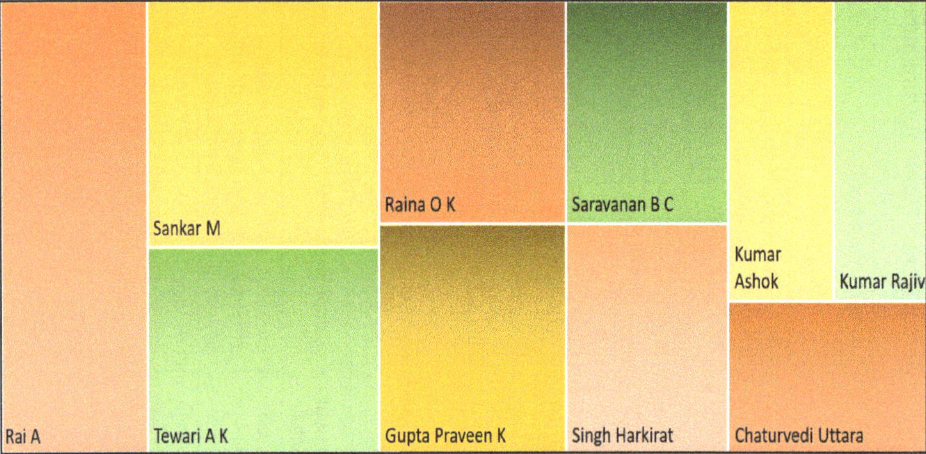

Figure 8.5: Top Ten Authors from UP on "Cloning" (2004-17).

An Analysis of Top Article in the Sector of "Cloning"

The citation of any article is generally referred as the article read and quoted in literature by an author. The number of citation of any articles represents the highest number of readability and weightage in that particular sector. In this study, top cited articles on the sector "Cloning" were identified and listed in Table 8.6. Here, an article published in Indian Journal of Urology in a year 2009 titled "Legal and ethical aspects of organ donation and transplantation" was cited 11 times by various authors.

An Analysis of Top Journal in the Sector of "Cloning"

The selection of journal for publication by author is majorly depends on the kind of articles it publishes and the institute/society from where the journal is

Table 8.6: Top Cited Articles on the Sector "Cloning" (2004-17) Observed from Indian Citation Index

Sl.No.	*Title*	*Total Citations*	*Total Citations per Year*	*Year*	*Publication Name*	*Author*	*State*
1	Legal and ethical aspects of organ donation and transplantation	11	1.22	2009	Indian Journal of Urology	Shroff Sunil	Tamil Nadu
2	Phylogenetic analysis of classical swine fever virus (csfv) by cloning and sequencing of partial 5' non-translated genomic region	9	0.64	2004	Indian Journal of Animal Sciences (The)	Singh V K, Saikumar G, *et al.*	Uttar Pradesh
3	Biodegradation of polymers	8	0.62	2005	Indian Journal of Biotechnology	Premraj R, Doble Mukesh	Tamil Nadu
4	Functional genomics of drought stress response in rice: Transcript mapping of annotated unigenes of an indica rice (*Oryza sativa* L. cv.	7	0.54	2005	Current Science	Gorantla Markande, Babu P R, *et al.*	Telangana
5	Production of cloned trees of *Populus deltoides* through *in vitro* regeneration of shoots from leaf, stem and root explants and their field cultivation	7	0.50	2004	Indian Journal of Biotechnology	Chaturvedi H C, Sharma A K, *et al.*	Uttar Pradesh
6	*In vitro* cloning of female and male *Carica papaya* through tips of shoots and inflorescences	6	0.43	2004	Indian Journal of Biotechnology	Agnihotri S, Singh S K, *et al.*	Uttar Pradesh
7	*In vitro* cloning of apple (*Malus domestica* Borkh) employing forced shoot tip cultures of M9 rootstock	6	0.50	2006	Indian Journal of Biotechnology	Dalal M Amin, Das B, *et al.*	Jammu and Kashmir
8	Polyamine biosynthetic pathway as a novel target for potential applications in plant biotechnology	6	0.50	2006	Physiology And Molecular Biology of Plants	Kumar S Vinod, Sharma M L, *et al.*	Delhi
9	Cloning, high-level expression and enzymatic properties of an intracellular serine protease from *Bacillus* sp. WRD-2	5	0.36	2004	Indian Journal of Biochemistry and Biophysics	Sun-Young An, Ok Min, Kim Ji-Youn, *et al.*	Korea
10	*In vitro* cloning of ornamental species of *Dianthus*	5	0.36	2004	Indian Journal of Biotechnology	Pareek Aparna, Kantia Archana, *et al.*	Rajasthan

published. Based on this study, top journals were identified for publication of the articles related to "Cloning" (Table 8.7). Here, Indian Journal of Biotechnology journal was top journal for the publication related to "Cloning" (Figure 8.6).

Table 8.7: Top Journal on "Cloning" (2004-17) identified from Indian Citation Index

Sl.No.	*Publication Name*	*Record Counts*	*Percent (per cent) Proposition*	*ISSN*	*NAAS rating (2017)*	*Publisher*
1	Indian Journal of Biotechnology	49	16.44 per cent	0972-5849	6.29	Natl Inst Science Communication-Niscair
2	Journal of Plant Biochemistry and Biotechnology	40	13.42 per cent	0971-7811	7.35	Scientific Publishers
3	Research Journal of Biotechnology	37	12.41 per cent	2278 -4535	6.24	Research Journal Biotechnology
4	Indian Journal of Animal Sciences (The)	34	11.41 per cent	2394-3327	-	Indian Council of Agricultural Research
5	Indian Journal of Microbiology	26	8.72 per cent	0046-8991	7.14	Springer
6	Journal of Biosciences	25	8.39 per cent	0250-5991	7.42	Indian Acad Sciences
7	Journal of Genetics	24	8.05 per cent	0022-1333	7.11	Indian Acad Sciences
8	Current Science	22	7.38 per cent	0011 -3891	6.97	Indian Acad Sciences
9	Indian Journal of Experimental Biology	21	7.04 per cent	0019-5189	7.17	Natl Inst Science Communication-Niscair
10	Indian Journal of Biochemistry and Biophysics	20	6.70 per cent	0301-1208	6.96	Scientific Publishers

An Analysis of Top Subject in the Sector of "Cloning"

The contribution of authors related to "Cloning" was classified into various subject category (Table 8.8). Here, Biological Science, Biotechnology, and Veterinary Science was top most subject category with highest number of record counts as 50 per cent coverage (Figure 8.7).

An Analysis of Top Type of Document in the Sector of "Cloning"

From Indian Citation Index, the following are the document type generated on the selected topic: Research Article, Short Communication, Review Article, and others (Table 8.9). Among all document type, the majority of articles were grouped a form of research articles (n=657; 82 per cent) (Figure 8.8).

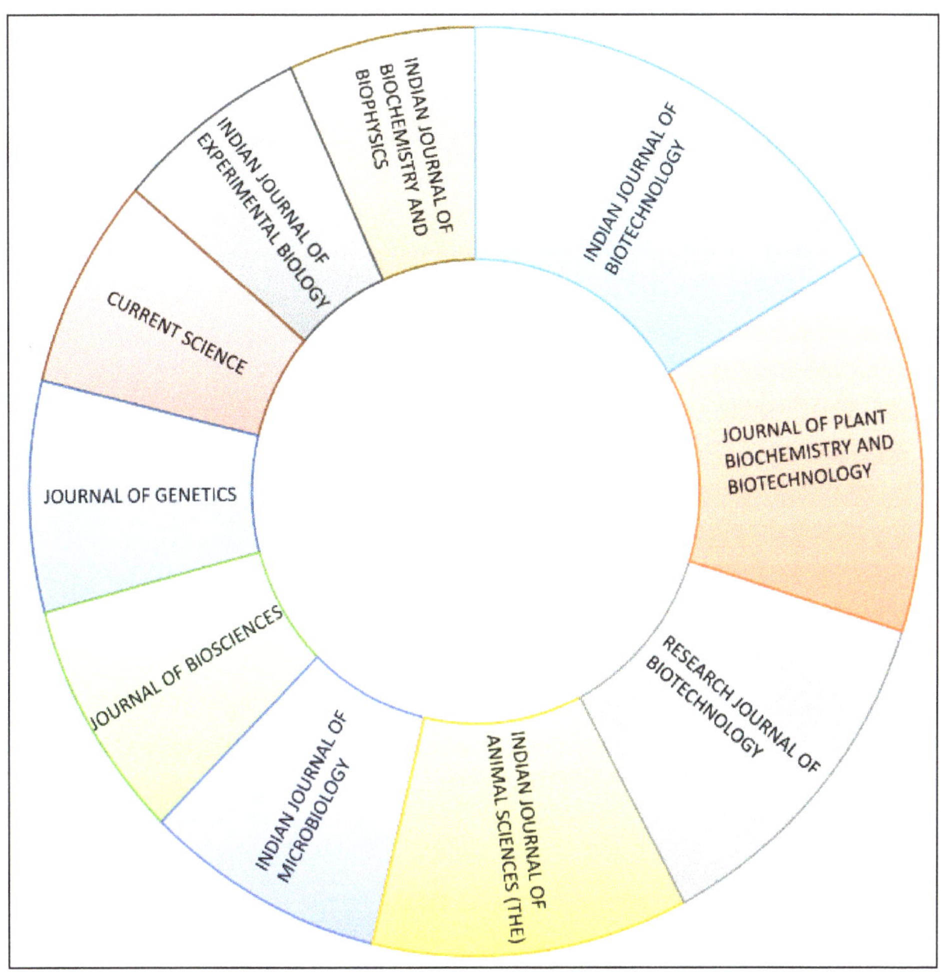

Figure 8.6: Top Journal Preference by Authors on "Cloning" identified from Indian Citation Index (2004-17).

Table 8.8: Subject-wise Categorization of the Work Related to "Cloning" Inherited from Indian Citation Index (2004-17)

Sl.No.	*Subjects*	*Record Counts*	*Percent (per cent) Proposition*
1	Biological Science	240	23.53 per cent
2	Biotechnology	167	16.37 per cent
3	Veterinary Science	104	10.20 per cent
4	Chemistry	90	8.82 per cent
5	Botany	89	8.73 per cent
6	Agriculture	81	7.94 per cent
7	Zoology	69	6.76 per cent

Sl.No.	*Subjects*	*Record Counts*	*Percent (per cent) Proposition*
8	Pharmacology and Pharmaceutical Science	67	6.57 per cent
9	Health Science	65	6.37 per cent
10	Dairying, Dairy, Animals and Animals Produce	48	4.71 per cent

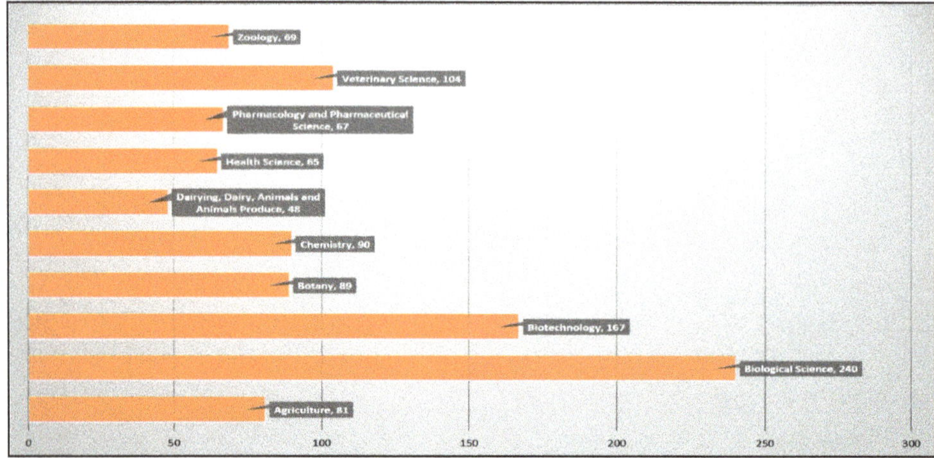

Figure 8.7: Categorization of the Work Related to "Cloning" from Year 2004-17 in Subject Category Derived from Indian Citation Index.

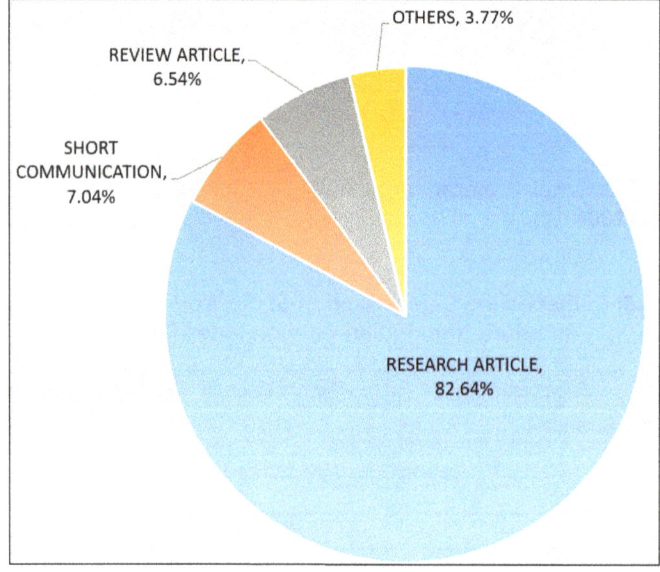

Figure 8.8: Per cent Proposition of Types of Documents on "Cloning" Prepared Based on Indian Citation Index (2004-17).

Table 8.9: Top Document Types Based on Record Counts in "Cloning" Derived from Indian Citation Index (2004-17).

Sl.No.	*Documents Type*	*Record Counts*
1	Research Article	657
2	Short Communication	56
3	Review Article	52
4	Others	30

Conclusions

The research work on cloning is increasing day by day in various fields of life science, agriculture science, medicine, pharmaceuticals and so on. This study has identified the current status of research on cloning. The total record count in various forms like research article, short communication, review article, and others observed was 798 articles from various countries in Indian journals. The highest number of contribution was observed from China. While studies related to contribution from state/UTs from India shown that Uttar Pradesh, Delhi, and Tamil Nadu were the top most State/UTs for contribution on "Cloning". This study will help the readers, academicians, students and authors to get the current research status in cloning globally.

Authors' contributions

R Mathakia has complied the dataset from IndianCitationIndex.com and VB Mandaliya has prepared the manuscript.

Chapter 9

Climate-Smart Agriculture: Mitigating Climate Change and Increasing Farm Income through Raising Off-Seasonal Seedlings of Papaya (*Carica papaya* L.) in Protected Environment–A Novel Approach

V.P. Joshi and P.M. Chauhan

Department of Renewable Energy and Rural Engineering,
College of Agricultural Engineering and Technology,
Junagadh Agricultural University, Junagadh-362001 (Gujarat).
e-mail: viraljoshi2088@gmail.com

ABSTRACT

As effect of climate changes due to rising concentrations of greenhouse gases in the atmosphere, agriculture is one of the key human activities affected. Projections show that while overall global food production in the coming decades may keep pace with the food requirements of a growing world population, climate change might worsen existing regional disparities because it will reduce crop yields mostly in lands located at lower latitudes where many developing countries are situated. Developing countries will have more difficulty in adapting, as the changes will have a greater impact there than in developed countries. Agricultural risk may be local, impacting crops, or global, impacting food security. Major difficulty of raising papaya seedling in tropical country like India is mortality of seedling, among abiotic factors of environment like unfavorable microclimate; especially temperature restricts raising off-season fruit nursery under open field condition in arid region. Papaya (*Carica papaya L.*) is widely grown fruit crop in tropics and India is the largest producer in the world. Papaya Seedling are fetching very high price during off-season availability.In this study a low tunnel greenhouse (S_1) and black Shade net house (S_2) were taken as protected structures for growing of papaya seedling. The variety of papaya seedlings were Madhubindu and soil + FYM was taken as growing media for this study. Survival and growth of seedling were monitored for 30-60 days. The environmental and morphological data were recorded and computed and response of papaya seedling growth was evaluated in terms of germination percentage, seedling height, collar diameter, no. of leaves, diameter of shoot, fresh and dry weight of aboveground and underground biomass, sturdiness, root shoot ratio, vigour index length and vigour index mass in root media. The result of this study revealed that the environmental factor during the entire study period was found significant in black shade net structure compared to greenhouse. Variation in seedling growth in different microclimatic conditions may be due to the differences in growth behavior under given set of environmental conditions. The minimum time taken for days of germination, germination percentage, and seedling height, collar and shoot diameter was found highest inblack Shade net house (S_2) with Variety *i.e.* Madhubindu and Soil + FYM as growing media. Economically black shade net house with net profit 513.27 Rs/m^2, BCR 3.94 and payback period 0.59 found highly suitable for raising seedling of papaya off seasonally and mitigating climate change in arid region.

Keywords: *Black shade net house, Climate change, Cost economics, Environmental parameters, Greenhouse, Growth dynamics.*

Introduction

Climate change impacts on agriculture are being witnessed all over the world. However, countries like India are more vulnerable in view of the high population depending on agriculture and excessive pressure on natural resources. Rainfall is the key variable influencing crop productivity in rainfed farming. Intermittent and prolonged droughts are a major cause of yield reduction in most crops. Climate change is a significant driver of change for agriculture practice in the developing world, because it threatens food production and its stability as well as other aspects of food systems such as storage, food access and utilization (Wheeler and Von-Braun, 2013). Climate change will impact on social, economic and environmental systems and shape prospects for food, water and health security (Steffen *et al.*, 2004; WHO 2003).Agriculture is the riskiest profession in the world. Among abiotic factors of environment like unfavorable microclimate, especially temperature restricts raising off-season nursery under open field condition.Facing these uncertainties are actor groups operating in different sectors and at multiple levels, with often widely divergent interests (Ingram *et al.*, 2010). The challenges around ensuring sustainable food security are systemic, and therefore require system-wide actions from decision-makers (Ericksen *et al.*, 2009; Vermeulen *et al.*, 2013). Similarly, a lack of local-level mechanisms and resources for adaptation and innovation can make large-scale policies or investments ineffective (Bourgeois *et al.*, 2012). Quality seedlings are essential for good growth and performance of crops. Hence, the practice of seedling production is emerging as a profession and commercial activity. Papaya (*Carica papaya L.*) is widely grown in tropics and India is the largest producer in the world. Maximum area under papaya is in Andhra Pradesh state, followed by Gujarat. In Gujarat, area and production is about 19.59 thousand ha with the production of 1185.47 M.T. grown in different districts of Gujarat state (Anon., 2015 a). Due to unfavorable environmental condition there is almost 10 month of lean season for papaya cultivation in Gujarat (Annon, 2015 b). Major difficulty of raising papaya seedling is mortality of seedling, which is a very serious problem in open field condition as global climate change scenario. It is difficult to maintain outside temperature as variable shift. Emphasize on protected cultivation like greenhouse and shade net house (Moller and Assouline 2007; Akabari and Chauhan, 2011) are supposed to be a better option for arid region to counter climatic effect (Behera *et al.*, 1990). The media should be reaching enough to sustain seedling for about a year (Srivastava *et al.*, 1998). A good potting medium is characterized by light weight, friable, easy blendable, excellent water capacity, porosity, drainage, low bulk density, free from fungal spores and insects and low inherent fertility *etc.* (Chakrabarti *et al.*, 1998) also strong pot size effects on biomass and photosynthesis are generally also observed when density is specifically controlled. (Endean and Carlson, 1975; Robbins and Pharr,1988; Nesmith *et al.*, 1992; Climent*et al.* 2011).

Materials and Methods

Design of Structures for Protected Cultivation

The one single span low tunnel naturally ventilated greenhouse of (6.08m x 30.4 m x 2.4m) structure was used for the experiment purpose. Structure was made of 1.0″ diameter G.I (Galvanized Iron) pipe and 200 micron UVS (Ultra violate stabilized) diffused light polyethylene sheet of good quality to be fixed appropriately over all sides of the greenhouse. The black shade net house was constructed by using 1.0″ diameter G.I pipe with 75 per cent black shade net covering all sides of the structure. The care was taken that shadow of one structure do not fall on other structure as well as wind do not interrupted by one structure for other. The construction detail of greenhouse and shade net structure is shown in Table 9.1 and Figure 9.1.

Table 9.1: Details of different Structures

Details	Low tunnel Greenhouse	Black shade Net house
Type	Single Span low tunnel	Black shade net 75 per cent shading
Floor Area	6.08 m x 30.4 m	3 m x 3 m
Ridge height	2.4 m	2.4 m
Ventilation	Natural ventilation and fogging	Natural ventilation
Orientation	North-South	North-South
Cooling mechanism	Natural ventilation and fogging	Natural ventilation
Covering	200 micron UVS diffused light polyethylene sheet of good quality to be fixed appropriately over all sides of the greenhouse.	-

Experimental Details

Parameter Considered

(A) Structure (S) with two levels *viz.*

(1) Low tunnel greenhouse (S_1)

(2) Black shade net house (S_2)

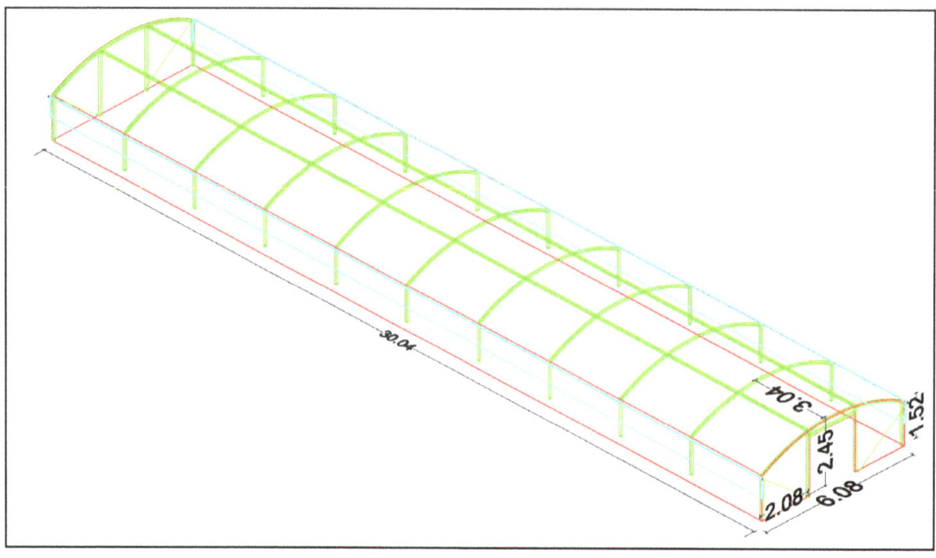

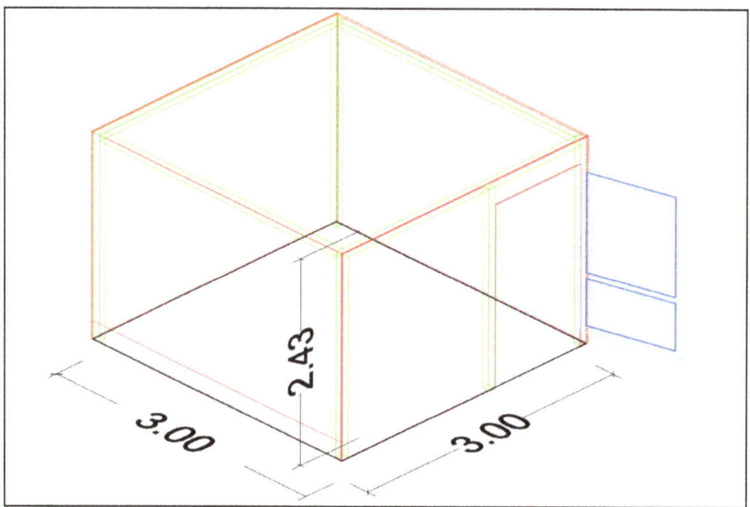

Figure 9.1: Constructional Details and Isometric View of Greenhouse and Shade Net House.

(B) Variety: Madhubindu, Taiwan (Red Leady 786)

(C) Media: Soil+Sand+FYM (Farm Yard Manure) (1:1:1)

Details of Observations Recorded

Environmental Observations

The environmental parameters like temperature and relative humidity were continuously recorded by digital recorders placed middle of the structure as well as in open field also. Light intensity was measured with digital lux meter and recorded from 8 AM to 16 PM for greenhouse, black shadenet house on daily basis. These data were used to calculate the monthly average data, which were used for observing variation in microclimate during the day.

Morphological Observations

Germination percentage were calculated based on total number of germinated seeds under each treatment, right from the first emergence of the seed up to the period of completion of seed germination. Seedling height, collar diameter and diameter of shoot were measured in centimeter with the help of digital vernier calipers at 15, 30, 45 and 60 days after sowing (DAS) and mean was calculated. Number of leavesentire seedling in each structure was counted at 15, 30, 45 and 60 days after sowing (DAS) and mean number of leaves per seedling was calculated.

Biomass Production

Fresh and Dry Weight of Above and Below Ground Biomass

The fresh weight of above and below ground biomass was recorded for the same seedling that was used for measuring the seedling height in each treatment and weights of sample biomass were calculated in Kg. Samples was then oven dried at 70 °C till constant weight dry weight of above and below ground biomass of seedling was achieved.

Quality Oarameters

Sturdiness, root shoot ratio and vigour index were measured. Sturdinessof plant was measured by using height to diameter ratio of seedling. Root shoot ratioof plant was measured by use of biomass of roots and biomass of shoots of seedling (Chauhan and sharma 1997).Vigour index length (Vigour index I) was calculated as follow:

Vigour index-I = Germination Per cent x Seedling length (cm)

Vigour index mass (Vigour index II)was determined by multiplication of germination percentage with seedling dry weight on the day of final count as per procedure prescribed by Abdul-Baki and Anderson (1973), as follow:

Vigour index- II = Germination Per cent x Seedling Dry Weight (g).

Economic Evaluation

The various cost component *i.e.* capital investment, fixed cost, maintenance cost, seasonal salvage value, operational cost were calculated and discussed. The maintenance cost of the structures during the entire crop season was considered as 5 per cent of the cost of the structures. The operational cost includes seed cost, soil treatment, bag feeling and manure cost,irrigation cost, labour cost. Seasonal salvage value was calculated on the basis of average salvage value divided by season, here 6 seasons were considered.

Benefit Cost Ratio (BCR)

This ratio was obtained when the present worth of the benefit stream was divided by the present worth of the cost stream. The mathematical benefit-cost ratio (Kothari and Mathur, 2006) can be expressed as:

$$\mathrm{BCR} = \frac{\sum_{t=1}^{t=n} \frac{B_t}{(1+i)^t}}{\sum_{t=1}^{t=n} \frac{C_t}{(1+i)^t}}$$

Payback Period (PBP)

The payback period is the length of time from the beginning of the project until the net value of the incremental production stream reaches the total amount of the capital investment. Here, the payback period was calculated for recommended treatment. Payback period can be expressed by the following equation.

$$\text{Payback Period(PBP)} = \frac{\text{Capital Investment (Rs)}}{\text{Net profit(Rs per year)}}$$

Results and Discussion

Detailed Analysis of Effect of different Structures on Microclimate

Temperature

Temperature is a critical environmental cue that affects seedling establishment. The diurnal variations in monthly average temperature for March to April months for open field, greenhouse and black shade net house were depicted in Figure 9.2. Air temperatures tended to be lower under the black net comparing with other covers, due to the interception of radiation which is greater than the gain of temperature caused by the use of nets due to their role in the interception of air circulation. Higher differences were recorded in the growing seasons. The highest temperature

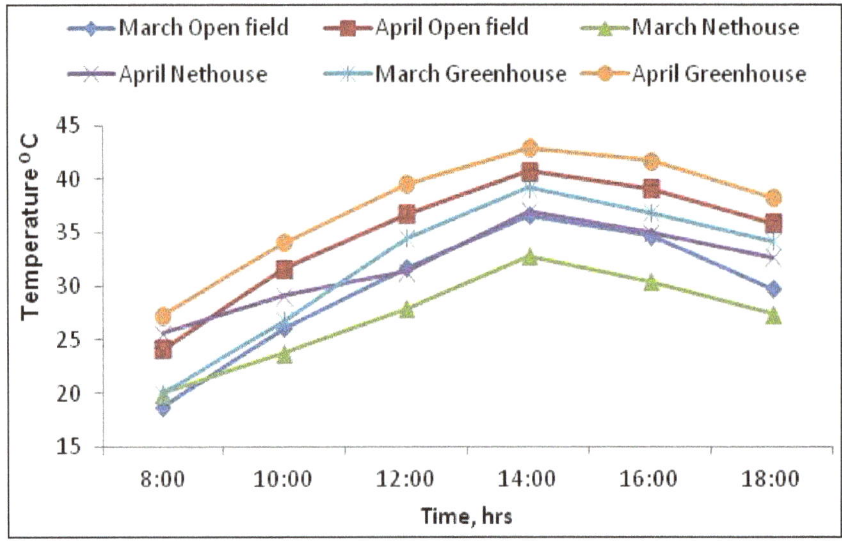

Figure 9.2: Diurnal Variation of Temperature in Greenhouse, Black Shade Net House and Open Field for March and April Month.

were recorded in greenhouse 42.9 °C while lowest temperature was recorded in black shade net house 20.0 °C.Very low temperature showed a strong delay in root growth (Badowiec and Weidner, 2014).

Relative Humidity

The diurnal variations in monthly average RH for March to April months for open field, greenhouse and black shade net house are depicted in Figure 9.3, which shows that average relative humidity was increased by the use of polyethylene sheet cover by 3–8 per cent as compared with black shadenet. These results were in line with those reported by Iglesias and Alegre (2006), indicating a 3–9 per cent increase in humidity associated with the use of nets. Campen and Bot (2003) pointed out that pressure difference over the openings was one of the driving forces for ventilation, which could be either due to the wind outside the greenhouse or due to the temperature difference over the openings.

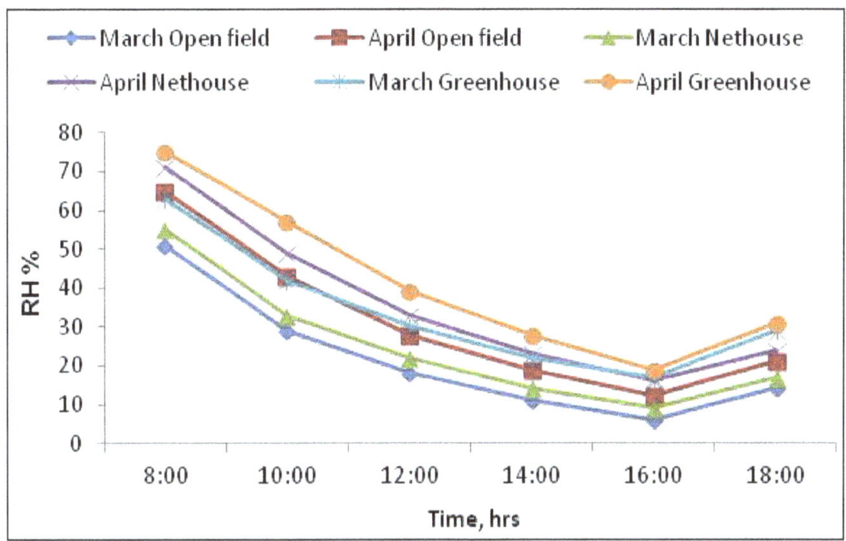

Figure 9.3: Diurnal Variation of Relative Humidity in Greenhouse, Black Shade Net House and Open Field of March and April Month.

Light Intensity

Light quality has been demonstrated to influence many aspects of plant growth and morphology (Smith,1982; 1995). The variations in monthly average light intensity for March to April months for open field, greenhouse and black shade net house are depicted in Figure 9.4. In summer both the day length and the light intensity provide abundant light to earth. In fact, excess light becomes a limiting factor in such cases. Coupled with high air temperature, high light intensities will adversely affect the growth of seedling. Greater average values for interception were recorded between 13:00 and 15:00, the period when the incidence of sunlight is most vertical. Due to 75 per cent black shade net in shade net house, it allows only 25 per cent of light to pass through it. Absolute values of PAR and the effects of nets on light interception were similar to those reported by Peano *et al.* (2001).

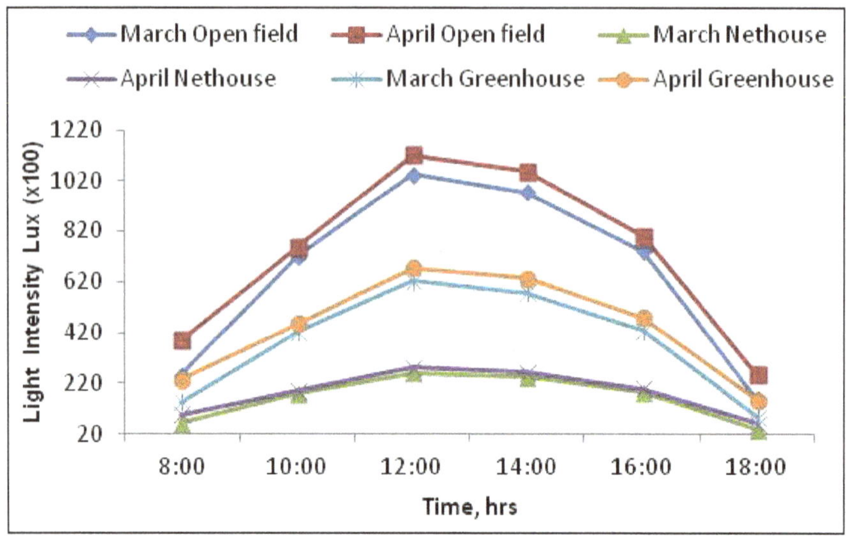

Figure 9.4: Diurnal Variation of Light Intensity Lux(x100) in Greenhouse, Black Shade Net House and Open Field of March and April Month.

Effect of Structures and Microclimate on Morphology of Papaya Seedling

Germination Percentage

Germination percentage of papaya seedling was significantly influenced by different structures and microclimate (Pedro and Isolde, 1999). The observation found that higher germination was found in structure S_1 (96.50 per cent) followed by structure S_2 (95.38 per cent). The soil media was provided high mixture of organic matter and responsible for the better growth environment. Due to off season environmental conditions germination was not found in open field condition.

Seedling Height

It is apparent from graph shown in Figure 9.5 that the plant height of papaya seedling was significantly influenced by different structures. Temperature difference 4-7 °C and microclimatic difference was found in structures compared to ambient condition. Thisinfluence the growth dynamic of plant height, which is associated with lower light regime (Khattak and Pearson, 2005). Higher plant height was observed in structure S_2 (38.75cm) and lower in S_1 (29.56 cm).

Collar Diameter (cm)

A perusal of data presented in Figure 9.6 indicated that the collar diameter of papaya seedling was significantly influenced by different structures and microclimatic conditions (Saikia and Khan, 2012).However, due to favorable

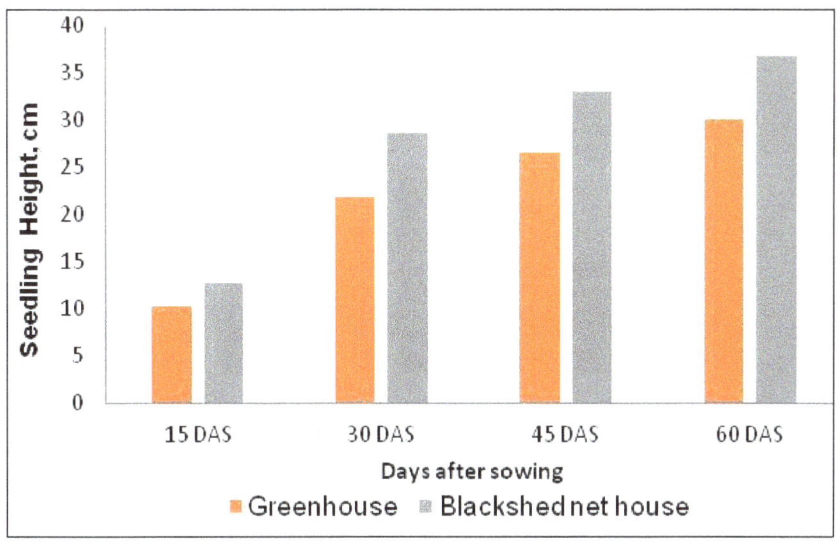

Figure 9.5: Variation of Seedling Height in Greenhouse and Black Shade Net House.

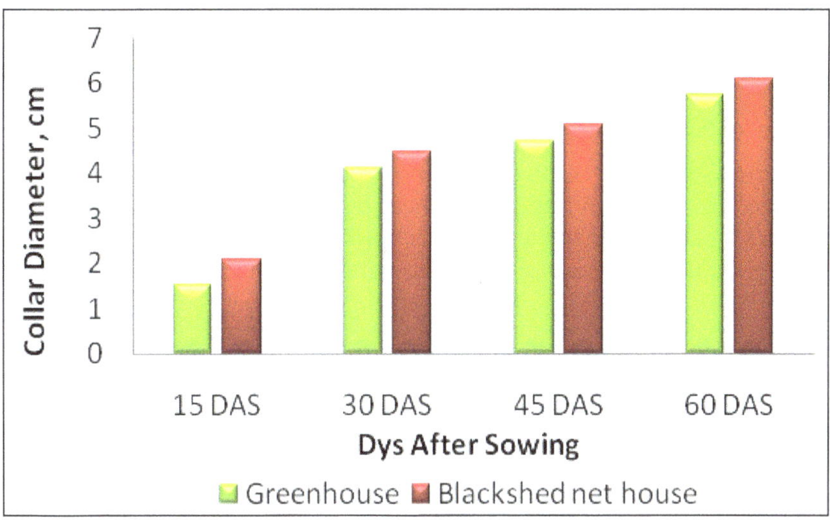

Figure 9.6: Variation of Collar Diameter in Greenhouse and Black Shade Net House.

environmental conditions, *i.e.*light intensity and relative humidity, highest collar diameter was observed in structure S_2 (6.06 cm) and lowest in S_1 (5.73 cm).

Number of Leaves

It has been suggested that rigid or flexible plastic greenhouse/shade net house covers with specific spectral qualities, would enable growers to use light quality to regulate the growth of crops in protected environment. (Rajapkse and Kelly, 1993). It is apparent from graph shown in Figure 9.7 that the number of leaves of papaya

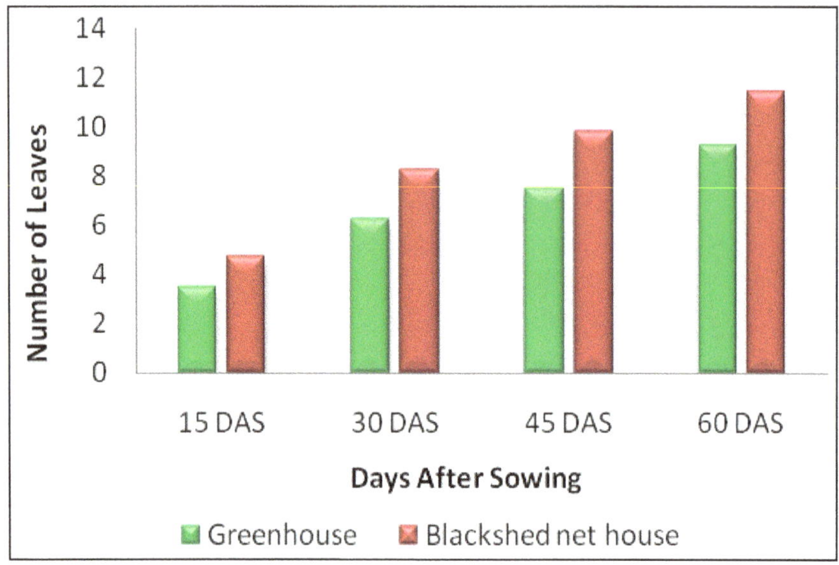

Figure 9.7: Number of Leaves of Seedling in Greenhouse and Black Shade Net House.

seedling was significantly influenced by different structures. Structure S_2 gave significantly higher number of leaves compared to structure S_1.

Diameter of Shoot (cm)

A perusal of data presented in Figure 9.8 indicated that the shoot diameter of papaya seedling was significantly influenced by different structures, growing media and microclimate. Black shade net house provided favorable condition in terms of light penetration to seedling and temperature limited to 32-35 °C for growth of

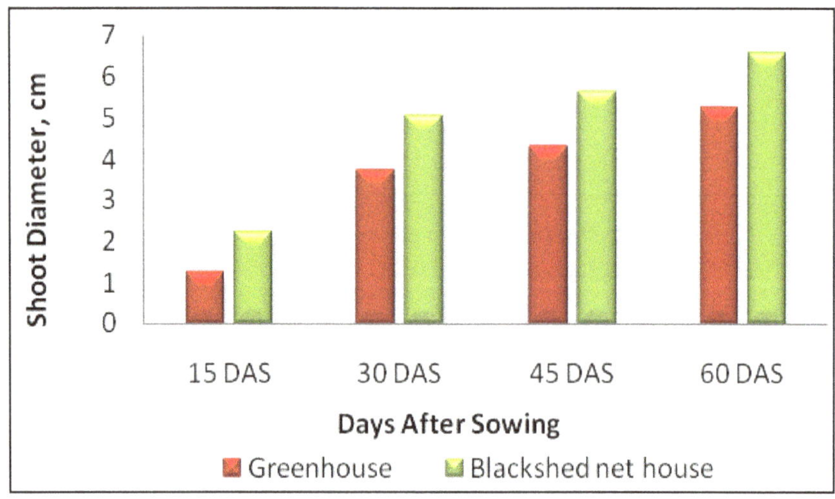

Figure 9.8: Shoot Diameter of Seedling in Greenhouse and Black Shade Net House.

seedling with media having mixture of soil, sand and FYM,s shoot diameter was observed higher in structure S_2 (5.70 cm) followed by structure S_1 (5.22 cm).

Effect on Biomass Production

Fresh and Dry Weight of Above and Below Ground Biomass

A perusal of data presented in Figure 9.9 indicated that the fresh and dry weight accumulation of above and below ground biomass of papaya seedling was significantly influenced by different structures, and its microclimate. Structure S_2 gave significantly higher fresh (21.89 g) and dry weight (4.16 g) of above, below ground, fresh (19.54 g) biomass and dry (3.33 g) biomass as compared to structure S_2.

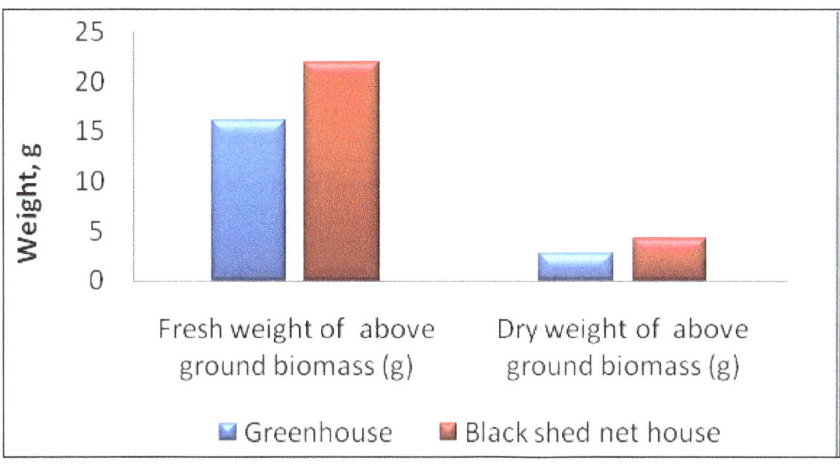

Figure 9.9: Fresh and Dry Weight of Above Ground Biomass in Greenhouse and Black Shade Net House.

Quality Parameter Analysis

Seedling quality can be reflects by sturdiness which is the stocky or spindly nature of the seedlings, although it is a good indicator of the ability to withstand physical damage in all stock-types. From Figure 9.10 it revealed that structure $S_1$was prove to be have better sturdiness (6.6) as compared to structure S_2 (6.0).

Root-shoot ratio is an indication of healthier plant. Here structure S_2 indicates higher root-shoot ratio as compared to structure S_1 presented in Figure 9.11.This result is in agreement with the findings of Rathore *et al.* (2004) that more sturdiness and root-shoot ratio was noted in *Casuarina equisetifolia* seedling with higher amount of soil and FYM in the media mixture.

Vigour index length (Vigour index I) is a growth indication of healthier plant. Structure S_2 indicates higher vigour index I (4777.7) as compared to structure S_1 (3934.6) as shown in Figure 9.12. These proprieties were very significantly with the effect of interactive influence of biotic and abiotic factors and evident from present investigation.

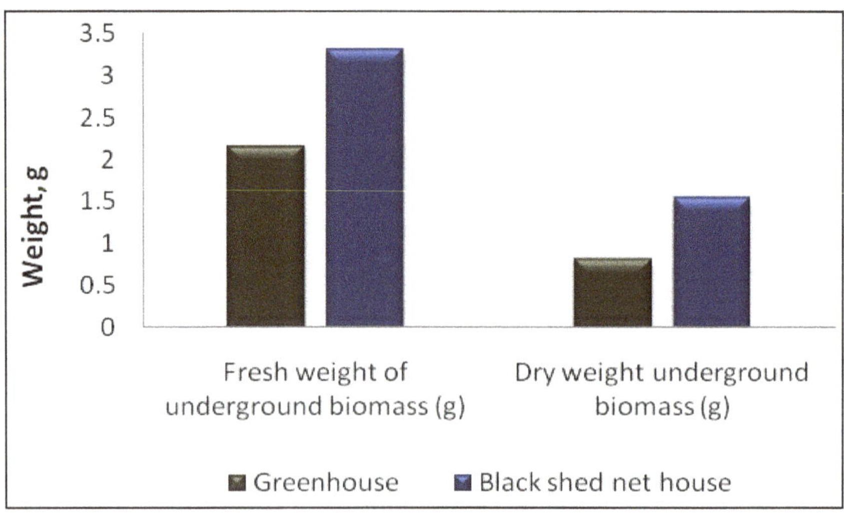

Figure 9.10: Fresh and Dry Weight of Below Ground Biomass in Greenhouse and Black Shade Net House.

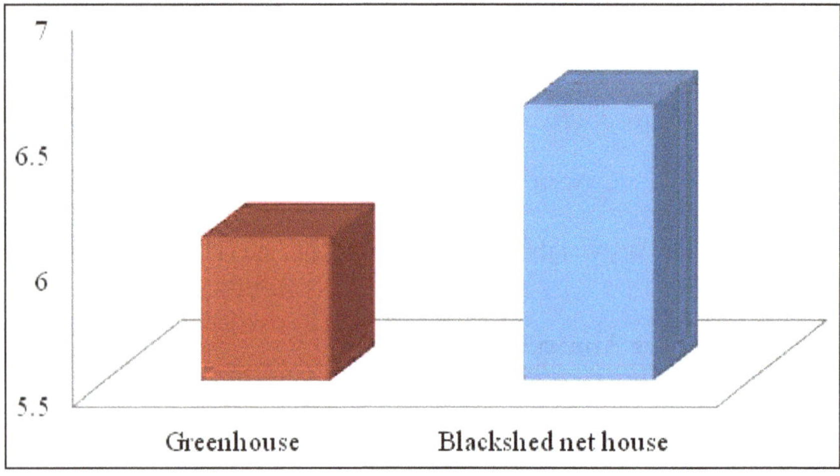

Figure 9.11: Sturdiness of Seedling in Greenhouse and Black Shade Net House.

Vigour index mass (Vigour index II) is also a growth indication of healthier plant. As discuss in material and methods it is measured accordingly.Structure S_2indicates higher vigour index II(439.36) as compared to structure S_1 (336.16) presented In Figures 9.13 and 9.14. These investigation revealed that environmental factors and physiological ability directly relate to the way in which seedling can adjust to their morphological and physiological characteristics of the environment.

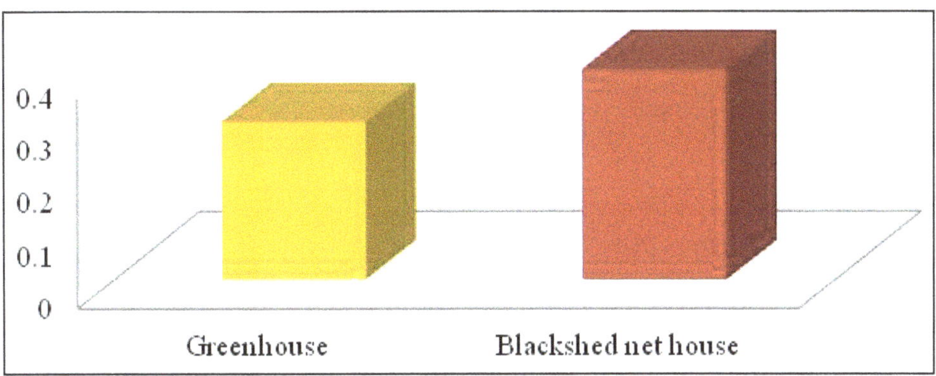

Figure 9.12: Root-Shoot Ratio of Seedling in Greenhouse and Black Shade Net House.

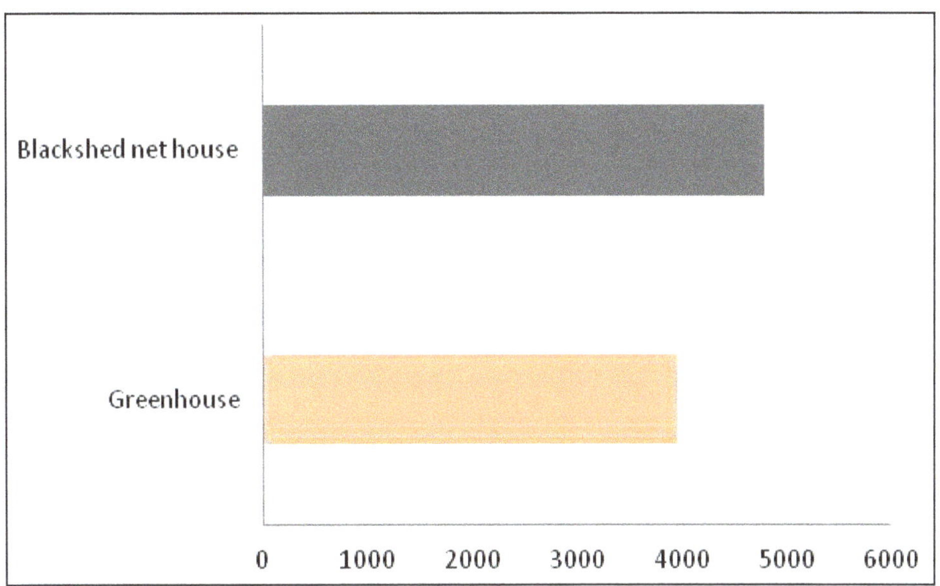

Figure 9.13: Vigour Index Length of Seedling for Greenhouse and Black Shade Net House.

Cost-Economic Analysis

The quantity of materials required and the details of the cost of construction for 180 m^2 greenhouse and 250 m^2 black shade net house is given in Tables 9.2 and 9.3. The total cost of construction including polythene sheet is Rs 1,05,240/- and for black shade net Rs. 81,141.5/-. The cost of cultivation includes expenditure incurred for field preparation, fertilizers, pesticide, insecticide, irrigation, routine maintenance. The temperature conditions inside the greenhouse restrict the growth of insects and pests and therefore, no insecticides or pesticides were used inside the greenhouse and black shade net house. To carry out economic feasibility of greenhouse and black shade net house for farmer, it was considered that each crop was grown at a time

Table 9.2: Constructional and Operational Cost of Greenhouse per square meter for Madhubindu Variety

Sl. No.		Name of Component	Cost for 180 m² Size			Cost Rs/m²
			Quantity for 180 m²	Rate (Rs)	Cost (Rs)	
A	Cost of structure without plastic					
	1	Square GI pipe 47mm	264 m	160/m	42,240	
	2	Clamp, hooks, rivets, nut bolts, *etc.*	-	-	20,000	
	3	Door (size 2m X 2m)	One	-	5,000	
	4	Insect proof whiet screen	60 sqm	30/m	1,800	
	5	Foundation	-	-	5,000	
	6	Labour	-	-	15,000	
	Total cost				89,040	495
B	Cost of UV Stabilized 200 microns plastic sheet @ Rs 60/m² X 270 sqm				16200	90
C	Cost of greenhouse structure					
	1	Greenhouse (A+B), CiG			1050240	585
D	Operating Cost					
	1	Seed Cost A (Madhubindu Rs.24/10 g/m²)			3/m²	3
	2	Soil treatment and manure			3/m²	3
	3	Irrigation cost			4/m²	4
	4	Labour cost/supervision			10/m²	10
	5	Transport and marketing cost			8/m²	8
	Total operating cost					28

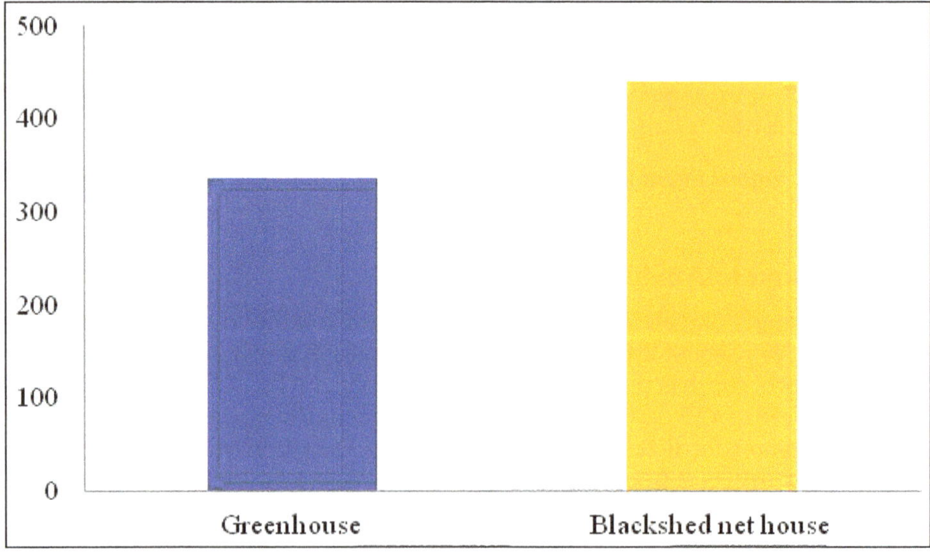

Figure 9.14: Vigour Index Mass of Seedling for Greenhouse and Black Shade Net House.

inside the greenhouse with full capacity. The details of the total cost and benefit for selected crops grown inside the greenhouse and black shade net house are given in Tables 9.2 and Table 9.4. Table 9.3 and Table 9.5 shows economic indicator of raising papaya seedling in protected structures, which shows that production cost for greenhouse and shade net house was 177.92 and 174.73 Rs/m^2 respectively. BCR for greenhouse and shade net house was 3.87, 3.94 and Payback period was 0.92, 0.59 respectively. It found similar results with Sengar and Kothari (2008) for raising of rose nursery in greenhouse in winter season.

Table 9.3: Economics of Raising of Papaya Seedling in Greenhouse for Madhibindu Variety

Treatment	*Variety*	*Revenue (Rs/m^2)*	*Economic Indicators*			
			Production Cost (Rs/m^2)	*Net Profit (Rs/m^2)*	*BCR*	*PBP*
Greenhouse	Madhubindu	688	177.92	510.08	3.87	0.92

Table 9.4: Constructional and Operational Cost of Black Shade Net House per square meter for Madhubindu Variety

Sl. No.		*Name of Component*	*Cost for 180 m^2 Size*			*Cost Rs/m^2*
			Quantity for 180 m^2	*Rate (Rs)*	*Cost (Rs)*	
A	Cost of structure without shade net					
	1	GI pipe 25mm B –class	280 m	165/m	46,200	
	2	GI pipe 50mm B –class	44 m	305/m	13,420	
	3	Door (size 1m X 2m)	one	-	1,500	
	4	Strings/wire, accessories *etc.*	-	-	3,000	
	5	Labour (Construction)	250 m^2	60/m^2	15,000	
	Total cost				81,120	324
B	Cost of 75 per cent UVS shading net @ Rs 25/m^2 X 2.15*				21.5	54
C	Cost of net house structure					
	1	75 per cent shade net (A+B), Ci_{75}			81141.5	378
D	Operating Cost					
	1	Seed Cost A (Madhubindu Rs.2.4/g)			3/m^2	3
	2	Soil treatment and manure			3/m^2	3
	3	Irrigation cost			4/m^2	4
	4	Labour cost/supervision			10/m^2	10
	5	Transport and marketing cost			8/m^2	8
		Total operating cost				28

Table 9.5: Economics of Raising of Papaya Seedling in Black Shade Net House for Madhibindu Variety

Treatment	*Variety*	*Revenue (Rs/m²)*	*Economic Indicators*			
			Production Cost (Rs/m²)	*Net Profit (Rs/m²)*	*BCR*	*PBP*
Black Shade net house	Madhubindu	688	174.73	513.27	3.94	0.59

Conclusion

There was a significant effect of structure and media on morphological parameter like maximum germination, seedling height, collar diameter, number of leaves, shoot diameter and fresh and dry weight of above and below ground biomass. Variation in seedling growth in different microclimatic conditions wasfound due to the differences in growth behavior under given set of environmental conditions. Due to off season raising seedling of papaya there was no germination in open field condition. Higher inside air temperature was found in greenhouse structure as compared to black shade net house and open field condition and relative humidity was found lower for greenhouse and higher in black shade net house. The microclimate for seedling emergence to groeth dynamics was found significant under black shade net house S_2than greenhouse S_1.The quality parameter like sturdiness, root: shoot ratio, vigour index I and vigour index II was recorded superior under black shade net house than greenhouse. It is therefore revealed that 75 per cent black colour shade net was the most effective for the raising papaya seedling and combating climate change in arid region during off season period.

Acknowledgements

The Authors acknowledge the department of Renewable Energy and Rural Engineering, College of Agricultural Engineering and Technology, Junagadh Agricultural University, Junagadh for all the support in terms of infrastructure as well as manpower for conducting the research.

References

Abdul-Baki Aand Anderson JD. 1973. Vigour determination in Soybean by multiple criteria. *Crop Science*.**13**: 630-637.

Akabari P D and Chauhan P M. 2011. Studies on micro climate and plant growth performance of capsicum under different types of shade net. Ph.D. Thesis. Junagadh Agricultural University.

Anonymous.2015a. National Horticulture Board, Sector 18, Gurgaon (Haryana). http//www.nhb.gov.in.

Anonymous.2015b. The Reports from Director of Horticulture, Gujarat State, Ganghinagar, http://agri.gujarat.gov.in.

Badowiec A and Weidner S. 2014. Proteomic changes in the roots of germinating Phaseolus vulgaris seeds in response to chilling stress and post-stress recovery. *J. Plant Physiol.***171**: 389–398.

Behera P C, Rao KA and Mitra B N.1990. Design, development and management of plastic house for nursery raising. Proceedings of XI International Congress of use of plastic in agriculture, New Delhi, India. P: E 91.

Bisla S S, Singhrot R S and Chauhan S S. 1984. Effect of growing media on seed germination and growth of Ber.*Haryana Journal Horticulture Science.***13**:118-122.

Bourgeois R, Ekboir J, Sette C, Egal C, Wongtchowsky M and Baltissen G. 2012. The State of Foresight in Food and Agriculture and the Roads Toward Improvement. GFAR, Rome.

Campen JB and Bot G P. 2003. Determination of green-house specific aspects of ventilation using three dimensional computational fluid dynamics. *Biosystem Engineering*.**84 (1)**:69–77.

Chakrabarti K, Azam Z and Siddhartha B. 1998.Compost for container nursery. *Indian forester*.**124(1)**:17-30.

Chauhan S K and Sharma R. 1997."Seedling quality evaluation: Important in afforestation", *advances in Forestry Res. In India*. **XVII**:59-27.

Climent J, Chambel MR, Pardos M, Lario F and Villar P. 2011. Biomass allocation and foliage heteroblasty in hard pine species respond differentially to reduction in rooting volume. *European Journal of Forest Research* **130**:841–850.

Endean Fand Carlson L. 1975. The effect of rooting volume on the early growth of lodgepole pine seedlings. *Canadian Journal of Forest Research* **5**:55–60.

Ericksen PJ, Ingram JS and Liverman D M. 2009. Food security and global environmental change: emerging challenges. *Environ. Sci. Policy*.**12**:373–377.

Iglesias I and Alegre S. 2006. The effect of anti-hail nets on fruit protection, radiation, temperature, quality and profitability of 'Mondial Gala' apples. *J. Appl. Hort.* **8(2)**: 91–100.

Ingram J, Ericksen P and Liverman D. 2010. Food Security and Global Environmental Change. Routledge, Oxford.

Khattak A M and Pearson S. 2005 Light quality and temperature effects on antirrhinum growth and development. *Journal of Zhejiang University Science.* **6(2)**:119-124.

Kothari, S K and Mathur AN. 2006. Greenhouse technology for protected cultivation a text book, Khana Publication. Udaipur. **18(3)**: 115-119.

Moller M and Assouline S. 2007. Effects of a shading screen on microclimate and crop water requirements,.*Journal of irrigation science*.**25**:171–181.

Nesmith DS, Bridges DC and Barbour JC. 1992. Bell pepper responses to root restriction. *Journal of Plant Nutrition* **15**, 2763–2776.

Peano C G, Giacolone A, Bosio G V. and Bounous G. 2001.Infl uenza delle reti antigrandine sulla qualita delle mele. *Rivista di Frutticoltura*, **9**: 61-64.

Pedro M M and Isolde D K. 1999. Effect of temperature on seed germination and seedling morphology *Maquira sclerophylla*(Ducke) CC Berg. *Brazilian journal of botany*. **22(2)**:303-307.

Rajamanickam C, Balasubramanyan S and Natarajan S. 2010. Studies on nursery management in papaya (*carica papaya l.*) var. co_2. *Acta Hort.***851**:307-312.

Rajapakse NC and Kelly J W. 1993. Spectral filters influence transpiration water loss in chrysanthemum. *Hort Sci.***28(10)**:999–1001.

Rathore T S, Annaourna D, Joshi G, and Srivastava A.2004. Studies on potting mixture and size of containers on the quality of seedling production in Casurina equisetifolia frost"*Indian Forester*.**130(3)**: 323-332.

Robbins NS and Pharr DM. 1988. Effect of restricted root growth on carbohydrate metabolism and whole plant growth of *Cucumis sativus L. Plant Physiology* **87**, 409–413.

Saikia P and Khan M L. 2012. Seedling survival and growth of *Aquilaria malaccensis* in different microclimatic conditions of northeast India. *Journal of Forestry Research*. **23(4)**: 569–574.

Sengar S H and Kothari S. 2008. Economic evaluation of greenhouse for cultivation of rose nursery. *African Journal of Agricultural Research.***3(6)**:435-439.

Smith H. 1982. Light quality, photoperception, and plant strategy. *Ann. Rev. Plant Physiol.***33**:481–518.

Smith H. 1995. Physiological and ecological function within the phytochrome family. *Annu. Rev. Plant Physiol. Plant Mol. Biol.* **46**:289–315.

Shrivastava R, Nanhorya R and Upadhyay J K., 1998. "Selection of proper potting mixture for root trainer of eucalyptus hybris",*Indian Forester*, **124 (7)**: 503-510.

Steffen W, Sanderson A, Tyson PD, Jager J, Matson P A, Moore B, Oldfield F, Richardson K, Schellnhuber H J, Turner B Land Wasson R J. 2004. Global change and the Earth system: a planet under pressure. Berlin, Heidelberg, New York: Springer-Verlag.

Srivastava R, Nahorya R and Upadhyay J K. 1998. Nursery studies on potting mixture, mulching and fertilizer requirement of chilgoza pine (*Pinus gerardiana Wall.*). *Indian J. of of Forestry*. **17(3)**:225-229.

Vermeulen S, Zougmore R, Wollenberg E, Thornton P, Nelson G, Kristjanson P, Kinyangi J, Jarvis A, Hansen J, Challinor A, Campbell B and Aggarwal P. 2012. Climate change, agriculture and food security: a global partnership to link research and action for low-income agricultural producers and consumers. *Curr. Opin. Environ. Sust.* **4**:128–133.

WHO 2003. Climate change and human health—risks and responses. Geneva: WHO

Wheeler T and Von-Braun J., 2013. Climate change impacts on global food security. *Science.***341**:508–513.

Chapter 10

Phenology, Taxonomy, Ethnobotany and their Relationship with Other Plant Studies: A Mini Review from Gujarat State, India

R.N. Nakar

Department of Botany, Sheth PT Arts and Science College, Shri Govind Guru University, Godhra - 389001, Gujarat, India
e-mail: rupeshnakar@gmail.com

ABSTRACT

Taxonomy is identification, classification and nomenclature of plants. Plants are unique gift of nature to human beings and other animals, are source of food, fodder and daily requirements. Plant diversity is the major research area in sciences. As India is having great diversity in plants with near about 4 lackh species, with diversity spots like Western Ghats, Deserts and Himalayas. Plant diversity is one of the priority research approaches for researchers throughout the world. In Gujarat state of India, also occurs diversity in vegetation with Pavagadh mountain, Girnar Mountain, Runn of Kuchchh along with sea coastal line of 1600 km which serves best chance to study plants in different habitats. Current review insights on different publications including books, thesis's, research articles and reviews on floristic diversity, taxonomy and phenology since 1900. It is matter of concern that specialist on the taxonomy and related subjects are not in much numbers but here is an effort to attract people towards old but very handful science which is in the centre of all branches of plant sciences.

***Keywords**: Gujarat, Taxonomy, Phenology, Ethnobotany, Floristic diversity, Review.*

Introduction

Plants are essential for human wellbeing as they provide food, fodder, medicines, fibres, fuel, building material and many such things that we use in our daily lives in one or other way. They are not only usefull for rain purpose but also for ecosystem services. Plants are main source of oxygen and are responsible for recycling of carbon dioxide which we inhale. India has distinct identity because of great diversity of natural ecosystem and forest which are main source for diversity. Biodiversity clearly means abundance distribution and interaction of genotypes, species, communities and ecosystem.

Flowering plants are by far the most numerous, diverse, and "successful" extant plant group, containing well over 95 per cent of all land plant species alive today (Simpson, 2006). Hooker (1904), commented that the Indian flora is more varied than that of any other country of equal area in the eastern hemisphere, if not on the globe. Among major and diverse hot spots of world, India shares very important place as having such diversity centers like Himalaya region, Western Ghats along with other marine diversity of sea. In India, there are about 45,000 plant species (Khoshoo, 1994, 1995; Sharma *et al.*, 1997), which includes 17,500 angiosperms, 23,000 fungus, 25,000 species of algae (fresh water and marine), 1600 different types of lichens, 1800 bryophytes and 30 microorganisms. In India, dicots are represented by 2,282 genera and 12,750 species whereas monocots are represented by 702 genera and 4,250 species. Dicots account for 75 per cent of flowering plants in terms of both genera and species. On the other hand, remaining 25 per cent is contributed by monocots. Such a beautiful gift of diversity is given by Nature to Indian sub-continent. In case of Gujarat, about 3200 flowering plants have been recorded yet. Such diversity gives chance of exploring research on floristic studies, as many species are still to be identified.

Floristic Study is in the Center of All Studies in Plant Science

Identification, classification and nomenclature of plant can be termed as taxonomy. Taxonomical study is in the center of all studies as physiological, biochemical or morphological. But if plant is in the proper form or stage like flowering or fruiting, identification becomes easy process. Identification in seedling stage, reproductive stage has specific traits pertaining present status of that plant. Furthermore, floristic study along with proper identification characters makes work more worthy as it deals directly with structure and function of particular plant or ecosystem. Physiological studies like water relation, photoperiod, transpiration, water use efficiency, chlorophyll florescence, photosynthesis, rain, temperature, vernalization *etc.* can never be studied without proper identification of species and family of that plant in wild. For any research work in the plant science related with Morphology, Anatomy, Physiology, Biochemistry, Biotechnology, Agriculture, Ecology and Environment, Genetics, Cell biology and others, needs through knowledge of plant systematic and taxonomy. Figure 10.1 indicates that floristic study in in the center of all studies.

Morpho-Geography and Forest Types

Panorama of Indian forest ranges from evergreen tropical to rain forests in Andaman and Nicobar Islands, Western Ghats and North eastern state to dry Alpines scrub high Himalaya evergreen rain forests, deciduous monsoon forests, thorn forest, sub-tropical pine forest in lower mountain zone and temperate

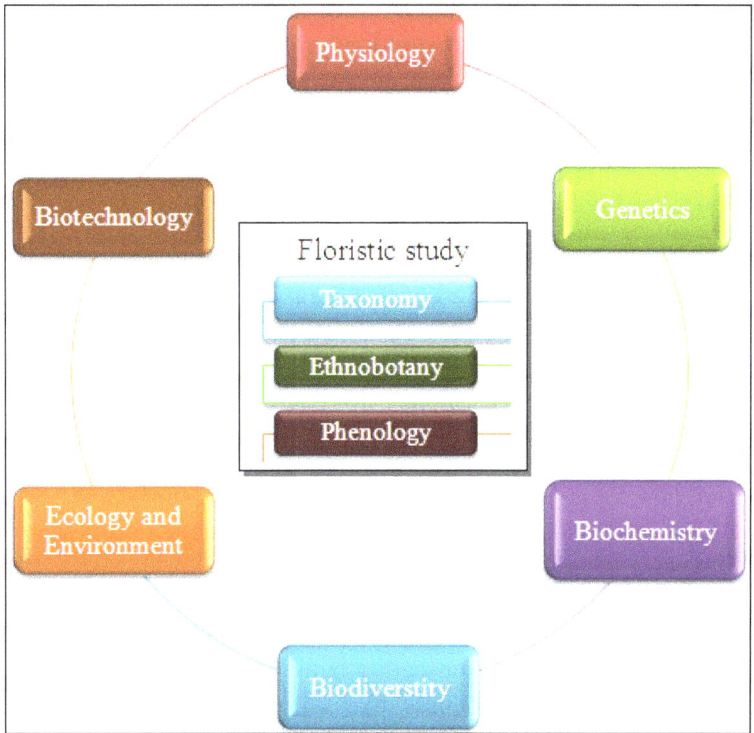

Figure 10.1: Floristic Study is in the Centre of all Studies.

mountain forest. Chowdhery and Murti (2000), have recognized 11 phytogeographic regions for India, each of which has its uniqueness in ecosystem, vegetation and floristic composition. These phytogeographic regions are: Western Himalaya, Eastern Himalaya, Gangetic plains, North East India, Semi arid and arid regions, Deccan Plateau, Western Ghats, Eastern Ghats, Andaman and Nicobar Islands, Lakshadweep and Coastal regions.

If we talk about Gujarat, there are three distinct geomorphologic divisions, *viz.* (1). Gujarat main land (2). Saurashtra Peninsula and (3). Kutch Peninsula

1. Gujarat Main land: It rises from estuarine tracts between Narmada and Tapi rivers, and goes North side, about 400 km and merge into desert of Rajasthan and Runn of Kutch. Eastern side is surrounded by Aravalli, Vindhya, Satpura and Sahyadri
2. Saurashtra Peninsula: It slopes towards all direction forming an elevated table land.
3. Kutch Peninsula: It is greatly isolated by great Rann on the north and east, and little Rann, on the south east side. During November it is barren tract of dry bed of salt encrusted mud, presenting aspects of inconceivable desolation. While during other half, it is flooded with waters of rivers that are held back owing to rise of sea by south west monsoon gates.

As there is lot of variation in geography of area, vegetation also shows diversity in Gujarat. Forest of Gujarat can be divided into, (I). Tropical dry moist deciduous forest- Hilly regions in south parts in Bulsar, Dangs and Surat districts. (II). Dry deciduous forest- It is subdivided into (a) Dry teak forest and (b) Non dry teak forest. Former occurs in Rajpipla, later occurs in Chota Udepur, Panchmahal, Sabarkantha in North Gujarat. While in Gujarat, Scrub forests occur only in Kutch, in mangrove forest which is mostly found along sea.

Major Families and Endemism

India represents about 11 per cent of world's flora in just about 2.4 per cent of total land mass. Out of the 25 biodiversity hotspots identified in the world, India has two, namely Eastern Himalaya and Western Ghats. On the basis of different climatic condition and physiognomy, India has rich collection in terms of floral diversity with high degree of endemism. India has great Himalaya peninsular region which is surrounded by ocean, hence Indian flora is isolated, which helps in large extent in endemism development. Among 17,500 total angiosperm plants, 28 per cent of the total Indian flora and about 33 per cent of angiosperms occurring in India are endemic (Nayar, 1996).

Nayar (1980), reported 141 endemic genera in India, as out of 34 global biodiversity hotspots in the world, Western Ghats ranks fifth. Among all flora, Poaceae and Acanthaceae are dominating families in Indian flora, also having 17 endemic species. There are approximately 17,000 plant species with 5,725 endemic plants, presenting about 33.5 per cent Indian flora. Total number of taxa, for Orchidaceae (1100), Asteraceae (1052), Rubiaceae (500), Cyperaceae (446), Labiateae (420), Acanthaceae (380), Scrophulariaceae (354), Rosaceae (250), Umbelliferi (209), Liliaceae (203), Ranunuculaceae (180), Balsaminaceae (180), Ericaceae (168), Primulaceae (165) and Lauraceae (163) express highest values. Ahmedullah and Nayar (1987), showed 58 genera with endemism among all to peninsular India. In case of great Himalaya, near about 72(71) genera, are found to be restricted,

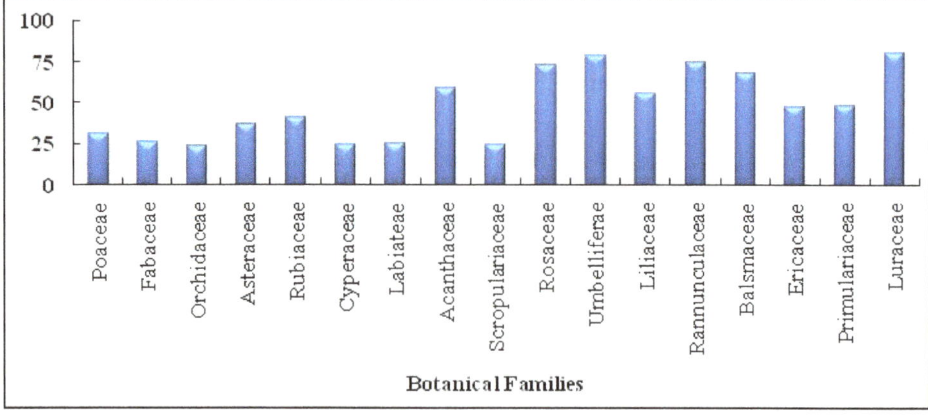

Figure 10.2: Family-wise Per cent Endemism in Indian Sub-continent (Nagar and Daniel, 2010).

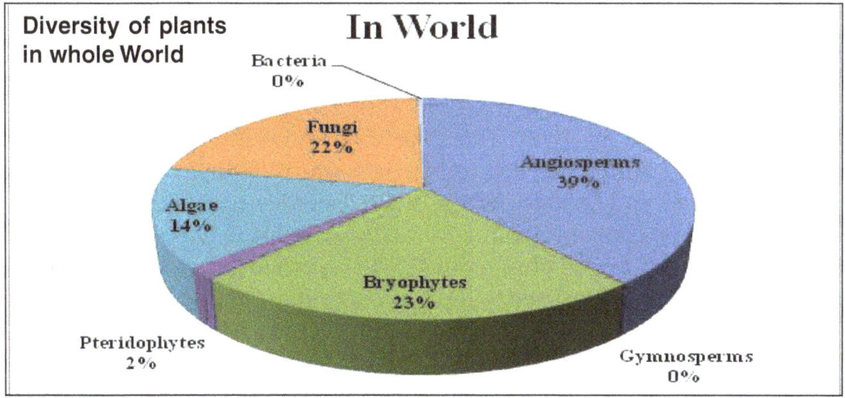

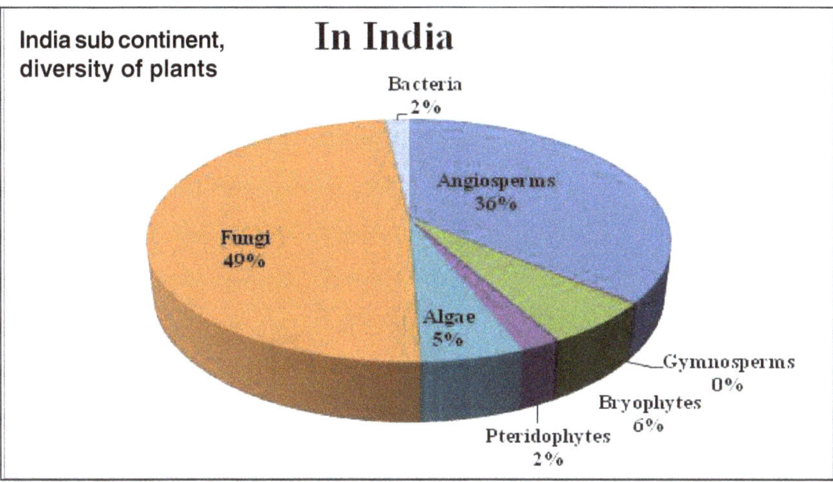

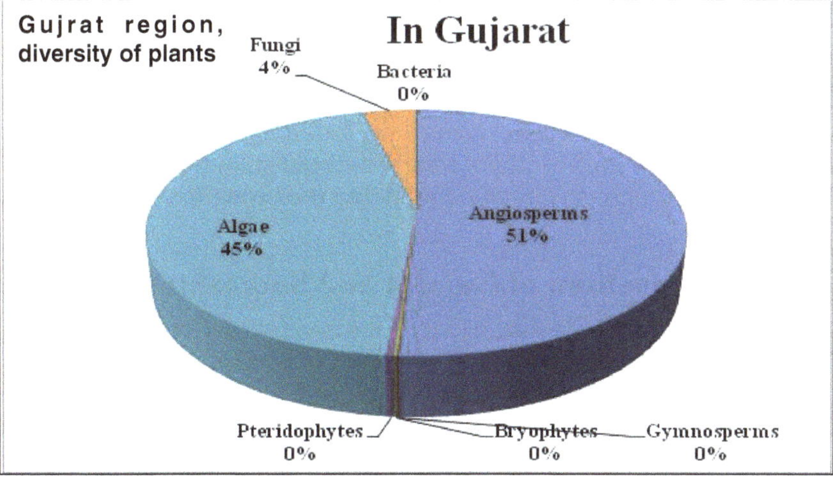

Figure 10.3: Per cent Species Identified among all Species for World, India and Gujarat (Nagar and Daniel, 2010).

but recently about 42 genera are confirmed to Eastern Himalaya and 12 belong to Western Himalaya (Rau, 1975). At species level, there are about 3,471 endemics restricted to Himalayas. Indian flora has as many as 6,100 species belonging to over 140 genera and 47 families which are endemic to Indian region (Chatterjee, 1939; Nayar, 1980; Balakrishnan, 1996). There are 2,500 endemics belonging to North east region and Eastern Himalaya, 800 to North western Himalaya, 200 to Andaman and Nicobar Island and 2600 for Western Ghat peninsula which itself says about endmism in Western Ghat. In Gujarat, Kathiyavad and Kutch region both contribute 8 endemic species. Mitra and Mukherjee (2006), recorded 267 genera and 782 species belonging to 80 families restricted to India and its adjoining areas. Of these restricted taxa of flowering plants, 72 families belong to dicots and 8 belongs to monocots. Dicot families comprise 213 genera and 622 species whereas monocots include 54 genera and 160 species. Endmism for individual families has been shown in Figure 10.2. Respective figures includes amount of per cent flora regions wise (Figure 10.3), also shows amount per cent of literature obtained for current topic (Figure 10.4).

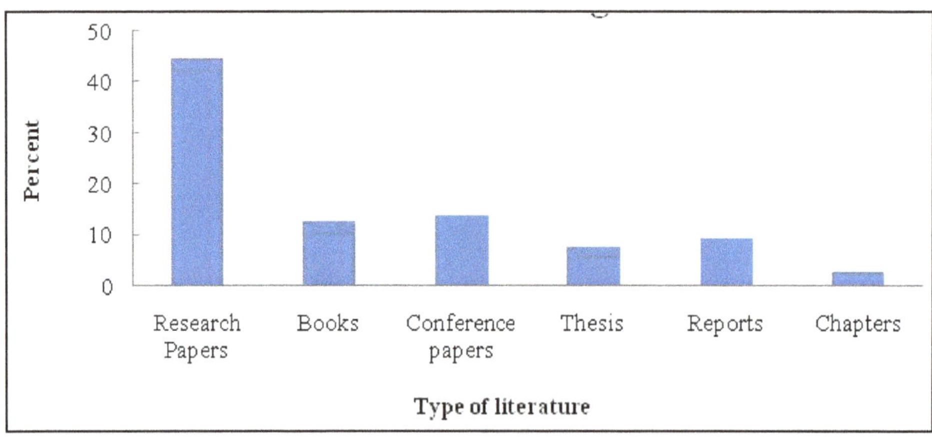

Figure 10.4: List of Literatures Studied for Review.

Highest per cent of research papers were found for floristic, phenological and other related studies, however there were some books, conference papers, thesis's, reports and book chapters were also found, but they were few compared to other literature.

Floristic Composition of Gujarat and Saurashtra Region

History of floristic study for Gujarat region is very old. Gujarat flora along with Sind flora was studied for Flora of the Presidency of Bombay (1901-1908). 450 plants species were identified at that time for Gujarat and 176 species were identified for Sind. Flora of Kutch and Saurashtra was studied (Blatter, 1908-09; Thakar, 1910;1926). But work of Santapau (1958) is well known among all.

Santapau produced important survey based book, flora of Saurashtra (Part-1), which covered Rannunculaceae to Rubiaceae family. Although work was incomplete, but Santapau and Janardan (1966), gave checklist of plants occurring in Saurashtra with 1,136 species under 591 genera of 126 families. During 1926, Santapau came with 'Kutch ane Saurashtra ni vanaspatio ane teni Upyogita '(Plants of Kutch and Saurashtra along with their utility) which had 10 chapters along with picture outlines. During second page of sanctuary, Botanical survey of Nawanagar which is now known as Jamnagar now, was carried out. Further research was done by adding 71 new species, published as "Vanaspati Shastra, Barda dungar ni jadibuti teni parikhsa ane upyog". In latest work, G.L. Shah (1978) published Flora of Gujarat, which contained list of 684 species. Important publications/contributions for floristic study, ethnobotany and phenology along with other important related work of Gujarat have been included in Table 10.1.

Table 10.1: Major Floristic, Taxonomic, Ethnobotanic and Phenological Studies in Gujarat State from Initial Level Starting from 1900

Sl.No.	*Title of work*	*Reference*
1.	Flora of presidency of Bombay	Cooke, 1908
2.	The flora of Kutch and Saurashtra	Blatter, 1909
3.	Vanaspatisastra ane Barda dungarni jadibuti tani parikhsa ane upyog. (A compete and comprehensive accout of the flora of Barda Mountain Kathiyavad).	Thaker, 1910
4.	Plants of Northern Gujarat	Saxton and Sedgwick,1918
5.	Katchni sawrathani Vanaspatiyo ane teni upyogita. (Plants of Kutch and their utility- An elaborate treatise containing ten chapters and litho figure).	Thaker, 1926
6.	Notes on Dwarka with reference to Raunkiaer's life forms and statistical methods.	Borgensen, 1929
7.	Notes on some grasses from Junagadh	Kapadia, 1945
8.	A note on Porbandar grasses.	Kapadia, 1947
9.	Forest wealth of Gir and Girnar in Junagadh District of Saurashtra.	Kapadia, 1951
10.	Flora of Saurashtra	Santapau, 1953
11.	Contribution to the Flora of the Gir Forest in Saurashtra	Santapau and Raizada, 1954
12.	Iter Kathiwarense: Being notes on a botanical tour in Nawanagar State,	Santapau, 1945
13.	Iter Kathiawrense: Being notes on a botanical tour in Nawangar state.	Santapau, 1952 a
14.	Report of the work done under the subspecies of the Saurashtra Research Society, for the botanical exploration of Saurashtra.	Santapau, 1952 b
15.	Reports of the second field season in the botanical exploration of Saurashtra, Rajkot	Santapau, 1952 c
16.	Reports of the third field season in the botanical exploration of Saurashtra, Rajkot	Santapau, 1952 d
17.	Plants of Saurashtra- a preliminary list, Rajkot	Santapau, 1952 e
18.	Contribution to the flora of Gir Forest in Saurashtra.	Santapau and Raizada, 1954
19.	Contribution to the Botany of Dangs Forest in Gujarat	Santapau, 1955
20.	La esploraccien botanica de Saurashtra en el No. de la India.	Santapau, 1956

Sl.No.	Title of work	Reference
21.	Contribution to the flora of Gir Forest in Saurasthra.	Santapau and Raizada, 1957 a
22.	Glimpses of the vegetation of Okhamandal	Raizada and Vaidya, 1957
23.	Flora of the presidency of Bombay	Cooke, 1958
24.	Medicinal plants of Jamnagar	Ahluwalia, 1964-1965
25.	Further contribution to Botany of Dangs Forest	Santapau and Shah, 1965
26.	Grasses of Gujarat state.	Patel, 1965
27.	Cyperaceae of Dangs	Chavan and Sabnis, 1966
28.	Addition to the flora of Dang Forest	Shah and Subranarayana, 1967
29.	Contribution to the flora of Gir Forest.	Raizada, 1967
30.	Contribution to the flora of Dangs forest	Chavan and Oza, 1967
31.	The flora of Baroda and Environs.	Sabnis, 1967
32.	Ecological studies of Saurashtra Coast and neighboring islands.	Rao, 1968-74
33.	A contribution to the flora of Dangs forest, Gujarat	Subranarayana, 1968
34.	Forest flora of Gujarat State	Patel, 1968
35.	Vegetation of Dangs District in Gujarat	Jain, 1968
36.	Further contribution to the flora of Dangs Forest	Shah and Subranarayana, 1969
37.	New plants records for Bombay collected from Dangs forest.	Shah and Subranarayana, 1969
38.	Addition to the flora of Dangs forest	Shah and Subranarayana, 1969
39.	Flora of Valsad,	Patel, 1971
40.	A contribution to the flora of North Gujarat	Yogi, 1970
41.	*Common Trees*.-Book	Santapau, 1971
42.	Working plant for Junagadh forest division.	Sinha *et al.*,1972
43.	Studies on the botany of Jamnagar District.	Malahotra and Wadhawa, 1973
44.	A contribution to the flora of Bansada Forest	Desai, 1976
45.	Flora and vegetation of Saurashtra	Pandya, 1976
47.	Flora of Gujarat. Part I and II.	Shah, 1978
48.	Studies on Botany of Jamnagar District	Malhotra and Wadhava,1978
49.	Floristics and phytosociological studies on some parts of Saurashtra	Menon, 1979
50.	Biological spectrum of the Flora of Shetrunjaya Hills, Palitana.	Patel *et al.*,1981
51.	Grasses of Western India.	Toby and Patrick, 1982
52.	An ethnobotanical profile of the Dangies.	Shah and Gopal, 1982
53.	Observation on some rare or endangered endemics of Southern Kutch. An assessment of threatened plants of India. Botanical Survey of India, Culcutta. Pp:71-77	Sabnis and Rao,1983
54.	Rare species with restricted distribution in South Gujarat.	Shah, 1983

Sl.No.	*Title of work*	*Reference*
55.	Floristic phytosociology and Ethno botanical study of Vapi and Umargaon area in South Gujarat.	Contractor, 1986
56.	Contribution to the flora of Surat district, Surat	Mac, R.N., 1986
57.	Biological flora of Rajkot	Thakrar, 1987
58.	Contribution to the ethnobotany of Khedbrahma region of North Gujarat.	Bhatt, *et al.*, 1987
59.	Flora of Dharampur Forest	Reddy, A.S.,1987
60.	Flora of Saurashtra. Part II and III.	Bole and Pathak, 1988
61.	Forest wealth of Kutch, its Utility and Potencials.	Pandya, 1989
62.	Red data book of Indian plants, Vol-I to III.	Nayar and Shastry, 1990
63.	Taxonomical and ecological studies of the flora of and around Bhavangar	Oza, 1991
64.	Vegetational and wildlife studies in Gir	Chavan, 1993
65.	Flora of Gir-report submitted to Department of Forest, Gujarat, India	Asari, 1994
66.	Flora of Girnar-report submitted to Department of Forest, Gujarat, India	Asari, 1994
67.	Biological diversiy of Gujarat-Current knowledge.	Pilo and Pathak, 1996
68.	Taxonomical study of angiosperms of Palitana	Mehta, 1997
69.	Plants used by the tribe Rabari in Barda Hills of Gujarat.	Jadeja, 1999
70.	Ethnomedicinal plants of Shetrunjaya Hills of Palitana, Gujarat	Bhatt *et al.*,1999
71.	Biodiversity of Barda Hills	Nagar, 2000
72.	Ethnobotanical studies of Angiosperms of Aravalli Hills (District Banaskantha, Gujarat State)	Ant, 2000
73.	Ethnobotanical aspects of some plants of Arravalli Hills in North Gujarat	Punjani, 2002
74.	*Stylosanthes hamatus* (Linn.) Taub.(Papilionaceae), A New record to the flora of Gujarat. (With one text figure).	Nagar and Pandya, 2002
75.	Addition to the flora of Saurashtra, Gujarat, India.	Nagar and Pandya, 2002
76.	*Cleome scaposa* D.C. (Capparidaceae). A rare species of Saurashtra	Nagar and Pandya, 2002
77.	Rediscovery of *Tephrosia jamnagarensis* (Fabaceae), an endangered and narrow endemic plant species of Saurashtra Side.	Nagar *et al.*,2003
78.	Floristic diversity of Barda Hills and their surroundings, Saurashtra, Gujarat.	Nagar and Pandya, 2003
79.	Status of some regionally threatened species of Saurashtra, Gujarat, India.	Nagar, 2004
80.	Floristic Diversity of Barda Hills and its surroundings	Nagar, 2005
81.	Asthetic values of selected floral elements of Khatana and Waghai forests of Dangs, Western Ghat.	Nirmal Kumar, 2005
82.	Phenological studies of Reserve Forest (Victoria Park) near Bhavanagar	Gohil, 2005
83.	Medicinal Plants- Chemistry and Properties	Daniel, 2006

Sl.No.	Title of work	Reference
84.	Floristic and ethnobotanical studies of Ambaji and Gorakhnath mountains of Girnar.	Makad, R.S., 2007
85.	Studies on plant species used by tribal communities of Saputara and Purna Forest, Dangs District, Gujarat.	Nirmal Kumar *et al*, 2007
86.	Herbal technology: Concept and Approaches.	Daniel, M., 2008
87.	Households and house of tribals of Gujarat – an ethnobotanical study	Jadeja *et al.*,2008
88.	Plant used in traditional phytotherapy for indigestion in Gujarat, india	Jadeja *et al.*,2008
89.	Study of some medicinal plants of vijapur taluka of Mahesana district of Gujarat, India.	Jadeja and Modhvadia, 2008
90.	Phenological observations on some dry deciduous forest trees at Barda hills, Gujarat.	Jadeja *et al.*,2008
91.	Study on medicinal Plant diversity in Arboretum.	Tadvi, D., 2009
92.	Ethnobotany of Maher Tribe In Porbandar District, Gujarat, India,	Odedara, 2009
93.	Study on morphology, ethnobotany and phenology of *Prosopis* in Girnar Forest Junagadh, Gujarat.	Nakar and Jadeja, 2009
94.	Plant Biodiversity: Collection, characterization and conservation. (on Motibaug Botanical Garden, Junagadh)	Dhaduk *et al.*, 2010
95.	Floristic diversity of Gujarat.	Nagar and Daniel, 2010
96.	Herbal folk medicines used for urinary complaints in tribal pockets of Northeast Gujarat.	Punjani, 2010
97.	Floristic status and its conservation in the Forests of North Gujarat Region, Gujarat India.	Rajendra Kumar, 2010
98.	Pictorial Floristic Diversity of Grasses and Associated Vegetation from Three Grasslands of Randhikpur Forest Range, Dahod, Gujarat	Tyagi *et al.*, 2010
99.	A soujoun to the herbal treasures of MSU., M.S. University	Daniel and Nagar, 2010
100.	Phenological studies of some tree species from Girnar Reserve Forest, Gujarat, India.	Jadeja and Nakar, 2010
101.	Study on ethno-medico botany of weeds from saurashtra region, Gujarat, India.	Jadeja and Nakar, 2010
102.	Issues Relating to Medicinal Plant Cultivation, Processing and Marketing. Workshop souvenir.	Mandavia *et al.*, 2010
103.	Floristic diversity of the stream and riparian zone of the Vishwamitri rivers Vadodara.	Patale and Parikh, 2010
104.	Uncommon tree resources to the ethnobotany from Ambaji Forest of Banashkantha district[North Gujarat]	Patel *et al.*, 2010
105.	Vegetational diversity in the land of Bhey (Garbada).	Gandhi *et al.*, 2010
106.	A contribution to the ethnobotany of Vijaynagar Forest of Sabarkantha District.	Bamna *et al.*,2010
107.	Taxoethnobotanical significance of some plants from Ambaji forest (North Gujarat).	Dave *et al.*, 2010
108.	Observation on tree species of Danta Range Forest of North Gujarat.	Patel *et al.*,2010

Sl.No.	*Title of work*	*Reference*
109.	Ethnobotany of *Lannea coromandlica* (Hautt). Merril. From Aravalli Forest areas of North Gujarat.	Patel *et al.*,2010
110.	Plants used in preparation of musical instruments and agricultural impliments of Ambaji forest in Banashkantha District (North Gujarat).	Patel *et al.*,2010
111.	A review on some medicinal plants of Gujarat College campus, Ahmedabad, Gujarat.	Gondalia *et al,* 2010
112.	Studies on some ethnomedicinal plants from Khanpur Forest Range in Panchmahal District, Gujarat.	Punjani *et al*, 2010
113.	Plant diversity and its life forms of Visnagar Taluka, North Gujarat.	Solanki *et al*, 2010
114.	Traditional aboriginal knowledge of the flora in the Girnar Holy hills areas, Gujarat.	Solanki *et al*, 2010
115.	Survey of ethnomedicinal plants of Anjar Taluka used in Anemia.	Sorathiya, 2010
116.	Medicinal uses of some plant species found around Navasari District of Gujarat state.	Yadav *et al,* 2010
117.	Biodiversity management and conservation by nature education at Hingolgadh Sanctuary	Gohil, 2011
118.	Study on density and Biomass of sea weeds at Port Okha, Gujarat-A case study	Nakar *et al.*,2011
119.	Floristic diversity of Isari zone, Megharj range forest District Sabarkantha, Gujarat, India	Vediya and Kharadi, 2011
120.	Floristic analysis of flora of Bhanvad, Jamjodhpur and LalipurTalukas of Jamnagar district, Gujarat	Jadeja *et al.,* 2011
121.	Socioeconomic Study of Grasses and egumes in Baria and Godhra Forest Division,Gujarat	Gandhi *et al.*,2011
122.	Floristic studies of Dadra and Nagar Haveli.	Nair, 2011
123.	Importance and conservation values of disturbed lands of North Gujarat region (NGR), Gujarat, India.	Rajendra Kumar *et al*, 2011
124.	Ecology and conservation of threatened plants in Tapkeshwari Hill ranges in the Kachchh Island, Gujarat, India	Joshi *et al.,* 2012
125.	In depth studies on some of the floristic components of Baroda and Panchmahal Districts with reference to Bioprospecting and speciation.	Gohil, 2012
126.	Floristic diversity of the Ahmedabad city	Jadeja and Patel, 2012
127.	Floral and avifaunal diversity of the Thol lake, wild life sanctuary of Gujarat State, India	Kariya, 2012
128.	Biological spectrum of Taluka Modasa, District Sabarkantha (Gujarat), India	Jangid, 2012
129.	Study of plant diversity in vadali range forest district Sabarkantha, North Gujarat, India	Desai and Ant, 2012
130.	Floristical and Ecological assessment of Joint Forest Management Plantations and Natural Forests	Bariya, and Sandhyakiran, 2012
131.	Observation on some energy plants among the rural people in Jambudia of Saurashtra region, Gujarat, India	Dave and Patel, 2012

Sl.No.	*Title of work*	*Reference*
132.	Taxonomic status and utilization of Halophytes in coastal Kutchh District, Gujarat.	Shah and Thivakaran, 2012
133.	Observations on folk medicinal plants used by inhabitat tribals in Bhiloda Forest Range of Sabarkantha, North Gujarat	Tintisara and Prajapati 2012
134.	Floristic studies on scared grooves sitated near Utkantheswar in Kheada District, Gujarat	Patel and Patel, 2012
135.	Floristic and ethnobotanical study of Palanpur and Dantiwada, Gujarat.	Patel and Patel, 2012
136.	Studies on phenology of some shrubs from Girnar Reserve Forest, Gujarat.	Nakar and Jadeja, 2013
137.	Comparision of phenology of *Cassia siamea* Lam. From Girnar Reserve Forest and GIDC polluted area from Junagadh, Gujarat.	Nakar and Jadeja, 2013
138.	Studies on phenological patterns of Girnar Reserve Forest, near Junagadh, Gujarat.	Nakar, 2013
139.	Biodiversity conservation through urban green spaces: a case study of Gujarat university campus in Ahmedabad.	Modi and Dudani, 2013
140.	Plant diversity assessment at land scape level in Jamnagar District, Gujarat using satellite remote sensing and geographic information system	Bhatt, 2013
141.	Plant richness modeling in South Gujarat using remote sensing and geographic information system	Bhatt *et al.*, 2013
142.	Floristic diversity and ecological studies in forest areas of Idar and Vadali Talukas, District Sabarkantha.	Desai, 2013
143.	Ethnobotanical survey of some medicinal plants in Jatashankar region of Girnar Forest, Gujarat, India.	Dhaduk and Raval, 2013
144.	Floristic study of Kaprada's hilly forest in South Gujarat	Rao *et al*, 2013
145.	Ethnobotanical survey of some parasitic plants growing in Girnar Forest of Junagadh District of Gujarat, India.	Sallaudin *et al*, 2013
146.	Phenological studies of two bombacacean members from Girnar Reserve Forest, Junagadh, Gujarat, India.	Nakar and Jadeja, 2014a
147.	Seed pattern, germination and viability studies on some forest tree species seeds from Girnar Reserve Forest of Gujarat	Nakar and Jadeja, 2014b
148.	Standardization of wild forest seeds for morphology and viability studies	Nakar and Jadeja, 2014c
149.	Qualitative and quantitative seed characteristics diversity from Girnar Reserve Forest, Gujarat, India.	Nakar and Jadeja, 2015a
150.	Study on the floristic diversity of two newly recorded sacred groves from Kachchh District of Gujarat, India	Patel *et al*, 2014d
151.	Phenological attributes of seven tree species in association with climate from Girnar Reserve Forest, Gujarat.	Nakar and Jadeja, 2014e
152.	Studies on phenological behavior of two *Cassia* species from Girnar Reserve Forest, Gujarat, India.	Nakar and Jadeja, 2015b
153.	Phenology and productivity of forest flora of Gujarat.	Nakar, Jadeja and Singh, 2015c
154.	Germination and viability studies in two undershrubs *Cassia* species from Girnar Reserve Forest, Gujarat.	Nakar and Jadeja, 2016

Sl.No.	*Title of work*	*Reference*
155.	Medicinal Plants: Cultivation and Uses	Nakar, Dhaduk and Chovatia, 2016
156.	Traditional knowledge of some Ethenomedicinal plants in Hariyawada village of Banaskantha district, North Gujarat.	Patel and Mali, 2016
157.	Status, Distribution And Phytosociologicalstudies of tree Halophytes In Kachchh District (Gujarat), India	Shah and Ant, 2016
158.	Studies on prevalence of Coastal Halophytes from semi-arid region, Kachchh, Gujarat	Jayanthi *et al.* (2016)
159.	Study Of Different Plant Species Uses On Dental Diseases In Aravali Sabarkantha District Of Gujarat, India	Vediya *et al.* (2016)
160.	Ethnomedicinal Study Of Some Selected Plants Of Euphorbiaceae Family Of Modasa Taluka,District Arvalli, Gujarat, India	Jangid *et al.* (2016)
161.	Biological Spectrum of Vagpur Range Forest District Aravalli Gujarat, India.	Kharadi *et al.* (2016)
162.	A Preliminary Survey of Lichens in Forest Area of Taranga, District Mehsana, Gujarat	Raval *et al.* (2016)
163.	Observation On Lichen Mycota in Coastal Area of Alang, District Bhavnagar, Gujarat	Punjani and Raval (2016)
164.	Uses and Harmful Effects of Differents Alkaloids From Laticiferous Plants in Vividhlaxi Vidyamandir Campus, Palanpur Banaskanta, North Gujarat	Chauhan, *et al.* (2016)
165.	Seedling morphology of selected species from Girnar Reserve Forest, Gujarat, India.	Nakar and Jadeja (2016)
166.	Cistaceae: a new family record from India	Patel and Gosavi (2016)
167.	Assessment of phonological diversity of GIDC polluted area, from Junagadh, Gujarat, India.	Nakar and Jadeja (2017)
168.	Distribution, morphology and floristic characters of selected Asclepiadaceae members from Saurashtra region, West-South India.	Jadeja and Nakar (2017)

6. Threatened and Endangered Plants

Plants are getting threatened as one or few reasons like urbanization, deforestation, pollution, overgrazing *etc.* Almost 10 per cent vascular plants fall into one or other category of threatened plant species. In 1980, Botanical Survey of India started working on rare and endangered species, came with list of threatened plants. Despite our reliance on plants, it is though that approximately 60,000 to 1,00,000 plants are under threat, may extinct in near future. Due to climate change, habitat change, invasive species, overexploitation, plants are getting disappeared at the rate 3 order magnitude, will increase in near future. From different parts of the country Jain and Shastry (1980), enlisted many species of rare plants. Finally red data book, with 4 volumes, including 620 plants was published. Nayar and Sastry (1987-90), published list of rare and endangered plants into various categories. According to him, there were 62 species of 22 families, in extinct group, 128 species with 43 families came in endangered list while 110 species of 50 families were in endangered list. 110 species of 50 families belonged to Vulnerable, 71 species of 37 families were into insufficiently known family. IUCN (1995), has given following categories of threatened plants on the basis of geographical range, populations and fragmentation of population.

1. Extinct- When species is no more, has become extinct
2. Critically endangered- When species has high risk of extinction in near future
3. Endangered- Although it will not disappear quickly, but soon it will disappear.
4. Vulnerable-When it doesn't come under Extinct, Critically endangered, Rare, Endangered, but still facing risk of extinction
5. Conservation dependent- When species are focused of a continuing taxon specific or habit specific conservation programme targeted towards the taxon in question, and cessation of which would result in taxon qualifying for one of the threatened categories above within period of five years.
6. Low risk- Species having very low risk of extinction.
7. Not evaluated- A taxon is not evaluated when it has not yet been assessed against criteria.
8. Data deficient- those species whose data are not available.

In India, it is presumed that out of 17,000 species of 3,000 plants come under category of threated plants which also includes several medicinal plants. The list is in support of four volumes of Red data book of India (Jain and Shashtry, 1984; Nayar and Shashtry, 1987-1990). Recently published popular article, by Sudhi (2012), gave details regarding latest figures of plants and animals which are in merge of extinction. In the article it is stated that International Union for Conservation of Nature (IUCN), has listed 132 species of plants and animals as Critically Endangered, the most threatened category, from India. In Plants, 60 species are listed as critically endangered while 141 was declared as endangered species. Two plant species were reported to be extinct in the wild, including the *Euphorbia mayuranthanii* of Kerala. A leaf frog species and six plants were recorded as extinct, according to the latest assessment.

Of the total 63,837 species globally assessed, the IUCN classified 3,947 as Critically Endangered, 81 as Extinct, 63 as Extinct in the Wild. In the lower risk categories, there were 5,766 species in Endangered, 10,104 in Vulnerable and 4,467 in near threatened categories. Scientific data regarding 10,497 species was not available and hence classified as Data Deficient, the report said. Some endangered plants of Gujarat and India are, *Aegle marmelos, Adhatoda vasica, Andrographis paniculata, Aristolochia bracteota, Artemisia nilagirica, Balanites aegyptica, Commiphora whightii, Cycus circinalis, Emblica ribes, Garcinia indica, Gardenia gummifera, Firmiana colorata, Gloriosa superba, Moringa cocanensis, Merremia turpethum, Leptadenia reticulata, Oroxylum indicum, Piper longum, Piper nigrum, Puerreria tuberosa, Rauvolfia quaticne, Saraca asoca, Schrebera swietenoides, Vernonia anthelmintica, Wood fordia fruticosa.*

Invasive Flora, Insectivorous Plants, Aquatic Plants and Mangroves

Due to climatic condition and internal competition between endemic species, outer plants have established their place in regional flora. They have been able to maintain their place permanently in Indian flora although they have arrived from outside. Many common plants like *Lantana camera, Ageratum conizoides, Jetropa gossipifolia, Opuntia elatior, Stellaria media, Spergula arvensis, Sagina apetala, Anagallis arvensis, Convolvulus arvensis, Trigonella corniculata, Euphorbia prostrata, Amaranthus spinosus, Argemone Mexicana,* and many others came to India as impurities with seeds of cultivated plants and established. Some plants depends on other insects for nitrogen supply, are called insectivorous plants. Total 450 species of insectivorous plants have been recorded among which India shares 30 species. Some common insectivorous families are: Droseraceae (3 spp.), Nepenthaceae (1 spcies) and Lentibulariaceae (36 spp.). The parasitic plant species are prominent in Loranthaceae (46 spp.), Santalaceae (10 spp.), Balanophoraceae (6 spp.), Rafflesiaceae (1 spp.), Cuscutaceae (12 spp.) and Orobanchaceae (54 spp.). In deep forest, of Dangs, Panchmahals, Barda Hills, Girnar Reserve Forest, of Gujarat we can easily find Cuscutacean members and Santalacean member along with other plants.

Among total aquatic plants of the world, almost 50 per cent resprent to India. (Lavania *et al.*, 1990). An aquatic plant performs an important role as water purifier by absorbing heavy metals, *e.g. Ceratophyllum demersum* (chromium), *Bacopa monnieri* (copper and cadmium). *Limosella quatic, Hippuris vulgaris* occur in subalpine-alpine lakes. Indian aquatics are highly diversified comprising free-floating forms (*Eichhornia crassipes, Lemna perpusila, Nymphoides hydrophylla, Trapa natans var. bispinosa, Pistia stratiotes, Wolffia microscopia, W. globosa*), rooted aquatics with their foliage floating (*Nymphaea nouchali, N. stellata, Euryale ferox, Nelumbo nucifera*), submerged aquatics (*Vallisnaria natans, Hydrilla verticillata, Najas graminea, Potamogeton pectinatus*) emergent aquatics (*Scirpus maritimus, Cyperus articulates, Sagittaria trifolia, S. guayanensis subsp. Leppula*) and marsh plants (*Ranunculus scleratus, Hydrolea zeylanica, Panicum paludosum, Polygonum barbatum, P. glabrum*). Gujarat has 1,600 km sea coast which is perfect for research work on sea weeds and mangroves also. Because mangrove species propagates well in marshy land, Indian coast with length of 6,700 km^2, favors mangroves species which ranks 7th place in world. Most of mangroves grow in Sundar bans (West Bangal), which is followed by other areas like Andhra Pradesh, Tamil Nadu, Orissa, Maharashtra, Gujarat, Goa and Karnataka. Some of the dominant mangrove species include *Avicennia marina, A. officinalis, Bruguiera gymnorrhiza, B. parviflora, Ceriops tagal, Heritiera fomes, Lumnitzera spp., Rhizophora mucronata, R. apiculata, R. stylosa, Sonneratia* spp., *Xylocarpus* spp., *etc.*

Ethno-Botanically Useful Plants

Since the time of Vedic ages, India has pride for her Ayurvedic medicines. Plants were thought to have vapons for combating ailments and as a preventive cure against diseases. Indigenous medicines are still practiced in all parts of the India traditionally and especially in rural and tribal belts. Plants are being major ingradient in almost all system of medicinal science. When he published "A catalogue of Indian medicinal plants and drugs". In 1813, Ainslie published "Materia medica of Hindustan". In 1969, Chunekar has published full glossary of Medicinal plants entitled "*Vanaspatika anusandhan Darsika*" which is included in ancient Indian literature like Charrak Samhita, Shushrut Shahita, Astangya haridham. These kinds of plants directly take part in Indian flora as they are important for economy of state and country also. Numbers of foresters, ethnobonists and other researchers have worked on medicinally important plants for specific region. National medicinal plants Board (NMPB) of India have listed 5,662 medicinal plants from different parts of Indian sub continent.

Religious Perspective

Since the time of Vedas and Upanishad, people have been worshiping plants in one or another way. Hindus worship and prevent some plants like, Tulsi (*Ocimum sanctum*), Pipal (*Ficus religiosa*), Bad (*Ficus glomerata*), Bilva (*Aegle marmelos*), Savan (*Gmelina arborea*), Chandan (*Santalum album*), Ashok (*Saraca indica*), Palash (*Beutia monosperma*), Neem (*Azadirechta indica*). Muslim families worship plants like Mahendi (*Lawsonia inermis*), Mulberry (*Morous alba*), Pomegranate (*Punica granatum*) and Fig (*Ficus glomerata*). Sikhs, believe that plants like, Bad (*Ficus benghalensis*), Aritha (*Sapindus laurifolios*), Sisam (*Dalbergia sissoo*), Ber (*Ziziphus* sp.) are very sacred and god is directly attached with these plants. In case of Buddhis, plants like Pipal (*Ficus religiosa*), Ginko (*Ginko biloba*), Chandan (*Santalum album*), Savan (*Gmelina arborea*), Sal (*Shorea robusta*), Rayan (*Manilkara hexandra*) are considered as sacred plants and they also believe that these are the way to reach to god. Religious concept is connected with sacred grove. Sacred groves are pockets of more or less climax vegetation which is preserved for religious perspective in remote areas and at home. In such remote areas, even picking twing is crime or sacrilege, even an offense, gives rise to deity anger. People of different cast protect their sacred plants for future, is very much helpful for social forestry, for reducing pollution as well as maintaining diversity.

Conclusion and Future Strategy

It is clear that floristic study is in the center of all studies and there is vast scope for plant systematic, floristic diversity, ethnobotany and region specific taxonomic studies. There is requirement or inventerization of diversity and distribution, phenology, reproductive biology, growth rate, nursery techniques, along with *In-situ* and *Ex-situ* preservations. (Pandey, 1995). According to Santapau (1958), when we are talking about preparing of National flora we should prepare district flora first as they are small unit which forms basis of compilation of State flora and National flora, which ultimately reaches global compilation. Taxonomists have main role to play for finding new species from different areas while those areas which are not surveyed yet, need to be explored in near future. In Gujarat, from the above analysis, there is good chance for angiosperm taxonomy and floristic survey based research as having different geographical conditions which involves hilly areas, desert, marine diversity also, in different areas of Saurashtra, Kutch and other parts of Gujarat.

Since last flora published, no accurate flora work has been done yet although, efforts are going on but there is ultimate requirement of revision of work and adding new species. Red data book also need to be reevaluated by adding different species with different categories. At Research institutes, University and College level, biodiversity calendar should be prepared along with arrangement of field trips for students, teachers and scientists. Collection of samples for herbariums should be done in proper way that it can be highly useful in future for further studies. Only floristic studies will not be enough but, DNA sequencing may be an useful idea for Gujarat and Indian Flora. People should be aware by current problem of conservation hence they should be encouraged by government for doing such work on conservation. Forest department of local, regional and National level should inspire people to participate more in such programmes.

References

Ainslie Whitelaw (1813) Materia medica of Hindustan, Madrash.

Ant, H. M. (2000). Ethnobotanical studies of Angiosperms of Aravalli Hills (District anaskantha, Gujarat State) Ph.D. Thesis Submitted to The Bhavnagar University, Bhavnagar.

Asari, (1994). Gir forest-report submitted to Gujart Government. Govt. of India.

Asari, (1994). Girnar forest-report submitted to Gujart Government. Govt. of India.

Bamna, R., Patel, R. S. and Patel, K. C. (2010). A contribution to the ethnobotany of Vijaynagar forest of Sabarkantha District. *International Journal of Bioscience Reporter*. 8, 59-65.

Bariya, P. and Sandhyakiran, G. (2012). Floristical and Ecological assessment of Joint Forest Management Plantations and Natural Forests. *Bulletin of Environmental and Scientific Research*. [ISSN: 2278-52105], 1, 11-17.

Bhatt, R.P. and Sabnis, S.D. (1987): ontribution to the Ethnobotany of Khedbrahma region of North Gujarat. *Jour. Eco and Tax. Bot.* 9 (1):139-145.

Bhatt, D.C., Mehta, S.K. and Mitaliya., K.D. (1999). Ethnomedicinal Plants of Shetrunjaya Hill of Palitana, Gujarat.

Bhatt G. D. (2013). Plant diversity assessment at land scape level in Jamnagar District, Gujarat using satellite remote sensing and geographic information system. International Journal of advancement in earth and environmental sciences. 1(1):23-25 [ISSN:2321-9149].

Bhatt G. D, Khushwaha, S. P. S., Nandy, S., Bargali, K., Tadvi, D., Nagar, P. S. and Daniel, M. (2013). Plant richness modeling in South Gujarat using remote sensing and geographic information system. *Indian Forester*, 139(9): 757-768.

Balakrishnan, N. P., Phytogeographic divisions: general considerations (1996). In: Flora of India (Introductory volume), Part I. (ed. P. K. Hajra *et al.*). BSI, Calcutta.

Blatter, E. (1908). Flora of Bombay presidency; Statistical and biological notes. *Journal of Bombay Natural Histroy Socety*. 18, 562-571.

Boergensen (1929). Notes on vegetation at Dwarka with reference to Raunkier's life forms and statistical methods. *Journal of Indian Botanical Society.*, 8, 1-18.

Bole and Pathak (1988). Flora of Saurashtra. Part II and III. Botanical survey of India, Culcutta, p. 545.

Contractor, B. J. (1986). Floristic Phytosociology and Ethno botanical study of Vapi and Umargaon area in south Gujarat. Ph.D. Thesis.

Cook, T (1908). The flora of the presidency of Bombay Vol I-III. Botanical survey of India. Culcutta, p. 649.

Chatterjee, D. (1939). Studies on the endemic flora of India and Burma. *Journal of Asiatic Society of Bengal.* 5, 19-68.

Chauhan, N. M., Chhaniyaniya, J. V. Chauhan, H. H., Dabgar, Y. B. (2016). Uses and Harmful Effects Of Differents Alkaloids From Laticiferous Plants In Vividhlaxi Vidyamandir Campus, Palanpur, Banaskanta, North Gujarat, *In Proceeding book of abstract, XXX Gujarat Science Congress,* KSKV Kachchh University, pp. 79.

Chavan, S. A. (1993). Vegetational and wildlife studies in Gir. Ph.D. Thesis, The Maharaja Sayajirao University of Baroda, Vadodara.

Chavan, A.R. and Oza, G. (1967). Contribution to the flora of Danga forest, Indian forester, 92:533-535.

Chowdhery, H. J. and Murti, S. K. (2000). Plant Diversity and Conservation in India- An Overview. Bishen Singh Mahendra Pal Singh, Dehra Dun.

Chunekar, K. C. (1969). Vanaspatika Anusandhan Darshika, Vidhya Bhavan, Varanashi.

Daniel, M. (2006). Medicinal Plants- Chemistry and Properties. Oxford and IBH Publishing Co. Pvt. Ltd., New Delhi, pp. 250.

Daniel, M (2008). Herbal technology: Concept and approaches. Satish Serial Publishers, New Delhi, pp. 580.

Daniel, M. and Nagar, P. S. (2010). A soujoun o he herbal treasures of MSU., M. S. University, Arihant offset Printers, Karelibaugh, Vadodara.

Dave, M., Patel, R. S., Patel, K. C. (2010). Taxoethnobotanical significance of some plants from Ambaji forest (North Gujarat). *International Journal of Bioscience Reporter*, 8(1): 67-70.

Dave, R. P. and Patel, R. S. (2012). Observations on some energy plants among the rural people in Jambudia of Saurashtra region, Gujarat, India. *Life Science Leaflets.* [ISSN:2277-4297], 5, 17-24.

Desai, M. J. (1976). A contribution to the flora of Bansda forests.

Desai, R. (2013). Floristic diversity and ecological studies in forest areas of Idar and Vadali Talukas, District Sabarkantha. PhD Thesis. Hemchandracharya North Gujarat University, Patan.

Desai, R. K. and Ant, H. M. (2012). Study of plant diversity in Vadali range forest District Sabarkantha, North Gujarat, India. *Life science leaflets*. [ISSN:2277-4297], 1, 32-43.

Dhaduk, H. L., Dhruj, I. U., Mandavia, C. K. and Chovatia, V. P. (2010). Plant Biodiversity: Collection, characterization and conservation. In souvenir of National Conference on Biodiversity Conservation, M. S. University, Vadodara, pp.110.

Dhaduk, H. L., Chovatia, V. P. and Mandavia, C. K. (2011). Aushdhiya vanaspatini Kheti (Gujarati) [Farming of medicinal plants]. Metro Offset Press, Junagadh,

Gandhi D, Susy A, Pandya N, Panchal K (2010). Vegetational diversity in the land of Bhey (Garbada). *International Journal of Bioscience Reporter*. 8(1):45-50.

Gandhi, D. J., Albert, S., Pandya, N. R., Panchal, K. R. (2011). Socioeconomic Study of Grasses and Legumes in Baria and Godhra Forest Division, Gujarat. *Notulae Scientia Biologicae*, 3, 53-61.

Gohil Deepa (2012). In depth studies on some of the floristic components of Baroda and Panchmahal Districts with reference to Bioprospecting and speciation. PhD Thesis. M. S. University, Baroda.

Gohil, K. S. (2005). Phenological studies of Reserve Forest (Victoria Park) near Bhavangar, PhD Thesis. Bhavangar University, Bhavangar.

Gohil, K. S. (2011). Biodiversity management and conservation by nature education at Hingolgadh Sanctuary. *Bioscience guardian*, 1, 329-337.

Gohil, T. G. (2005). A contribution to the floristics of Chikhi and Gandevi Talukas with emphasis on the cultivars and ethnobotany of the area.

Gondaliya, H., Patel, R. S., Patel, K. C. (2010). A review on some medicinal plants of Gujarat College campus, Ahmedabad, Gujarat. *International Journal of Bioscience Reporter*, 8(1): 71-73.

Hooker, J. D (1904). *A sketch of the Flora of British India*. London.

Jain, S.K. (1968). The Vegetation of Dangs District in Gujarat. *Ibid*. 5; (3 and 4); 351-361.

Jain, S. K. and Shastry, A. R. K. (1980). Threatened plants of India. A state of art report. Botanical survey of India. Hawra,

Joshi, P. N., Joshi, P. B. and Jain, B. K. (2012). Ecology and conservation of threatened plants in Tapkeshwari Hill ranges in the Kachchh Island, Gujarat, India. *Journal of threatened taxa*, 4, 2390–2397.

Jangid, M. S. (2012). Biological spectrum of Taluka Modasa, District Sabarkantha (Gujarat), India. *Life science leaflets*. [ISSN:2277-4297], 12, 77-98.

Jangid, M. S., Dholu B., Panchal J., Panchal K., Patel V., Patel P. (2016). Ethnomedicinal Study Of Some Selected Plants Of Euphorbiaceae Family Of Modasa Taluka,District Arvalli, Gujarat, India. *In Proceeding book of abstract, XXX Gujarat Science Congress*, KSKV Kachchh University, pp. 76.

Jadeja, B. A. (1999). Plants used by the tribe Rabri in Barda Hills of Gujarat. *Ethnobotany* 11: 42-46.

Jadeja, B. A., Bhatt, K. J. and Patel, A. (2008). Households and house of tribals of Gujarat – an ethnobotanical study. *Plant archieves*, 8, 1027-1028.

Jadeja, B. A. and Modhvadia, A. R. (2008). Study of some medicinal plants of vijapur taluka of mahesana district of gujarat, india. *Plant archieves*, 8, 719-721.

Jadeja, B. A., Kanjaria, K. V. and Odedara, N. K. (2011). Floristic analysis of flora of Bhanvad, Jamjodhpur and Lalipur Talukas of Jamnagar district, Gujarat. *Bio Nano frontiers*. 4, 294-296.

Jadeja, B.A., Odedara, N.K., Chavda, D.K., Bhatt, D.C. (2008) Plant used in traditional phytotherapy for indigestion in Gujarat, india, *Journal of Economic and taxonomic botany*, 32:186-193.

Jadeja, B. A., Odedara, N. K. and Singh, R. S. (2008). Phenological observations on some dry deciduous forest trees at Barda hills, Gujarat. *Journal of economic and taxonomic botany*, 32, 51-56.

Jadeja, B. A. and Nakar, R. N. (2010). Study on ethno-medico botany of weeds from saurashtra region, Gujarat, India. *Plant Archieves*,. 10, 761-765.

Jadeja, B. A. and Nakar, R. N. (2010). Phenological studies of some tree species from Girnar Reserve Forest, Gujarat, India. *Plant Archieves*, 10, 825-828.

Jadeja, B. A. and Nakar, R. N. (2017). Distribution, morphology and floristic characters of selected Asclepiadaceae members from Saurashtra region, West-South India. In Proceedings International Conference on Agriculture and allied sciences (GRISSAS-2017), Udaipur, Maharana Pratap Agricultural University, Rajasthan, India, December 2 to 4, pp. 350

Jayanthi G., Thivakaran, G. A., Chavda, H. H., Karthikeyan, K. (2016). Studies on prevalence of Coastal Halophytes from semi-arid region, Kachchh, Gujarat. *In Proceeding book of abstract, XXX Gujarat Science Congress*, KSKV Kachchh University, pp. 81

Joshi, M. C. (1983). A floristic and phytochemical survey of some important South Gujarat forests with special reference to plants of medicinal and ethnobotanical interest, Baroda.

Joshi, P.N., Joshi, E.B. and Jain, B.K. (2012). Ecology and conservation of threatened plants in Tapkeshwari Hill ranges in the Kachchh Island, Gujarat, India, *Journal of threatened taxa*, 4(2):2390-2397.

Kariya, J. P. (2012). Floral and avifaunal diversity of the thol lake, wild life sanctuary of Gujarat State, India. Biodiversity enrichment in the diverse world. Intech Publications, pp.1-34.

Kharadi, H. S., Patel, N., Damor, R., Sutariya, A., Katara S., Prajapati A. (2016). Biological Spectrum Of Vagpur Range Forest District Aravalli Gujarat, India. *In Proceeding book of abstract, XXX Gujarat Science Congress*, KSKV Kachchh University, pp. 77

Khoshoo, T. N. (1994). India's Biodivesity. Tasks ahead. *Current Science*, 67, 577-584.

Khoshoo, T. N. (1995). Census of Indian Biodiversity. Tasks a head. *Current Science*, 69, 14-17.

Mac R. N. (1986). A contribution to the flora of Surat district, Surat.

Mehta (1997). Taxonomical Study of Angiosperms of Palitana.

Mandavia, C. K., Dhaduk, H. L., Padaliya, P. and Nakar, R. N. (2010). *Issues Relating to Medicinal Plant Cultivation, Processing and Marketing.* Workshop souvenir. Department of Agricultural Botany, Junagadh Agricultural University, Junagadh.

Mankad, R. S. (2007). *Floristic and ethnobotanical studies of Ambaji and Gorakhnath mountains of Girnar.* Phd Thesis. Bhavanagar University, Bhavangar.

Malhotra, S. K. and Wadhava, B. M. (1978). Studies on Botany of Jamnagar District. *M.V.M. Patrika*, 8, 3-23.

Menon, A. R. R. (1979). Floristics and phytosociological studies of some parts of Saurashtra. Ph.D. Thesis. Sardar Patel University, VallabhVidyanagar.

Mitra, S. and Mukherjee, S. K. (2006). Diversity, reassessment and phytogeographical significance of angiospermic genera restricted in India and its adjoining areas. In: *Plant Taxonomy: Advances and Relevance* (ed. A.K. Pandey *et al.*), CBS Publishers and Distributors, New Delhi, pp. 145-162.

Modi, N. R. and Dudani, S. N. (2013). Biodiversity conservation through urban green spaces: a case study of Gujarat university campus in Ahmedabad. *International Journal of Conservation Science*, 4, 189-196.

Nayar, M. P. and Shastry, A.R.K. (1990). Red Data Book of Indian Plants. Vol I-III. Botanical Survey of India.

Nirmal Kumar, J. I., Soni, H., Kumar, R. N. (2005). Asthetic values of selected floral elements of Khatana and Waghai forests of Dangs, Western Ghat. *Indian Journal of Traditional knowledge*, 4, 275-283.

Nirmal Kumar, J.I., Kumar, R.N., Patil, N., Soni, H. (2007). Studies on plant species used by tribal communities of Saputara and Purna Forest, Dangs District, Gujarat, *Indian Journal of traditional knowledge*, 6(2): 368-374.

Nagar, P.S. (2000). Biodiversity of Barda hills, PhD Thesis, Saurashtra University, Rajkot.

Nagar, P. S. (2004). Status of some regionally threatened species of Saurashtra, Gujarat, India. *Journal of Current Biosciences*, 1, 238-247.

Nagar, P. S. (2005). Floristic Diversity of Barda Hills and its surroundings. Scientific Publishers, Jodhpur, pp. 325.

Nagar, P. S. and Daniel, M. (2010). Floristic diversity of Gujarat. In National conference on Biodiversity conservation. M. S. University, Vadodara, pp. 63-77.

Nagar, P. S. and Pandya, S. M. (2002). *Stylosanthes hamatus* (Linn.) Taub. (Papilionaceae), A New record to the flora of Gujarat. (With one text figure). *Journal of Bombay Natural History Society*, 99, 363-364.

Nagar, P. S. and Pandya. S. M. (2002). Addition to the flora of Saurashtra, Gujarat, India. *Journal of Economic and Taxonomic Botany*, 26, 75-77.

Nagar, P. S. and Pandya. S. M. (2002). *Cleome scaposa* D. C. Capparidaceae. A rare species of Saurashtra, Gujarat. *Journal of Bombay Natural History Society*, 99, 543-544.

Nagar, P. S. and Pandya. S. M. (2003). Floristic diversity of Barda Hills and their surroundings, Saurashtra, Gujarat. *Journal of Economic and Taxonomic Botany*, 27, 1166-1180.

Nagar, P. S., Sata, S. J. and Pathak, S. J. (2003). Rediscovery of *Tephrosia jamnagarensis* (Fabaceae), an endangered and narrow endemic plant species of Saurashtra Side. *Journal of Economic and Taxonomic Botany*, 20, 1701-1705.

Nair Rajeshwary (2011).Floristic study of dadra and nagar haveli, *Life sciences Leaflets*, 20:872-875.

Nakar, R. N. (2013). Studies on Phenological patterns of Girnar Reserve Forest, near Junagadh, Gujarat. PhD. Thesis. Saurashtra University, Rajkot.

Nakar, R. N., Jadeja, B. A. (2009). Study on morphology, ethnobotany and phenology of *Prosopis* in Girnar Forest Junagadh, Gujarat. *Proceedings of the National Symposium on Prosopis: ecological, economic significance and management challenges*. Gujarat Institute of Desert Ecology, Bhuj, pp. 51-53.

Nakar, R. N., Jadeja, B. A. (2010). Phenological studies of two tree species of Bombaceae from Girnar Reserve Forest, Gujarat. In Proceedings of National Conference on biodiversity conservation, M. S. University, Vadodara, pp. 133.

Nakar, R. N., Jadeja, B. A. (2013a). Studies on phenology of some shrubs from Girnar Reserve Forest, Gujarat. In National conference of medicinal and aromatic plants for rural development and prosperity, Ananad agricultural University, Ananad, pp.18.

Nakar, R. N., Jadeja, B. A. (2013b). Comparision of phenology of *Cassia siamea* Lam. From Girnar Reserve Forest and GIDC polluted area from Junagadh, Gujarat. In UGC sponsored State level seminar on conservation of biodiversity and environment-A challenge, KKSJ Maninagar Sci. College, Ahmadabad, pp. 41.

Nakar, R. N., Joshi, N. H., Jadeja, B. A. (2011). Study on density and Biomass of sea weeds at Port Okha, Gujarat-A case study. *Journal of Plant development Sciences*, 3, 217-224.

Nakar, R. N., Jadeja, B. A. (2014a). Phenological attributes of seven tree species in association with climate from Girnar Reserve Forest, Gujarat. In Proceedings of National Seminar SUSUP-2014, at Department of Botany, Gujarat University, Ahmadabad, 29-30 Sept, pp.40.

Nakar, R. N., Jadeja, B. A. (2014b). Phenological studies of two bombacacean members from Girnar Reserve Forest, Junagadh, Gujarat, India. *The Indian Forester*, 140 (1): 59-64.

Nakar, R. N., Jadeja, B. A. (2014c). Seed pattern, germination and viability of some tree species seeds from Girnar Reserve Forest of Gujarat. *Indian Journal of Plant Physiology*, 19(1): 57-64.

Nakar, R. N, Jadeja, B. A. (2014d). Standardization of wild forest seeds for morphology and viability studies. *Plant archives*, 14(1): 111-114.

Nakar, R. N., Jadeja, B. A. (2014e). Phenology of some herbs, shrubs and undershrubs from Girnar Reserve Forest, Gujarat, *Current Science*, 101: 111-118.

Nakar, R. N., B. A. Jadeja, V. P. Chovatia, C. K. Mandavia (2015 a). Qualitative and quantitative seed characteristics diversity from Girnar Reserve Forest, Gujarat, India. *Proceedings of National Academy of Science, Section-B.* pp. 1-13, [ISSN: 0369-8211]

Nakar, R. N., Jadeja, B. A. (2015b). Studies on phenological behavior of two *Cassia* species from Girnar Reserve Forest, Gujarat, India. *Proceedings of International Conference on Agriculture and Forestry*, 1:43-48, DOI:10.17507/icoaf2015-1106. [ISSN: 2362-1036 online]

Nakar, R. N., Jadeja, B. A., Singh, A. L. (2015c). Phenology and productivity of forest flora of Gujarat. In Recent Advances in Crop Physiology (Ed. Amrit Lal Singh), Daya Publishers (India), New Delhi, India. Vol. 2, pp: 261-294.

Nakar, R. N., Jadeja, B. A. (2016a). Germination and viability studies in two undershrubs *Cassia* species from Girnar Reserve Forest, Gujarat. In *Proceedings of XXX-Gujarat Science Congress*, February-2016, KSKV Kuchch University, Bhuj, Gujarat, pp. 137.

Nakar, R. N., Dhaduk, H. L., Chovatiya, V. P. (2016b). Medicinal Plants: Cultivation and Uses, Astral International Publication, New Delhi, pp: 1-555 [ISBN: 9789351247654 Hardbound, ISBN: 9789351309918 International Edition]

Nakar R.N. and Jadeja, B.A. (2016c). Seedling morphology of selected species from Girnar Reserve Forest, Gujarat, India. *Perception*, 2(2):31-45 [ISSN:2395-0129]

Nakar R.N. and Jadeja, B.A. (2017) Assessment of phonological diversity in GIDC polluted area of Junagadh, Gujarat, India. In Proceedings of International Conference on Agriculture and allied sciences (GRISSAS-2017), Udaipur, Maharana Pratap Agricultural University, Rajasthan, India, December 2 to 4, pp. 139.

Nayar, M. P. (1980). Endemism and patterns of distribution of endemic genera (angiosperms) in India. *Journal of Economic and Taxonomic Botany*, 1, 99-110.

Nayar, M. P. (1996). Hotspots of Endemic Plants of India, Nepal and Bhutan. TBGRI, Thiruvananthpuram,

Nayar, M. P. and Sastry, A.R.K. (1987-1990). Red Data Book of Indian Plants (3 vols). Botanical Survey India, Kolkata,

Nair, R. (2011). Floristic studies of Dadra and Nagar Haveli. *Life science leaflets*, 20:898-903 [ISSN: 0976-1098]

Nirmal Kumar, Rita Kumar, Patil, N., Soni, H. (2007). Studies on plant species used by tribal communities of Saputara and Purna Forest, Dangs District, Gujarat. *International Journal of Traditional knowledge*, 6(2): 368-374.

Oza, A. R. (1991). Taxonomical and ecological studies of the flora of and around Bhavnagar. Ph.D. Thesis. Saurashtra University, Rajkot.

Odedara, N. K. (2009). *Ethnobotany of Maher Tribe In Porbandar District, Gujarat, India*, PhD Thesis, Saurashtra University, Rajkot

Panchal, S. M. (2016). A Preliminary Survey Of Lichens In Forest Area Of Taranga, District Mehsana, Gujarat. *In Proceeding book of abstract, XXX Gujarat Science Congress*, KSKV Kachchh University, pp. 44.

Pandya, S. M. (1976). Flora and vegetation of Saurashtra. Souvenir: 45th session. *National Academy of Science, India*. Saurashtra University, Rajkot, pp. 22-24.

Pandya, S. M. (1989). Forest wealth of Kutch, its utility and potencials. In: All India symposiums. *Biology and Utility of Wild Plants*, Surat, pp. 175-189.

Pandey, A. K. (1995). Conservation of biodiversity: present status and future strategy. In: *Taxonomy and Biodiversity* (ed. A.K. Pandey), CBS Publishers and Distributors, Delhi, pp. 44-51.

Pareek, S. K. (2013). Harnesing oppurtunities in medicinal and Aromatic plants for lively hood security in India. In Natioanal Conference on Integration of Medicinal and Aromatic Plants for Rural development and Prosperity, Anand, pp: 1-4.

Patale, V. and Parikh, P. (2010). Floristic diversity of the stream and riparian zone of the Vishwamitri river Vadodara. *Bioscience guardian*, 1, 201-207.

Patel, A. M. and Patel, K. C. (2012). Floristic studies on scared groves situated near Utkantheswar in Kheda District, Gujarat State. *In National Conference on Plant Science: Changing pathways, Changing lives*, Talod, pp. 41.

Patel, B. B., Mali, M. (2016). Traditional knowledge of some Ethenomedicinal plants in Hariyawada village of Banaskantha district, North Gujarat. *In Proceeding book of abstract, XXX Gujarat Science Congress*, KSKV Kachchh University, pp. 144

Patel, B.K., Patel, B.P. and Vora, U.A. (1981). Biological spectrum of the Flora of Shetrunjaya Hills, Palitana. *Geobios*, 8: 234-235.

Patel, H. K., Patel, K. C., Patel, R. S. (2010). Plants used in preparation of musical instruments and agricultural impliments of Ambaji forest in Banashkantha District (North Gujarat). *International Journal of Bioscience Reporter*, 8(1): 81-63.

Patel, K. C. and Patel, R. S. (2010). Observation on trees species of Danta Range Forest of North Gujarat. *Electronic Journal of life Science leaf lets*, 5, 148-157[ISSN:0976-1098].

Patel, K. C., Patel, R. S., Shah, R. B., and Jangid, M. S. (2010). Ethnobotany of *Lannea coromandalica* (Houtt). Merrill. From Aravalli Forest areas of North Gujarat. *Plant Archieves*, 10, 729-731.

Patel, M. K., Patel, P. K. (2012). Floristic and ethnobotanical study of Palanpur and Dantiwada, Gujarat. Lap-Lambert Academic Publishing, pp:1-292 [ISBN: 978-3-659-12553-9]

Patel, R. I. (1968). Forest flora of Gujarat State. Forest Department, Gujarat State, pp. 381.

Patel, R.M. and Gosavi, K.V.C. (2016). Cistaceae, a new family record for India. *Rheedea*, 26(1): 21-25 [ISSN:0971-2313]

Patel, R., Roy Mahato, A. K., Vijay Kumar V. and Asari, R. V. (2013). Status of the medicinal plants in Tharawada-Gandher Reserve Forest of Kachchh, Gujarat and the ethnomedicinal practices of local community. *Journal of Medicinal Plants studies*. [ISSN: 2320-3862], 1, 1-10.

Patel, R., Roy, A. K., Patel, Y. S. (2014). Study on the floristic diversity of two newly recorded sacred groves from Kachchh District of Gujarat, India. *Indian Journal of Plant Science*, 1(1): 34-36

Patel, R. M. (1971). Flora of Valsad, Ph.D. Thesis, Sardar Patel University, VallabhVidyanagar, Gujarat.

Patel, R. S., Patel, K. C., Patel, N. B. and Shah, R. B. (2010). Uncommon tree resources to the ethnobotany from Ambaji Forest of Banashkantha District [North Gujarat], India. *Plant Archieves*, 10, 293-297.

Pilo, B. and Pathak, J. (1996). Biological diversity of Gujarat- Current knowledge. Gujarat Ecology Commission, Baroda, pp.329.

Punjani, B. L. (2002). Ethnobotanical aspects of some plants of Arravalli Hills in North Gujarat. *Ancient Life Sciencce*, 21, 268-280.

Punjani, B. L. (2010). Herbal folk medicines used for urinary complaints in tribal pockets of Northeast Gujarat. *Indian Journal of Traditional knowledge*, 9, 126-130.

Punjani, B. L., Vyas, V. C., Chaniyara, H. B., Pandya, A. V. (2010). Studies on some ethnomedicinal plants from Khanpur Forest Range in Panchmahal District, Gujarat. *International Journal of Bioscience Reporter*, 8(1): 85-89.

Punjani, B. L., Raval, J. (2016). Observation On Lichen Mycota In Coastal Area Of Alang, District Bhavnagar, Gujarat. *In Proceeding book of abstract, XXX Gujarat Science Congress*, KSKV Kachchh University, pp. 34.

Raval, N., Dhaduk, H. L. (2013). Ethnobotanical survey of some medicinal plants in Jatashankar region of Girnar Forest, Gujarat, India. *Global Journal of Research on Medicinal plants and indigenous medicines*. 2(12):830-841.

Raval, J. and Punjani, B.L. (2016). A Preliminary Survey Of Lichens in Forest Area Of Taranga, District Mehsana, Gujarat, *In Proceeding book of abstract, XXX Gujarat Science Congress*, KSKV Kachchh University, pp.44

Rajendra Kumar, (2010). Floristic status and its conservation in the Forests of North Gujarat Region, Gujarat India. *PhD Thesis*. Bharathidasan University, Tiruchirappalli-620 024.

Rajendra Kumar, S., Joshi, P. N., Joshua, J., Sunderraj, S.F.W., Kalawathy, S., Raghunathan, P. (2011). Importance and conservation values of disturbed lands of North Gujarat region (NGR), Gujarat, India. *Plant Sciences Feed* 1(8):121-141

Rao, V. H., Gohil, T. G., Thakor, A. B. (2013). Floristic study of Kaprada's hilly forest in South Gujarat, *International Journal of Plant Science*, 8(1):100-102.

Rau, M. A. (1975). High altitude flowering plants of Western Himalayas. Botanical Survey India, Kolkata

Reddy, A. S. (1987). Flora of Dharampur Forest, Ph. D. Thesis, S. P. University.

Sabnis, S. D. (1967). The flora of Baroda and Environs. Ph.D. Thesis. M. S. University of Vadodara

Sabnis, S. D. and Rao, K.S.S. (1983). Observation on some rare or endangered endemics of Southern Kutch. An assessment of threatened plants of India. Botanical Survey of India, Culcutta. pp. 71-77.

Salahuddin, K., Gor, S., Visavadiya, M., Soni, V., Tatamia, N. (2013). Ethnobotanical survey of some parasitic plants growing in Girnar Forest of Junagadh District of Gujarat, India. *International Research Journal of Biological Sciences*, 2(4): 59-62 [ISSN 2278-3202]

Santapau, H. (1950). Inter Kathiwrense: Being notes on a botanical tour in Nawagar State, Oct Nov 1945. *Gujarat Research Society*. 11-12, 226-237.

Santapau, H. (1952a). A note on the Jay Krishna Indraji Thaker collections of plants preserved in the Herbarium, Agricultural College, Poona. *Agri. Coll. Mag.* Poona, 42, 210-233.

Santapau, H. (1952b). Report of the work done under the auspices of the Saurashtra Research Society, for the botanical exploration of Saurashtra. *Annaul Report of Saurashtra Research Society*, pp. 9-20.

Santapau, H. (1952c). Report of the second field season in the botanical exploration of Saurashtra. Rajkot, pp. 16.

Santapau, H. (1952d). Report of the third field season in the botanical exploration of Saurashtra. Rajkot, pp. 16.

Santapau, H. (1952e). Plants of Saurashtra. A preliminary list. Rajkot, pp. 16.

Santapau, H and Raizada, M. B. (1954). Contribution to the flora of Gir Forest in Saurashtra. *Indian Forester*, 80, 379-389.

Santapau, H. (1956). La esploracien botanica de Saurashtra, India. *Anal. Inst. Bot. Cavanilles*, Madrid, 13, 423-454.

Santapau, H and Raizada, M. B. (1957a). Contribution to the flora of Gir Forest in Saurashtra, India. *For. Rec. n.s. Bot.*, 4, 105-170.

Santapau, H. (1958). The floristic study in India. *Mem. Indian Bot. Soc.*, 1, 117- 121.

Santapau, H. (1971). Common trees. National book trust of India, New Delhi.

Saxton, W. T. and Sedgwick, L. J. (1918). Plants of Northern Gujarat, 6, 209-323.

Shah, G. L (1978). Flora of Gujarat. Part I and II. Saradar Patel Univeristy, Vallabh Vidhyanagar. pp.1074.

Shah, G. L. (1983). Rare species with restricted distribution in South Gujarat. In: S.K. Jain and R.R. Rao(eds.) *An assessment of threatened plants of India*. Botanical survey of India. Cucultta. pp. 50-54.

Shah, G. L. and Gopal, G. V. (1982). An ethnobotanical profile of the Dangies *Journal of Economic and Taxonomic Botany*, 3, 355-364.

Shah, J. P. and Thivakaran, G. A. (2012). Taxonomic status and utilization of Halophytes in coastal Katch District, Gujarat. In National Conference on Plant Science: Changing pathways, Changing lives, Talod, pp. 20.

Shah, T. P., Ant, H. A. (2016). Status, Distribution And Phytosociologicalstudies of tree Halophytes In Kachchh District (Gujarat), India. *In Proceeding book of abstract, XXX Gujarat Science Congress*, KSKV Kachchh University, pp. 142

Shah G.L. and Subranarayana, B. (1967). Addition to the flora of Dangs forest. *Ibid.*, 64; 136- 138.

Shah G.L. and Subranarayana, B. (1967). Further contribution to the flora of Dangs forest in Gujarat. *Bull. Bot. Surv.* India. 11;209-300.

Shah G.L. and Subranarayana, B. (1967). New plants records for Bombay collected from Dangs forest, Gujarat. *J. Bombay. Nat. Hist. Soc.* 66; 412-414.

Sharma, J. R., Mudgal, V., and Hajra, P. K. (1997). Floristic diversity- Review, Scope and Perspective. Pp. 1-45. In: V. Mudgal and P.K. Hajra (eds.) Floristic Diversity and conservation Strategies in India. Vol. I. Botanical Survey India, Kolkata.

Simpson, M. G. (2006). Plant Systematics. Elsevier, Amsterdam.

Singh, H. S. and Nagar, P. S. (2005). Biodiversity of Barda Wildlife Sanctuary, GEER Foundation, Gandhinagar,

Sinha, S. K., Pinto, A. G., Patel, R. I. (1972). Working plant for Junagadh forest division. Printed at the Government Press, Baroda, pp. 167.

Solanki, H. A., Dabgar, Y. B., Mali, M. S., Khokhariya, B. P. (2010). Plant diversity and its life forms of Visnagar Taluka, North Gujarat. *International Journal of Bioscience Reporter*. 8(1):43-48.

Solanki, H. A., Bhatt, K. J., Naghera, B. D., Goswami, N. D., Sirdhvad, K. N. (2010). Traditional aboriginal knowledge of the flora in the Girnar Holy hills areas, Gujarat. *International Journal of Bioscience Reporter*, 8(1):91-96.

Sorathiya, K. D. (2010). Survey of ethnomedicinal plants of Anjar Taluka used in Anemia. *International Journal of Bioscience Reporter*, 8(1): 97-99.

Sudhi, K. H. (2012). Current status of endangered plants. The Hindu, Kotchi, June 21.

Subranarayana B. (1968) A Contribution to the flora of Dangs forest, Gujarat. Ph.D. Thesis.

Tadvi, D. (2009). Study on medicinal Plant diversity in Arboretum. Msc thesis, MS University, Baroda.

Thaker, (1910). Vanaspati sastraane Barda dungarni jadibuti teni parikhsa ane upyog. (A compete and comprehensive account of the flora of Barda Mountain (Kathiyavad). Gujrati printing Press) Bombay, pp. 717.

Thaker (1926). Katchni sawathani Vanaspatiyo ane tani upyogita. (Plants of Kutch and their utility- An elaborate treatise containing ten chapters and litho figure). Gujarati printing press and Nirnaya- Sagar Press. Bombay, pp.200.

Thakrar, N.K. (1987). Biological Flora of Rajkot. Ph.D. thesis. Saurashtra University, Rajkot.

Tintisara, M. P. and Prajapati, M. M. (2012). Observations on folk medicinal plants used by the inhabit tribals in Bhiloda Forest range of Sabarkantha, North Gujarat, Life science leaflets, 59, Doi: 10.1234/lsl.v59iO.215

Tobyo H., and Petric H. (1982). Grasses of Western India. Bombay Natural History Society.

Tyagi,S. N. Padhiar, A, Albert, S., Pandya, N., Gandhi, D., Panchal, K. (2010). Pictorial Floristic diversity of grasses and associated vegetation from three grasslands of Randhikpur Forest Range, Dahod, Gujarat. *Indian Forester*, 136, 1581-1592.

Vediya, S. D., Kharadi, H. S. (2011). Floristic diversity of Isari zone, Megharj range forest District Sabarkantha, Gujarat, India. *International Journal of Pharmacy and Life Science.* [ISSN: 0976-7126], 2, 1033-1034.

Vediya, S., Patel P., Chaudhary N., Chaudhary, R., Patel T. (2016). Study Of Different Plant Species Uses On Dental Diseases In Aravali Sabarkantha District Of Gujarat, India. *In Proceeding book of abstract, XXX Gujarat Science Congress*, KSKV Kachchh University, pp. 75

Venu, P. (1999). A review of floristic diversity inventory and monitoring methodology in India. *Proceedings of Indian National Science Academy*, 64, 281-292.

Yadav, M. K., Patel, N. L., Hazarika, A., Choudhary, M. (2010). Medicinal uses of some plant species found around Navasari District of Gujarat state. *International Journal of Bioscience Reporter*, 8(1): 101-103

Yogi, D. V. (1970). A contribution to the flora of North Gujarat. Ph.D. Thesis, S. P. University, Vallabh Vidyanagar.

Chapter 11

Legal Regime of Seed Regulations in India

Sanjeev Kumar Choudhary

Gujarat National Law University, Gandhinagar-382426, Gujarat, India
e-mail: schoudhary@gmail.com

ABSTRACT

Agriculture is the backbone of the economy of India. The major population of this country largely dependent on the agricultural sector for maintaining their livelihood. It also provides an opportunity for the highly marginalized population to sustain their life. Apart from the economic perspective, the betterment of agriculture is equally important to sustain the life of the huge population of the County. Food is one of the essential element of survival. Hunger problem in India is a matter of serious concern. We are very poorly placed on the global hunger index. It is, not only the quantity but also quality of agricultural produce, been the issue of debate in recent time. The farmer's suicide in our country is becoming a new normal. They are complaining that they are unable to recover the cost incurred in cultivation; profit is altogether a distant question. The solution to all these questions lie in, if not completely then at least partially, to high production. To have the greater yield; producing, procuring and regulating the distribution of tested and certified variety of seed is highly important. This paper tries to present the laws at one place which govern the seed production, quality control, distribution, marketing, import and export etc. in India. In fact, the short summary of the overall perspective of seed policy of India.

Introduction

The constantly growing hunger problem in India is a matter of serious concern. As per recent Global Hunger Index (GHI), 2017, India has further came down to 100th position out of 119 countries[1]. Despite having good production of verities

---

1 http://www.business-standard.com/article/current-affairs/global-hunger-index-india-slips-3-positions-to-100th-among-119-nations-117101200345_1.html.

of food, India continuously failing to resolve the issue of hunger problems. The State of Food Security and Nutrition in the World 2017 report, 14.5 per cent of the population of India is undernourished[2].

India has passed the National Food Security Act, 2013 with the objectives of providing food and nutritional security in human life cycle approach by ensuring access to adequate quantity of quality food at affordable price to people, especially the poor people.

In India, agriculture is main source of livelihood for majority of its population even today. Hence, performance of agriculture to ensure food security and to provide strong economic base is of utmost importance. Improved seeds have been widely recognized as a key ingredient for enhancing farm productivity and overall crop production and thereby attaining the goal of food security[3]. An efficient system for supply of these improved and quality seeds to farmers on timely manner is equally important for sustainable agricultural production and productivity.

In this context, the operational National Seed Policy and the various legal norms regulating the production and distribution of the quality seeds to the farming communities becomes very important for realization of UN Sustainable Development Goal of Zero Hunger by 2030.

This chapter is dedicated to the discussion pertaining to the National Seed Policy, applicable laws, rules and orders regulating seed production, storage and distribution in India. The various Acts, Bill, Policies, rules and orders will be summarily discussed in this chapter.

National Seed Policies

On recommendation of National Commission on Agriculture in the year 1971, private sector was given entry into the Indian Seed market[4]. Subsequently, National Seed Policy, 1988 was formulated to help privatize the Indian seed industry.

New Policy on Seed Development, 1988

The New Policy was formulated with an aim of encouraging seed production on commercial lines and to provide the farmer the best planting materials available in the world so as to increase productivity and thereby to increase farm income and export earnings. The Policy covers the import of selected seeds.

After a careful consideration of all the related aspects, such as; variety of agro-climate zones of the country, plant quarantine procedure to prevent entry of exotic

---

2 http://www.livemint.com/Politics/8BBA9K4GHvpSvXR0ps602O/India-home-to-234-of-worlds-hungry-51-women-are-anemic.html.

3 Promoting the Growth and Development of Smallholder Seed Enterprises for Food Security Crops, FAO, 2010 http://www.fao.org/docrep/013/i1839e/i1839e00.pdf.

4 V. Santhy P.R. Vijaya Kumari Anshu Vishwanathan R.K. Deshmukh, Legislations for Seed Quality Regulation in India, CICR Technical Bulletin No: 38, 2009.

pests, diseases and weeds detrimental to Indian agriculture *etc.*, this new policy evolved with special emphasis on:

1. The import of high quality seeds;
2. A time bound-programme to strengthen and to modernize plant quarantine facilities;
3. Effective observance of procedures for quarantine/post entry quarantine (PEQ); and
4. Incentives to encourage the domestic seed industry

The New Policy for the Import of Seeds covered categories, namely, seeds of Wheat and Paddy; seeds of coarse cereals, oilseeds and pulses; seeds of vegetables, flowers and ornamental plants; Tubers and bulbs of flowers; cuttings/saplings *etc.* of flowers; and seeds/planting materials of fruits.

Except for the National Seeds Corporation (NSC) and the State Seeds Corporation (SSC), the import of seeds of coarse cereals, pulses and oilseeds for sowing were allowed for a period not exceeding two years by companies which have technical or financial collaboration agreements for production of seeds with companies abroad, on the condition that the foreign supplier agreed to supply parent line seeds or nucleus or breeder seeds and technology to the Indian company within a period of two years from the date of import of the first commercial consignment. The authority for granting import license was given to the office of the Chief Controller of Import and Export (CCI and E) subject to the recommendations of the Departments of Agriculture and Cooperation (DAC) and to the provisions of the plants, Fruits, and Seeds (Regulation of import into India) Order, 1984.

The Indian Council of Agricultural Research (ICAR) was mandated to conduct trial and evaluation for one crop season and submit the report within three months of the season to DAC. After the receipt of the results of the ICAR trial/evaluation, an eligible importer may apply for the import of such seed to the DAC. DAC may, within 30 days of the receipt of the application, reject the application or recommend it to the CCI and E for grant of an import license to the importer. The CCI and E shall issue the import license within 15 days of the receipt of the recommendations from DAC.

All importers was mandated to make available a small but specified quantity of the imported seed to the ICAR at cost price, for testing and accession to the Gene Bank with the National Bureau of Plant Genetic Resources (NBPGR). The Plant Protection Adviser (PPA), within three weeks, after quarantine checks reject or clear the bulk import consignment of coarse cereals, oilseeds and pulses. The import of seeds of vegetables, flowers and ornamental plants, tubers and bulbs, cuttings, saplings, *etc.* of flowers will be allowed on Open General License (OGL).

The New Policy provided enough safeguards for strengthening of the quarantine facilities and plant quarantine procedures by authorizing the establishment of a National Plant Quarantine Advisory Committee (NPQAC) to advise the PPA on various technical matters in different disciplines of Entomology, Plant Pathology, Nematology, Virology, Bacteriology, Weed Sciences and for serological detection techniques of viruses. A proposed High Level Review Committee in the DAC was entrusted the task of monitoring the progress of the implementation of the Policy.

National Seed Policy 2002

No doubt, New Policy on Seed Development 1988 removed the obstructions in import of horticultural seeds and allowed import of limited quantity of seeds of course cereals, pulses and oilseeds, but flawed due to nonexistence of IPR laws and several restrictions on import and exports. Thus, the National Seed Policy 2002 was adopted to provide intellectual property protection to new varieties and to usher this sector into planned development protecting the interest of farmers and encouraging conservation of agro-biodiversity.

The policy identified the major thrust area namely - Varietal Development and Plant Varieties Protection; Seed Production; Quality Assurance; Seed Distribution and Marketing; Infrastructure facilities; Transgenic Plant Varieties; Import of seeds and planting material; Export of seeds; Promotion of Domestic Seed; and Strengthening of monitoring system.

Varietal Development and Plant Varieties Protection

Development of new and improved varieties of plants is vital for sustained agricultural productivity and hence, investment in research for developing new varieties of plant and to facilitate the growth of seed industry, the policy provides for the implementation of an effective *sue generis* system for intellectual protection. The policy conceptualize establishment of a Plant Varieties and Farmers' Rights Protection (PVP) Authority to undertake registration of new plant varieties on the basis of varietal characteristics based on the criteria of novelty, distinctiveness, uniformity and stability. Farmers' rights to save, use, exchange, share or sell farm produce of all varieties is protected, except for a sale under the brand name. A National Gene Fund will be established for implementation of the benefit sharing arrangement, and payment of compensation to communities for their contribution by sharing traditional knowledge and thus helping in the development and conservation of plant genetic resources. Suitable systems will be worked out to identify the contributions from traditional knowledge and heritage. Plant Genetic Resources will be permitted to be accessed by Research Organizations and Seed Companies from public collections as per the provisions of the 'Material Transfer Agreement' of the International Treaty on Plant Genetic Resources and the Biological Diversity Bill. The PVP Authority may resort to compulsory licensing of a protected variety in public interest.

Seed Production

Availability of superior quality of seeds in adequate quantity on timely manner is consequential to secure victuals security. Through Indian seed programme, which adheres to three generation system of seed multiplication – breeder, foundation and certified seed, public sector seed institution is inspirited and they perpetuates to have free access to breeder seed under the National Agriculture Research System. Private seed production agencies have also been given access to the breeder seed subject to terms and conditions as decided by the Government of India. ICAR and State Agriculture Universities (SAUs) have been assigned with the responsibility for production of breeder seed as per the requirements of the respective States. Further, it conceptualizes the establishment of seed banks for stocking specified quantities of seed of required crops, varieties for ensuring timely and adequate supply of seeds to farmers during adverse situations such as natural calamities, shortfalls in production, *etc.*

Quality Assurance

The National Seeds Board (NSB) is established as an apex body to perform the responsibility of executing and implementing the provisions of the Seeds Act and advising the Government on all matters relating to seed planning and development. It is also mandated to prescribe minimum standards (of germination, genetic characteristics, physical purity, seed health, *etc.*) as well as suitable guidelines for registration of seed and planting materials. It will accredit ICAR, SAUs, and public/private organizations to conduct VCU trials of all varieties for registration as per prescribed standards. It is also competent to take stringent measures to ensure the availability of high quality of seeds and check the sale of spurious or misbranded seeds.

Seed Distribution and Marketing

The availability of high quality seeds to farmers through an improved distribution system and efficient marketing set-up will be ensured to facilitate greater security of seed supply. For promoting efficient and timely distribution and marketing of seed throughout the country, a National Seed Grid will be established as a data-base for monitoring of information on requirement of seed, its production, distribution and preference of farmers on a district-wise basis. Distribution and marketing of seed of any variety, for the purpose of sowing and planting will be allowed only if the said variety has been registered by the National Seeds Board. National Seeds Board can direct a dealer to sell or distribute seeds in a specified manner in a specified area if it is considered necessary to the public interest.

Infrastructure Facilities

National Seed Research and Training Center will be set up to impart training and build a knowledge base in various disciplines of the seed sector. The Central Seed Testing Laboratory will be established at the National Seed Research and Training Center to perform referral and other functions as required under the Seeds Act. A computerized National Seeds Grid will be established to provide information on availability of different varieties of seeds with production agencies, their location, quality *etc.* State Governments, or the National Seeds Board in consultation with the concerned State Government, may establish Seed Certification Agencies.

Transgenic Plant Varieties

Biotechnology will play a vital role in the development of the agriculture sector. This technology can be used not only to develop new crops/varieties, which are tolerant to disease, pests and abiotic stresses, but also to improve productivity and nutritional quality of food. All genetically engineered crops/varieties will be tested for environment and bio-safety before their commercial release, as per the regulations and guidelines of the Environment Protection Act (EPA), 1986. Transgenic crops/varieties will be tested to determine their agronomic value for at least two seasons under the All India Coordinated Project Trials of ICAR before any variety is commercially released in the market. If the seed or planting material is a product of transgenic manipulation, it will be allowed to be imported only with the approval of the Genetic Engineering Approval Committee (GEAC), set up under the EPA, 1986.

Import of Seeds and Planting Material

All imports of seeds will require a permit granted by the PPA to the Government of India, which will be issued within the minimum possible time frame. All import of seeds and planting materials, *etc.* will be allowed freely subject to EXIM Policy guidelines and the requirements of the Plants, Fruits and Seeds (Regulation of import into India) Order, 1989 as amended from time to time.

Export of Seeds

Given the diversity of agro-climatic conditions, strong seed production infrastructure and market opportunities, India holds significant promise for export of seeds. Government will evolve a long term policy for export of seeds with a view to raise India's share of global seed export from the present level of less than 1 per cent to 10 per cent by the year 2020. Establishment and strengthening of Seeds Export Promotion Zones with special incentives from the Government will be facilitated. A data bank will be created to provide information on the International Market and on export potential of Indian varieties in different parts of the world.

Promotion of Domestic Seed Industry

Incentives will be provided to the domestic seed industry to enable it to produce seeds of high yielding varieties and hybrid seeds at a faster pace to meet the challenges of domestic requirements. Financial support for capital investment, working capital and infrastructure strengthening will be facilitated through NABARD. Tax rebate will be considered on the expenditure incurred on in-house research and development of new varieties. Unnecessary local taxation on sales of seeds will be encouraged to be removed to develop a competitive seed market.

Strengthening of Monitoring System

The Department of Agriculture and Cooperation (DAC) will supervise the overall implementation and monitoring of the National Seeds Policy. The technical capacity of DAC need to be augmented and strengthened to undertake the additional work relating to implementation of National Seeds Policy, implementation of PVP and FR Bill, Seeds Act, Import and Export of Seeds, *etc.*

Seed Acts, Rules and Order

Rationale of the Seed Act, 1966

This central legislation prima-facie empowers central government to regulate all essentials segment of seeds production, distribution and import as well for better, improved and sustainable quality of seeds for improving the agriculture as a whole and the economic condition of the farmers as well as the country. The important steps taken into consideration through this acts are:

1. Constitution of a Central Seed Committee (comprising eight members) to advise the Central and State Governments on matters arising out of the administration of this act and carry out other functions assigned to it by the Act.
2. Empowerment of the committee to fix the minimum limits of germination and purity of seed for a variety to be notified as well as for marking or labeling a seed lot to be sold commercially.
3. Establishing a Central Seed Laboratory as well as State Seed Laboratory to carry out seed analysis of notified variety and also constituting a certification agency for undertaking the process of certification.
4. Appointment of a seed analyst to undertake seed testing, and appointment of seed inspector to draw samples from any seller and verify the quality by sending samples to a seed analyst.
5. Restriction on import and export of seeds of notified varieties. Any variety imported or exported should meet the minimum limits of seed germination and purity marked or labeled on the container truly.
6. Penalty or punishment or both for those who do not comply with the provisions of the act. Forfeiture of property (seeds) belonging to any person convicted under this act due to contravention of the procedures under this act
7. Non-application of the act to the seed exchange by the farmers without any brand name
8. Power of Government to make rules to carry out various functions of Central Seed Committee, Central Seed Laboratory, Certification Agency and Seed Inspectors

Seed Rules, 1968

The major legislative measures involved under the Act are Seeds rules framed in 1968, the amendments made to the rules time to time and the Seeds (Control) order formulated in 1983 after including seeds as an essential commodity

The important development under seed rules are as follows:

1. Central Seed committee: The Committee entrusted with specific functions such as recommendation for Seed Testing fee, advice on the suitability of seed testing laboratory, recommendation for the procedure and standards for seed certification.

2. Central Seed Laboratory: The specific functions entrusted to the Laboratory are coordination with State Seed Laboratories for uniformity in test results and collection of data on quality of seeds available in the market.
3. Seed Certification Agency: The detailed procedure of seed certification starting from applying for certification till the grant of certificate has been provided under the rule. Outlining the procedure for submission of applications, growing, harvesting and processing and storage of seeds indented for certification, maintaining a list of recognized nucleus seed breeders, inspections of seed production fields, seed processing plant and seed stores, grant of certificates are the major task of the Agency.
4. Seed Analyst and Seed Inspectors: The specific duties of seed analyst and seed inspectors have been provided. Seed analyst shall analyze the seed samples according to the provisions of the Act.
5. Sealing, Dispatch and Analysis of Samples: The details of sampling, labeling, manner of packing and sealing the samples as well as its dispatch to the seed analyst has been provided.

Seeds (Control) Order, 1983

The Seeds (Control) Order came as a consequence of inclusion of seed as an essential commodity item under the Essential Commodity Act, 1955. The Essential Commodity Act, 1955 gives powers to State governments to regulate various aspects of trading in essential commodities under the supervision of Central Government.

It makes mandatory to have a license to carry on the business of seed and also gives right to detain the person adopting unethical practice in the business. The State Government is empowered with for appointing a licensing authority, inspectors and mode of action for supply regulation. The accountability of seed dealers such as essential display of seed stock, indicative price of different seeds, providing a cash or credit memorandum to the seed purchaser, cancellation of license in case of misrepresentation *etc.* are the important steps taken under the Order.

Protection of Plant Varieties and Farmers Right Act, 2001

With an aim to establish an effective protection of plant varieties, the rights of the breeders, to encourage the development of new varieties of plants and to give the effect to TRIPS agreement, the Protection of Plant Varieties and Farmers Rights Act, 2001 (PPV and FRA) was enacted.

Any variety that fulfills the Distinctive Uniform and Stable (DUS) criteria and that is "new" is eligible for this kind of protection under the Act. Plant varieties present in wilderness cannot be registered, under PPV and FR Authority. However, any traditionally cultivated plant variety which has undergone the process of domestication and improvement through human interventions can be registered and protected subjected to fulfillment of the eligible criteria of Novelty, Distinctive, Uniformity and Stability.

1. Novel: If at the date of filing an application for registration for protection, the variety has not been sold off in India earlier than one year or outside

India, in the case of trees or vines earlier than six years, or in any other case earlier than four years can be considered novel.

2. Distinct: A variety is said to be distinct if it is clearly distinguishable by at least one essential characteristic from any other variety whose existence is a matter of common knowledge in any country at the time of filing an application.
3. Uniform: A variety is said to be uniform, if subject to the variation that may be expected from the particular features of its propagation it is sufficiently uniform in its essential characteristics.
4. Stable: A variety is said to be stable if its essential characteristics remain unchanged after repeated propagation or, in the case of a particular cycle of propagation, at the end of each such cycle.

A new variety can be registered under the Act if it conforms to the criteria for novelty, distinctiveness, uniformity and stability. For an extant variety – a variety which is in public domain or about which there is a common knowledge, novelty is novelty is not considered for the protection. A detailed procedures for implementing the objectives of the Act was enacted in the name of Protection of Plant Varieties Rules, 2003.

Conclusion

Majority within the group of people who cultivates, produce and depend directly for their livelihood on agriculture are poor, not highly educated and less informed. Hence, governments are under obligation to regulate the agriculture sector in a way that their betterment could be achieved. Agricultural income depend a lot on high production and high production in turn depends upon the good quality of seed. Hence, law regulating the production, storage, distribution of seed and commercial selling needs to be regulated.

Therefore, the steps taken by the Government in the form of bringing Therefore Government of the Seed Act, Seed Rules, Seed (control) order, National Seed Policy, Plant quarantine order, PPV and FR Act to protect breeders, researchers and a common farmer is highly appreciable; but the responsibility does not come to an end here. Government must take all possible major to resolve any issue that surface pertaining to the seed. Some of the issues which could not get addressed through these existing measures, hopefully be resolved once the Seeds Bill, 2004 is passed.

Chapter 12

Microalgae Cultivation Strategies for Biofuel Production to Mitigating Climate Change through CO_2 Sequestration

V.P. Joshi, P.M. Chauhan and K.B. Joshi

Department of Renewable Energy and Rural Engineering, College of Agricultural Engineering and Technology, Junagadh Agricultural University, Junagadh-362001 (Gujarat).

e-mail: viraljoshi2088@gmail.com

ABSTRACT

The global energy demand especially petroleum derived fuels (PDF), has been increasing at an unprecedented rate with an increasing pressure on the utilities of fossil based fuels. Growing energy demand and water consumption have increased concerns about energy security. With growing concerns surrounding the continued use of fossil fuels, renewable biofuels have received a large amount of recent attention. While biofuels produced using oil crops and waste oils cannot alone meet the existing demand for fuel, microalgae appear to be a more promising feedstock option. Recently, the eyes of world are focusing on the microalgae biofuel development. Microalgae have several advantages over traditional crops, the lipid content of microalgae is usually in the range of 20 per cent to 50 per cent (dry base), and can be as high as 80 per cent under certain circumstances so as to suitable for biofuel production. Large-scale production of microalgae and the harvesting of microalgae in a way that allows for downstream processing to produce biofuels is major challenges to the implementation of an integrated system. Algae offer a diverse spectrum of valuable products and pollution solutions through different conversion routes. Although the majority of algal production systems use suspended cultures in either open ponds or closed reactors, the use of attached cultures may offer several advantages. One of the most prominent advantages of algae is their adaptability to grow in extreme conditions and even polluted environments.The most environmentally sustainable way to reduce greenhouse gas emissions associated with energy production is to generate energy from carbon-neutral or reduced-carbon-emission sources. Carbon dioxide, a Greenhouse Gas (GHG), is the one of the principle pollutant, warming earth. In the past 150 years, anthropogenic activities have pumped enough carbon dioxide into the atmosphere to raise its levels to 400 ppm, higher than they have been for hundreds of thousands of years. Microalgae have a higher CO_2 fixation ability compared to plants and produce value-added products *e.g.* micro algae carotenoids. This paper reviews microalgae cultivation system for biofuel production and also way forward to mitigation of climate change through CO_2 sequestration.

Keywords: *Microalgae cultivation, CO_2 sequestration, Biofuel, Climate change mitigation, Byproduct utilization.*

Introduction

There are dwindling growths in the economy of most oil producing nations due to instability in the global market oil prices. In addition, the constant depletion of oil reserves has intensified the worldwide demand for renewable energy resources. Microalgal cultivation has attracted much attention in recent years, due to their applications in CO_2 sequestration, biofuels, fees, food and bio-molecules production. The attendant consequences provoke environmental concerns in terms of increased greenhouse gases which also affects mitigating climate change strategies. Microalgae are microscopic photosynthetic organisms that are found in both marine and fresh water environments. These are current burning global issues for the climatic, economic and technological preferences for renewable energy technologies and resources. Their photosynthetic mechanism is similar to land-based plants, due to a simple cellular structure, and the fact that they are submerged in an aqueous environment, where they have efficient access to water, CO_2 and other nutrients; they are generally more efficient in converting solar energy into biomass. Estimates of the number of algal range from 350,000 to 1,000,000 species however only a limited number of approximately 30,000 have been studied and analyzed (Richmond 2004). Many of the microalgae studied are photosynthetic whilst only few of them are known to grow mixotrophically or heterotrophically (Lee 2004). The general requirements for successful microalgal cultivation include light (photosynthetic and mixotrophic), carbon, macronutrients such as nitrogen phosphorus, magnesium and silicates and several micronutrients (species dependant) for their successful cultivation.

Algae offer a diverse spectrum of valuable products and pollution solutions as given in Figure 12.1 such as food, nutritional compounds, omega-3 fatty acids, animal feed, energy sources (including jet fuel, aviation gas, biodiesel, gasoline, and bioethanol), organic fertilizers, biodegradable plastics, recombinant proteins, pigments, medicines, pharmaceuticals, and vaccines (Pulz, 2001; Pienkos and Darzins, 2009).

Algae for Biofuel Production

ALGAE FOR BIOFUEL PRODUCTION

Microalgae are unicellular photosynthetic microorganisms that are found naturally in freshwater and marine environments. There are about 200,000–800,000 algae species, of which around 50,000 species have been described (Richmond, A. 2004). The sizes of microalgae depend on their species and vary from micrometres to millimetres (Graham, *et al.*, 2009). Their position is at the bottom of food chains.

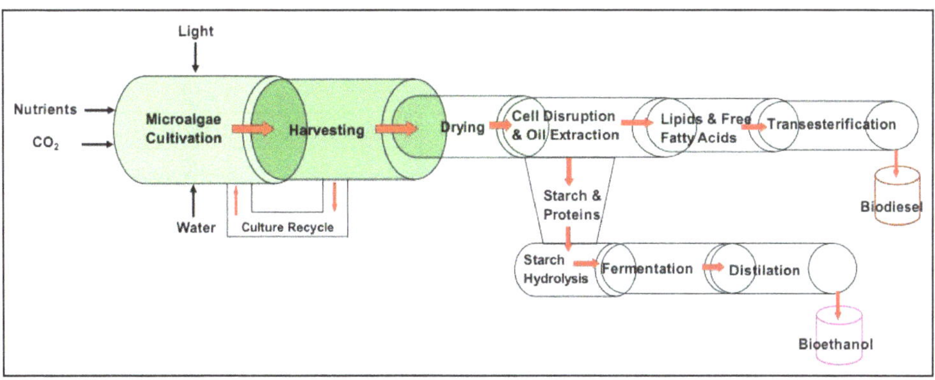

Figure 12.1: Biodiesel and Bioethanol Production Processes from Microalgae (Dragone *et al.*, 2010).

Microalgae are considered to be one of the oldest living organisms on our planet. While the mechanism of photosynthesis in these microorganisms is similar to that of higher plant s, microalgae are general ly more efficient converters of solar energy. The y can convert CO_2 and H_2O to biomass using sunlight (Ozkurt, I., 2009). The average photosynthetic efficiency of microalgae is 6–8 per cent (Aresta, *et al.*, 2005), which is much higher than that of terrestrial biomass (1.8–2.2 per cent). They may be grown in shallow lagoons, raceway ponds, closed ponds, photobioreactors and sea-based systems (Zhu, *et al.*, 2014). and are very efficient in utilizing the nutrients from wastewater, including nitrogen and phosphorus. Due to its rapid growth rate, the nutrients can be recycled back to the soil by fertilizing the waste by-products. Typical biofuel yields from various biomasses are shown in Table 12.1 (Najafi, *et al.*, 2011). The table clearly shows the huge potential of microalgae compared to other biomasses. The production rate (L/ha) of oil from microalgae (91 per cent) is much higher than other feedstocks such as oil palm (3 per cent), coconut (1.5 per cent), jatropha (1.2 per cent), vocado (1.4 per cent) and rapeseed/canola (1 per cent) (Maity, *et al.*, 2014).

Table 12.1: Typical Oil Yields from the Various Biomasses (Adapted from Najafi *et al.*, 2011).

Sl.No.	*Crop*	*Oil Yield (L/ha)*
1	Rubber seed	80–120
2	Corn	172
3	Soybean	446
4	Safflower	779
5	Chinese tallow	907
6	Camelina	915
7	Sunflower	952
8	Peanut	1,059
9	Canola	1,190

Sl.No.	Crop	Oil Yield (L/ha)
10	Rapeseed	1,190
11	Castor	1,413
12	Jatropha	1,892
13	Karanj	2,590
14	Coconut	2,689
15	Oil palm	5,950
16	Microalgae (30 per cent oil by wt)	**58,700**
17	Microalgae (70 per cent oil by wt)	**136,900**

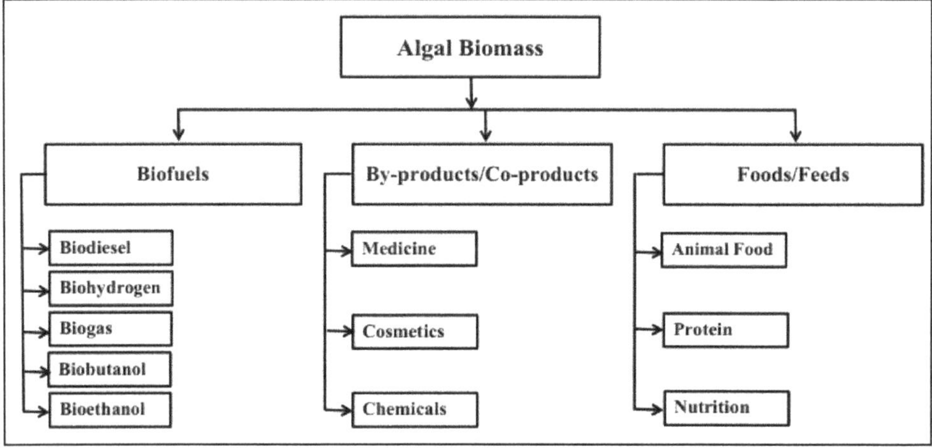

Figure 12.2: Potential Product from Algae (Adopted from Ramaraj, 2014).

Indian Energy Scenario

Biomass based energy was a major cradle of India domestic energy and has been extensively used since antiquity of energy applications in country. The biomass energy as a module of rural renewable energy policy was incorporated in 1970s. The biomass utilization policies have a branched approach from decades which includes " i) improving efficiency of the traditional biomass use (*e.g.* use of improved cook-stove programme), ii) improving the supply of biomass (*e.g.* social forestry, wasteland development), iii) technologies for improving the quality of biomass use (*e.g.* biogas, improved cook-stoves), iv) introduction of biomass based technologies (*e.g.* wood gasifiers for irrigation and biomass electricity generation) to deliver services provided by conventional energy sources, and establishing institutional support for programme formulation and implementation". These policies were implemented with the help of several government agencies, which were supporting the Biomass to Biofuel concept.

In India energy from biomass resources contributes to more than one-third of primary energy. Customarily biomass is used for cooking and heating in rural households of India, including small old-style handicrafts industries.

In India, energy from biomass is derived primarily from forest wood and self-owned sources like farm trees or cattle. Though India is currently a growing economy of the world, approximately 550-600 million tons of biomass is used every year as a primary energy need and more than 70 per cent of the country's population depends upon it for its energy needs (Ministry of New and Renewable Energy (MNRE) website http://mnre.gov.in/). It has also been observed that due to lack of proper synchronization between energy market of rural and urban areas, most of the biomass is not available for appropriate utilization and thus is not able to compete with commercial energy resources available in the market. Since biomass driven energy markets are weak in India, the conventional approaches did not play any role to endorsing biomass and biofuel supply to the market for its efficient uses.

The transportation fuel demand is increasing in India to fuel its rapid growth, thereby increasing the import expenditures. To reduce its reliance on imports, country through its policy regimes, now intends to promote eco-friendly options of biofuels. The new initiatives indicate the Government is keen in motivating production of biofuel within the country through its new policy measures and full R and D support commitments. The feedstock usually identified for the biofuel production are molasses (for ethanol production), while for biodiesel production the best options are oilseed which are non-edible like Jatropha and Pongamia. There are some exceptional benefits for India, in terms of land availability for plantation of oilseeds. India has enormous waste or unutilized land, and most of them are in the drought susceptible areas. For provide the required impetus in the biofuel sector, India government has brought in several actions plans like minimum support price for Jatropha seeds, minimum purchase price for fuel like bio-ethanol and biodiesel *etc*. There is also a focus on third generation biofuels, where in the strategic importance on its research and development is promoted. In present scenario, the country is dealing with the production of biofuel mainly form first and second-generation sources, which has to face the political disapproval in India, due to the fact that these raw materials sources are adequately use for human and animal consumption.

Bio-Mitigation of CO_2 Emission by Microalgae

One of the largely considered methods for CO_2 mitigation is the use of microalgae in biomass conversion in photo bioreactor (Fulke *et al.*, 2010). Marine and freshwater microalgae are microscopic photosynthetic organisms. Microalgae namely, Cyanobacterial (Cyanophyceae) and eukaryotic microalgae, green algae (Chlorophyta) and diatoms (Bacillariophyta) can be used to capture CO_2 from three different sources: atmospheric CO_2, CO_2 emission from power plants and industrial processes and soluble carbonate (Fulke *et al.*, 2013). In this context, possibly the transfer of CO_2 from the atmosphere to the microalgae through photosynthesis is fundamental route for CO_2 capture (Fulke *et al.*, 2010). However, 360ppm CO_2 concentration in atmospheric air makes what economically non-feasible (Stepan, 2002). In contrast, CO_2 capture from flue gas emissions from fossil fuel based power plants achieves better recovery because of, The higher concentration is in exhaust stream, raceway pond systems for microalgae production, and not in photobioreactor" (Bilanovic *et al.*, 2009). However, only a small number of algae are tolerant to the high levels of Sox and NOx present in flue gases. Further, the gases need to be cooled prior to injection into the growth medium. Some microalgae species can assimilate CO_2 from soluble carbonates such as Na2CO3 and NaHCO3 (Wang *et al.*, 2009) leading to high pH of the medium because of conversion of carbonate/bicarbonate alkalinity to hydroxyl alkalinity. Such a condition tends to control invasive species since only a very small number of algae can grow in such extreme conditions. The high cost of process technology and price competitiveness of biodiesel extraction from microalgae can be offset by bio-mitigation of CO_2 emissions which may be simultaneously exploited to reduce cost. The harvested biomass methods, include sun drying, low-pressure shelf drying, drum drying, spray drying, fluidized bed drying (Leach, *et al.*, 1998) freeze drying and refractance Window TM technology drying. Intracellular oils are extracted more easily from dried biomass. Fulke *et al.*, 2009, evaluated the photosynthetic ability of different microalgae leading to higher CO_2 fixation and calcite formation vis-a-vis their ability to synthesize biodiesel precursors. Further, Fulke *et al.*, 2010, observed the presence of Fatty Acid Methyl Esters (FAME) such as docosapentaenoic acid (C22:5), palmitic acid (C16:0) and docosahexaenoic acid (C22:6) and superior quality calcite production with simultaneous CO_2 mitigation using *Chlorella* species. Demirbas reported that microalgae could covert CO_2 into chemical energy via photosynthesis, subsequently leading to fuels biosynthesis. Thus, the photosynthetic potential of microalgae can be integrated with advance CO_2 sequestration and biodiesel production which is a new area of research interest.

Mechanism of CO_2 Fixation

Photosynthetic Pathway

Photosynthesis is the process in which CO_2 is fixed into carbohydrates using the light energy and water. Algae use this process to prepare their food for growth and survival. Chloroplast is the site of photosynthesis in the microalgae. Whereas, in cyanobacteria, photosynthetic apparatus is found in the cytoplasm. It has two stages: light dependent and light independent. Chlorophyll and light harvesting complex harness the light energy and conserve it in the form of energy currencies such as ATP and NADPH formed in the light dependent stage. In the light independent stage, ATP and NADPH are consumed during the synthesis of carbohydrates.

CO_2 is reduced as carbohydrates into the algal cells during the light independent phase through the process called Calvin cycle. Calvin cycle takes place in the stroma of chloroplast and all the participating proteins are found residing outside the thyla- koid membrane in the aqueous phase (Kumar and Das, 2014; Whitmarsh and Govindjee, 1999). Calvin cycle has broadly three steps: carboxylation, reduction and regeneration. Several complex reactions are involved in the Calvin cycle. However, only major reactions are shown in the diagram (Figure 12.3).

CO_2 Fixation through Algal Biomass Production

The CO_2 is fixed during algal growth through several processes such as biomass formation, mineralization (transformation of gaseous CO_2 into chemical species

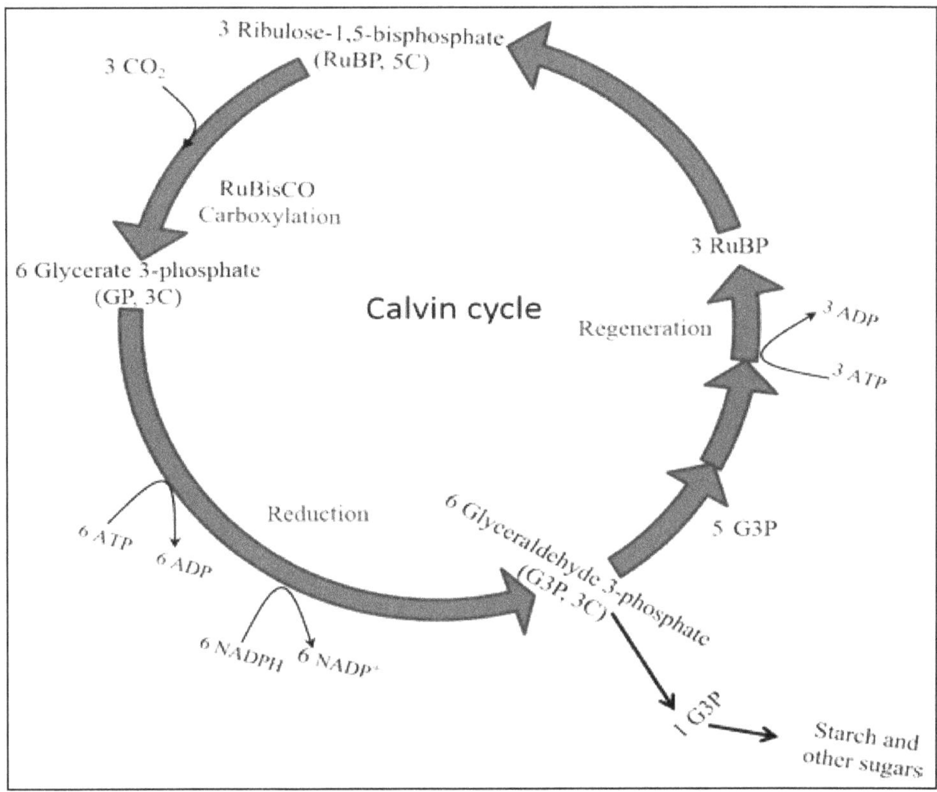

Figure 12.3: Schematic Diagram of the Calvin Cycle. Only major intermediates have been shown (Modified from Kumar and Das, 2014).

such as bicarbonates, carbonates) and production of extracellular products such as polysaccharides, volatile organic compounds, organ halogens, hormones *etc.*

Among them, biomass formation is the major factor, which was found to account for 70–88 per cent of total CO_2 fixation during algal cultivation (Sydney *et. al.*, 2014) as shown in Figure 12.3. CO_2 fixed during other processes are wasted or easily lost to the environment. Therefore, most of the researchers quantify the CO_2 fixation taking only biomass formation into account. The CO_2 fixation ability of microalgae and cyanobacteria varies as shown in Table 12.2.

The elemental composition of biomass of algal species such as *Chlorella* sp. changes depending upon experimental conditions such as the concentration of CO_2 used for growing algae. C, H, N and S were reported in the range of 46.1 per cent–50.1 per cent, 6.1 per cent–7.74 per cent, 6.7 per cent–8.52 per cent and <0.5 per cent (w/w), respectively (Kumar *et al.*, 2014; Rizzo *et al.*, 2013; Friis *et. al.*, 1998). The molecular formula of the algal biomass of microalgae can be determined from the relative percent of C, H and N present in the algal biomass and can be represented in the form of CHxNyOz. The corresponding molecular weight of algal biomass of

Table 12.2: Biomass Productivity and CO_2 Fixation Rate of different Microalgae in different Cultivation Techniques

Algal Species	*Photobioreactor (volume)*	*Biomass Productivity ($mg\ L^{-1}\ d^{-1}$)*	*CO_2 Fixation ($mg\ L^{-1}\ d^{-1}$)*	*References*
Anabaena sp. ATCC 33047	Bubble column	310	1450	Lopez *et al.*, 2009
Aphanothece microscopica	Bubble column (3.2 L)	301	562	Jacob-Lopes *et al.*, 2009
Spirulina platensis	BioFlowfermentor (11 L)	156	319	Sydney *et al.*, 2010
Spirulina sp.	Vertical tubular (1.8 L)	280	–	de Morais and Costa, 2007
Synechocystis aquaticlis	Vertical flat plate (24 L)	78	128	Zhang *et al.*, 2001
Botryococcusbraunii	BioFlowfermentor (11 L)	207	497	Sydney *et al.*, 2010
	–	27	–	Yoo *et al.*, 2010
Chlorella vulgaris	BioFlowfermentor (11 L)	129	252	Sydney *et al.*, 2010
Chlorella sorokiniana	Airlift reactor (1.4 L)	338	619	Kumar and Das, 2012
Chlorella sorokiniana	Airlift reactor (1.4 L)	338	619	Kumar and Das, 2012
Chlorococcum littorale	Vertical tubular (20 L)	530	900	Kurano *et al.*, 1995
	Vertical tubular (15 L)	120	200	Yang *et al.*, 2013
Scenedesmusobliquus	–	218	–	Yoo *et al.*, 2010
	Erlenmeyer flask (0.2 L)	142	253	Basu *et al.*, 2013
	Vertical tubular (1.8 L)	160	–	de Morais and Costa, 2007
Dunaliellatertiolecta	BioFlowfermentor (11 L)	143	272	Sydney et al., 2010
Nannochloropsisoculata	Cylindrical (0.8 L)	480	902	Chiu *et al.*, 2009

C. sorokiniana was in the range of 24–26 g (Kumar *et al.*, 2014). For example, 24.04 g per mole of biomass of *C. sorokiniana* was obtained, when the air was the sole carbon source. Material balance can be writ- ten in the form of Equation adopted from Kumar *et. al.*, 2014.

$$CO_2 + 0.92\ H_2O + 0.14\ NO^-_3 \rightarrow CH_{1.84}N_{0.14}O_{0.51} + 1.415\ O_2$$

Assuming 50 per cent carbon content in the algal cells, 1.83 kg of CO_2 from the air is fixed for the production of one kg of algal biomass along with the release of nearly 1.9 kg of oxygen (Kumar *et. al.*, 2014; Kumar and Das, 2012).

Challenges and Economics Associated with Microalgal CO_2 Sequestration

There are numerous hurdles that need to be overcome before microalgae can be employed to significantly reduce CO_2 emissions at a commercial level. Strain selection and design of the culturing system are key factors in maximizing CO_2 mitigation rates. Even though open systems are much more cost-effective compared to closed PBRs, it is difficult to maintain culture purity in such systems. Closed systems are efficient vessels for sustaining axenic cultures as well as minimizing CO_2 loss to the atmosphere. However, cleaning and sterilizing of large-scale PBRs is difficult, and this then poses a problem in the production of high value-added products. Land availability for set-up of propagation vessels also becomes a problem in developing countries. For example, Kadam (2001) demonstrated that 1,000 ha of land area will be required for the construction of open ponds to mitigate CO_2 emissions from a 50-MW power plant. Carbon-fixation rates for microalgal cultures differ under varying operational conditions. Preliminary ideas of these values are required so as to estimate space requirements for reactor implementation for effective CO_2 fixation. In this example a Portuguese cement industry annually produces ±450 kt of CO_2. If two types of reactors (open ponds and light-diffusing optical fiber reactors) are considered for the effective sequestration of CO_2 emitted from this industry, the estimated space required would be very different. Studies showed that under natural day/night cycles, a 4,000 m^3 pond could sequester up to 2.2 kt of CO_2 per year. If ponds were to be scaled up to a height of 30 cm (to prevent dark zones), open ponds occupying an area of 2.72 9 106 m^2 would be required to sequester almost all the CO_2 from this cement company. CO_2-fixation rates for light-diffusing optical fiber reactors were reported to be 4.44 g $L^{-1}d^{-1}$. Therefore, a reactor height of 1 m and a culturing area of 2.78 9 105 m2 would be needed to effectively sequester CO_2 from this cement plant (Stewart and Hessami 2005; Pires *et al.*, 2012).

Geographical considerations must also be taken into account: fluctuations in temperature and solar irradiation over the seasons. Tropical areas are often considered most suitable for microalgal cultivation. To maximize the overall economic and environmental efficiency of micro- algal CO_2 sequestration, culturing systems should be located as close as possible to the point source. Further- more, a comprehensive plan should be compiled for the large-scale production of microalgae. This scheme should encompass modeling and LCA of the overall process. Failure in doing so could render many algal production systems unsustainable. It should also be noted that potential leaks from large-scale algal systems could cause ecological damage by eutrophication (Pires *et al.*, 2012; Farrelly *et al.*, 2013).

Conclusion

Microalgae have attracted a great deal of attention for CO_2 fixation and biofuel production because they can capture and convert CO_2 into algal biomass by photosynthesis at much higher rates than other crops responsible for generating conventional biofuels. The fixation of CO_2 by a biological route could be the most effective carbon-capturing method on earth. Until now most of the work on biological carbon capture by microalgae has been on lower CO_2 concentrations (\20 per cent). There are few studies available regarding the influence of high CO_2 levels ([20 per cent) on the growth, CO_2 biofixation rate and the fatty acid composition of microalgae. There is a need to focus on this area as the concentration of CO_2 is rising globally. Most of the studies reported to date have been conducted on bench scale units under strictly controlled conditions. Certain factors, such as supply of adequate amounts of CO_2, nutrients and light should be investigated and optimized for the application of best parametric conditions in production of biodiesel commercially at large scale. The technical feasibility has been proven at small scale and, in fact, small samples of algal biofuel have been produced, but economic feasibility is unknown. To be economically feasible, microalgal biodiesel must be cost-competitive with petroleum-based fuels. The process of biofuel production from microalgae can be made cost-effective by combining the process with utilization of CO_2 from point source flue gas emissions, with remediation of wastewater or with the extraction of valuable compounds for application in other industries. The concept of a pond ulture is economical but there are certain major environmental conditions required for microalgal growth which can only be fulfilled by employing photobioreactors. Numerous works have been done on CO_2 bio-sequestration and biofuel production by microalgae but still much research is needed to meet the increasing demand for energy. We hope that in the future, biofuel will replace fossil fuel to a large extent and reduce the atmospheric CO_2 concentration combating global warming. Hence, it can be concluded that substantial investment in the development of this technology and technical expertise in this area is still required before biofuel can become a reality. The growth of biofuel industries will definitely be economically and environmentally beneficial and at the same time it will create a large number of jobs at different levels of the society as well as helpful to mitigate in climate mitigation.

References

Aresta, M., Dibenedetto, A., and Barberio, G. (2005). Utilization of macro-algae for enhanced CO2 fixation and biofuels production: Development of a computing software for an LCA study. Fuel ProcessingTechnology, 86, 1679–1693.

Bilanovic D, Andargatchew A, Kroeger T, Shelef G (2009) Freshwater and marine microalgae sequestering of CO at different C and N concentrations-Response surface methodology analysis. Energy Conversion and Management. 50:262-267.

Dragone, G., Fernandes, B., Vicente, A. A. and Teixeira, J. A. (2010). Third generation biofuels from microalgae in current research. In Mendez-Vilas, A. (Ed.) Technology and Education Topics in Applied Microbiology and Microbial Biotechnology. 1355-1366.

Farrelly DJ, Everard CD, Fagan CC, McDonnell KP (2013) Carbon sequestration and the role of biological carbon mitigation: a review. Renew Sustain Energy Rev 21:712–727.

Fulke AB, Chambhare K, Giripunje MD, Sangolkar L, Krishnamurthi K, *et al.* (2013) Potential of wastewater grown algae for biodiesel production and CO sequestration. African Journal of Biotechnology 12:2939-2948.

Fulke AB, Mudliar SN, Yadav R, Shekh A, Srinivasan N, *et al.* (2010) Bio-mitigation of CO, calcite formation and simultaneous biodiesel precursors production using Chlorella sp. BioresourTechnol 101: 8473-8476.

Friis, J.C., Holm, C. and Sorensen, B.H. (1998). Evaluation of elemental composition of algal biomass as toxical endpoint. *Chemosphere.*, 37(13), 2665–2676.

Graham, L. E., Graham, J. M., and Wilcox, L. W. (2009). Algae. California, USA: Benjamin-Cummings publishing Company. ISBN-13: 978-0321559654.

Kadam KL (2001) Microalgae production from power plant flue gas: Environmental implications on a life cycle basis. Technical report, National Renewable Energy Laboratory Contract No. DE-AC36-99-GO10337.

Kumar, K. and Das, D. (2014). Carbon Dioxide Sequestration by Biological Processes. *In:* Bhanage, B.M. and Arai, M. (eds), Transformation and Utilization of Carbon Dioxide. Springer, pp. 303–334.

Leach G, Oliveira G, Morais R (1998) Spray-drying of Dunaliellasalina to produce a dippa-carotene rich powder. Journal of Industrial Microbiology and Biotechnology 20: 82-85.

Maity, J. P., Bundschuh, J., Chen, C.-Y., and Bhattachary, A. P. (2014). Microalgae for third generation biofuel production, mitigation of greenhouse gas emissions and wastewater treatment: Present and future perspectives—a mini review. Energy, 78, 104–113.

Najafi, G., Ghobadiana, B., and Yusaf, T. F. (2011). Algae as a sustainable energy source for biofuel production in Iran: A case study. Renewable and Sustainable Energy Reviews, 2011 (15), 3870–3876.

Ozkurt, I. (2009). Qualifying of safflower and algae for energy. Energy Education Science and Technology Part A, 23, 145–151.

Pienkos, P. T. and Darzins, A. (2009) The promise and challenges of micro-algal derived biofuels. *Biofuel Bioproducts Biorefinary.***3**:431–440.

Pires JCM, Alvim-Ferraz MCM, Martins FG, Simo˜ es M (2012) Carbon dioxide capture from flue gases using microalgae: engineerin aspects and biorefinery concept. Renew Sustain Energy Rev 16:3043–3053.

Pulz, O. (2001) Photobioreactors: production systems for phototrophic microorganisms. Applied Microbiology Biotehnology. 57:287–293.

Ramaraj, R., and Dussadee, N. (2014). Biological purification process for biogas using algae culture: A review. International Journal of Sustainable and Green Energy, 4, 20–32.

Richmond, A. (2004). Handbook of microalgal culture: Biotechnology and applied phycology. Blackwell Science Ltd.

Rizzo, A.M., Prussi, M., Bettucci, L., Libelli, I.M. and Chiaramonti, D. (2013). Characterization of microalga Chlorella as a fuel and its thermogravimetric behavior. Appl. Energy, 102, 24–31.

Singh S, Singh D. Biodiesel production through the use of different sources and characterization of oils and their esters as the substitute of diesel: a review. Renew Sustain Energy Rev 2010;14(1):200–16.

Stewart C, Hessami MA (2005) A study of methods of carbon dioxide capture and sequestration—the sustainability of a photosynthetic bioreactor approach. Energy Convers Manag 46:403–420

Stephens E, Ross IL, Mussgnug JH, (2010) Future prospects of microalgal biofuel production systems. *Trends Plant Sci*. 15(10):554–64.

Stepan DJ, Shockey RE, Moe TA, Dorn R (2002) Carbon dioxide sequestering using microalgae systems.US Department of Energy, Pittsburgh, PA.

Sydney, E.B., Novak, A.C., de Carcalho, J.C. and Soccol, C.R. (2014). Respirometric balance and carbon fixation of industrially important algae. *In:* A. Paney, D.-J. Lee, Y. Chisti and C.R. Soccol (eds.), Biofuels from algae. Elsevier, MA, USA, pp. 67–84.

Wang B, Li Y, Wu N, Lan CQ (2008) CO bio-mitigation using microalgae. ApplMicrobiolBiotechnol 79: 707-718.

Whitmarsh, J. and Govindjee (1999). The photosynthetic process. *In:* Singhal, G.S., Renger, G., Sopory, S.K., Irrgang, K.-D., Govindjee (eds), Concepts in Photobiology: Photosynthesis and Photomorphogenesis. Narosa Publishers, New Delhi and Kluwer Academic, Dordrecht, pp 11–51.

Zhu, L. D., Hiltunen, E., Antila, E., Zhong, J. J., Yuan, Z. H., and Wang, Z. M. (2014). Microalgal biofuels: Flexible bioenergies for sustainable development. Renewable and Sustainable Energy Reviews, 30, 1035–1046.

Chapter 13

CRISPR-Cas: A Potential Tool in Plant Genome Editing

R.K. Kalaria

ASPEE Shakilam Biotechnology Institute, Nau, Surat (Gujarat) 395 007
e-mail: risheekal@nau.in

ABSTRACT

CRISPR-Cas is a genome editing tool that quicker, cheaper and more precise than previous techniques of editing DNA and has a wide range of potential applications in crop improvements. Genetic diversity is a vital source for trait improvement in crops. Creating genetic variations in the gene pool is the prime requirement for developing plant varieties. Once the desired modifications are achieved, transgenes can be transfer out from the improved plant variety. Crop improvement has been done for years via conventional plant breeding techniques or through various mutations methods. This chapter discuses types, CRISPR-CAS mechanism and application of CRISPR.

Keywords: *Cas, Cas9, gRNA, epigenomics and crRNA*

CRISPR stands for Clustered Regularly Interspaced Short Palindromic Repeats while Cas is a associated protein. CRISPR was not an innovation, but a breakthrough during the whole genome sequencing in the 1980s, when researchers at Osaka University sequenced the genomes of common bacteria *E.coli*. In few bacteria and archaea, the functions of CRISPR and CRISPR-associated (Cas) genes are crucial in adaptive immunity that enabling the organisms to respond and eradicate foreign genetic material[7]. They found the repeating DNA sequences in many species but did not recognize its biological function until 2007 by Barrangou and colleagues, who confirmed that *S. thermophilus* can obtain resistance by integrating a small fragment of an infectious virus into its CRISPR locus against a bacteriophage[1,2].

CRISPR-Cas is a genome editing tool that quicker, cheaper and more precise than previous techniques of editing DNA and has a wide range of potential applications in crop improvements. CRISPR-Cas is a unique technology that enables geneticists and researchers to edit parts of the genome by removing, adding or altering sections of the DNA sequence[4]. It is currently the simplest, most versatile and precise method of genetic manipulation in crop improvement and is therefore causing a boom in the scientific cummunity. These genome-editing technologies use programmable nucleases to increase the specificity of the target locus[3].

Genetic diversity is a vital source for trait improvement in crops. Creating genetic variations in the gene pool is the prime requirement for developing plant varieties. Once the desired modifications are achieved, transgenes can be transfer out from the improved plant variety. Crop improvement has been done for years via conventional plant breeding techniques or through various mutations methods. The beginning of site-specific nucleases (SSNs) highlighted the importance of site directed mutagenesis over random mutagenesis [12,16].

Types of CRISPR

The system is categorized into three distinct types, type I, II, and III on the basis of the presence of the specific signature Cas protein. Out of these three types of CRISPR mechanisms, of which type II is the most studied. All three types have Cas1 and Cas2 proteins in common. However, the effector complex that binds to crRNA (CRISPR RNA) and triggers cleavage, differs among different CRISPR–Cas systems. The type I system is found in both bacteria and archaea and targets DNA sequences with the help of the endonuclease activity of Cas3 protein. The type III system is recognized by the presence of Cas10 and Cas6 proteins in addition to repeat-associated mysterious proteins RAMPs.

The type II CRISPR–Cas system has been reported only in bacteria. In type II, invading DNA from viruses or plasmids is cut into small fragments and incorporated into a CRISPR locus amidst a series of short repeats (around 20 bps). The loci are transcribed, and transcripts are then processed to generate small RNAs (crRNA), which are used to guide effector endonucleases that target invading DNA based on sequence complementarily. It involves several proteins *viz.*, Cas1, Cas2, Cas9, and Cas4/Csn2 among which Cas9 is most efficient, signature, multifunctional protein[3,7,15].

CRISPR-CAS Mechanism

The CRISPR-Cas9 system consists of two key molecules that introduce a change into the DNA. These are: an enzyme called Cas9 and guide RNA (Figure 13.1). Cas9 acts as a pair of 'molecular scissors' that can cut the two strands of DNA at a specific location in the genome so that fragment of DNA can then be added or removed. A piece of RNA called guide RNA (gRNA). This consists of a small piece of pre-designed RNA sequence (about 20 bp) located within a longer RNA scaffold. The scaffold part binds to DNA and the pre-designed sequence 'guides' Cas9 to the specific part of the genome. This makes sure that the Cas9 enzyme cuts at the specific point in the genome[3,7].

Here the guide RNA could be designed to find and bind to a specific sequence in the DNA. The guide RNA has RNA bases that are complementary to those of the target DNA sequence in the genome of organism.

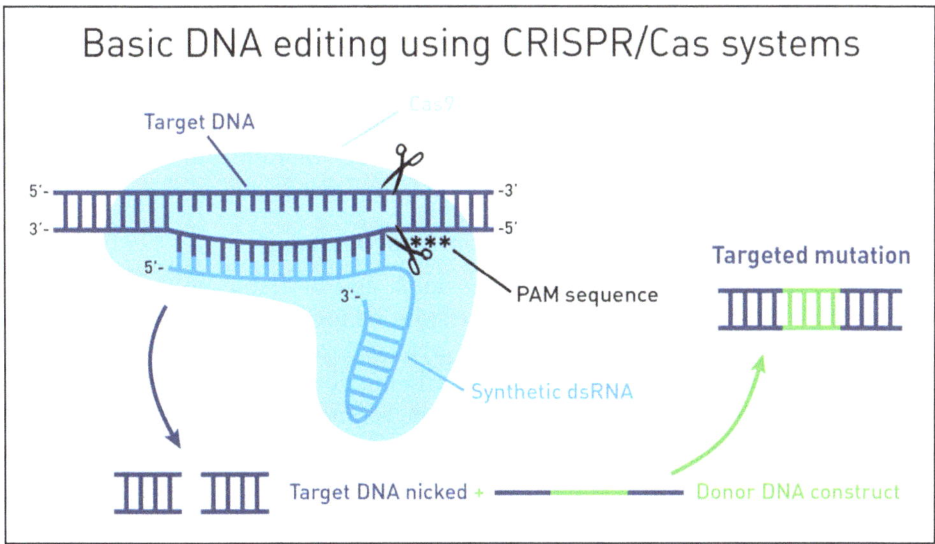

Figure 13.1: General Mechanism of CRISPR-Cas (https://www.jax.org/news-and-insights/jax-blog/2014/march/pros-and-cons-of-znfs-talens-and-crispr-cas).

Application

The CRISPR–Cas system couples several desirable features, including simplicity, competence, minimal off-target effects, and amenability to multiplexing, thus seems to be extremely promising in plants and animals. The ease and multiplicity have shown the potential in three dimensions of plants functional genomics, *i.e.*, genomics, transcriptomics, and epigenomics. This can allow simultaneous induction as well as repression of certain sets of genes and at the same time aid in reprogramming the epigenome[2].

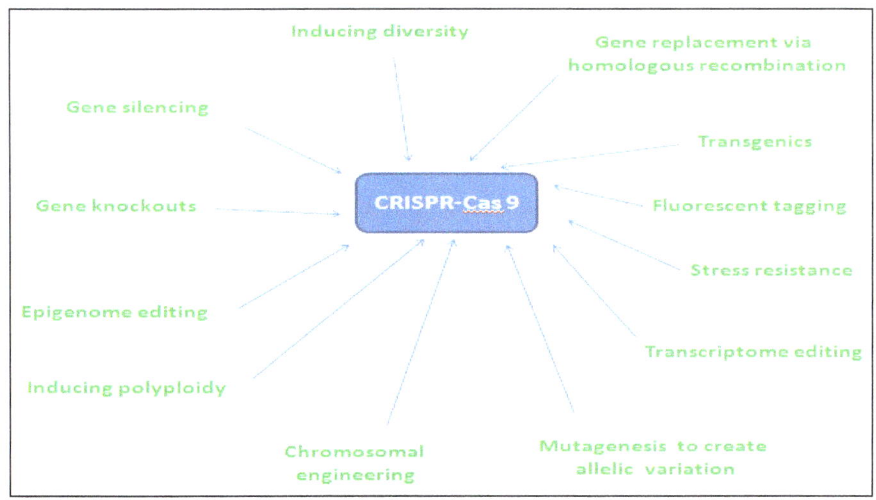

Figure 13.2: Various Application of CRISPR-Cas.

Targeted Genome Modification in Crops

Over past few years, the biotic (bacteria, fungi, insects, and viruses) and abiotic (salinity, drought, flooding, heavy metal toxicity, high temperature) stresses have negatively affected crop productivity. Recent researches in plant biotechnology focuses on developing new varieties in crops to tolerate harsh agro climatic conditions and to meet the needs of the ever-growing human race[8].

Genome Modification for Nutrition Improvement

CRISPR/Cas9 system can generate stable and heritable mutations without affecting the existing valuable traits. This results in the development of homozygous modified transgene free plants in only one generation and it's stable transmission to successive generations[4,13]. Classic works are being done for producing acrylamide free potatoes[5], non-browning apples[11], mushrooms and potatoes by mutating Polyphenol oxidase (PPO) genes[5,6,17] and low phytic acid in maize [9]. Genetic improvement of citrus is limited due to its slow growth, pollen incompatibility, polyembryony and parthenocarpy[8].

Biotic and Abiotic Stress Resistance via CRISPR/Cas9

Multiple disease resistance plants have been obtained using CRISPR/Cas9 technology. Wang and his colleagues in 2014 introduced mutations using site-specific endonucleases in homeoalleles encoding Mildew-resistance locus (MLO) proteins of hexaploid bread wheat [14]. Peng and his colleagues targeted citrus canker caused by Xanthomonas citri subsp. Xcc in *Citrus sinensi*[8,17]

CRISPR System in Metabolic Engineering

Further applications of CRISPR/Cas9 include extensive research in the field of metabolic engineering where plant cells are targeted for production of specific metabolites. Li and his colleagues targeted diterpene synthase gene (SmCPS1), involved in tanshinone biosynthesis in Salvia miltiorrhiza, Chinese herb well-known for vasorelaxation and antiarrhythmic effects [10]. SmCPS1 is the entry enzyme that uses GGPP (geranylgeranyl diphosphate) as its substrate for generating tanshinones. GGPP also acts as a precursor for taxol.

Advancements in Genome editing technologies have revolutionized the fields of functional genomics and crop improvement. Targeted genome editing using engineered nucleases has rapidly gone from being a niche technology to a mainstream method used by many biological researchers. This widespread adoption has been largely fuelled by the emergence of the clustered, regularly interspaced, short palindromic repeat (CRISPR) technology, an important new approach for generating RNA-guided nucleases, such as Cas9, with customizable specificities[15]. CRISPR-Cas9 has a lot of potential as a tool for treating a range of potential conditions that have a genetic component in plants and animals. Much research is still focusing on its use in models organism, with the aim to eventually use the technology to routinely treat biotic and abiotic factor. CRISPR-Cas9 is not alternative to conventional breeding, but help this techniques permit breeders to meet their breeding goals for introgress the specific trait into elite breeding lines. Many of the countries already believed that the Genetic modification (GM) regulations and CRISPR regulations are different, after testing the thorough effects it is needed to be encouraged rapidly, because it is a tool of one time investment which makes quick changes and several crop-related problems can be solved within a short span of time and can attain the food demand of ever growing population in terms of quality as well as quantity[8,19]. Many companies are also engaged in using this technology for the production of elite food and feed crops[19]. The products, which are obtained by editing through CRISPR-Cas9, have no exogenous DNA and furthermore editing can be done in such a way, which abides by all the rules and regulations that are complaisant to withstand against Genetically Modified issues and can get an easy approval by the competent authorities in respective countries.

References

1. Barrangou, R., Fremaux, C., Deveau, H., Richards, M., Boyaval, P., Moineau, S., Romero, D.A., Horvath, P. (2007) CRISPR provides acquired resistance against viruses in prokaryotes. *Science* 315(5819):1709-12.
2. Barrangou, R. and Doudna, J. A. (2016) Applications of CRISPR technologies in research and beyond. *Nature Biotechnology* 34:933-941
3. Burstein, D., Harrington, L. B., Strutt, S. C., Probst, A. J., Anantharaman, K., Thomas, B. C., Doudna, J. A. and Banfield, J. F. (2016). New CRISPR-Cas systems from uncultivated microbes. *Nature*: 22:1-8.
4. Feng, Z., Mao, Y., Xu, N., Zhang, B., Wei, P., Yang, D. L., Wang, Z., Zhang, Z., Zheng, R., Yang, L., Zeng, L., Liu, X., Zhu, J.K. (2014). Multigeneration analysis reveals the inheritance, specificity, and patterns of CRISPR/Cas-induced gene modifications in Arabidopsis. *Proc. Natl. Acad. Sci. U.S.A.* 111:4632–4637.
5. Halterman, D., Guenthner, J., Collinge, S., Butler, N., Douches, D. (2015). Biotech Potatoes in the 21st Century: 20 years since the first biotech potato. *Am. J. Potato* 93:1–20.
6. Ishino, Y., Shinagawa, H., Makino, K., Amemura, M., Nakata, A. (1987) Nucleotide sequence of the iap gene, responsible for alkaline phosphatase isozyme conversion in Escherichia coli, and identification of the gene product. *J. Bacteriol.* 169(12):5429-33.
7. Jinek, M., Chylinski, K., Fonfara I, Hauer M, Doudna JA, Charpentier E. (2012) A programmable dual-RNA-guided DNA endonuclease in adaptive bacterial immunity. *Science*. 337(6096):816-21.
8. Leena Arora and Alka Narula (2017) Gene Editing and Crop Improvement Using CRISPR-Cas9 System Front. *Plant Science*, 08:1-21.
9. Liang, Z., Zhang, K., Chen, K. and Gao, C. (2014). Targeted mutagenesis in Zea mays using TALENs and the CRISPR/Cas system. *J. Genet. Genomics* 41:63–68.
10. Li, B., Cui, G., Shen, G., Zhan, Z., Huang, L., Chen, J. and Qi, X. (2017). Targeted mutaGenesis in the medicinal plant Salvia miltiorrhiza. *Sci. Rep.* 7:43320–43329.

11. Nishitani, C., Hirai, N., Komori, S., Wada, M., Okada, K., Osakabe, K., Saika, H. and Toki, S. (2016). Efficient genome editing in apple using a CRISPR/Cas9 system. *Sci. Rep.* 6:31481

12. Osakabe K., Osakabe Y. and Toki S. (2010). Site-directed mutaGenesis in Arabidopsis using custom-designed zinc finger nucleases. *Proc. Natl. Acad. Sci. U.S.A. 107*:12034–12039.

13. Pan, C. T., Ye, L., Qin, L., Liu, X., He, Y. J., Wang, J., Chen, L., Lu, G. (2016). CRISPR/Cas9-mediated efficient and heritable targeted mutagenesis in tomato plants in the first and later generations. *Sci. Rep.* 6:24765.

14. Peng, A., Chen, S., Lei, T., Xu, L., He, Y., Wu, L., Yao, L. and Zou, X. (2017). Engineering canker-resistant plants through CRISPR/Cas9-targeted editing of the susceptibility gene CsLOB1 promoter in citrus. *Plant Biotechnol. J.* 15(12):1509-1519

15. Quétier, F. (2016). The CRISPR-Cas9 technology: Closer to the ultimate toolkit for targeted genome editing, *Plant Science* 242: 65–76.

16. Sikora, P., Chawade, A., Larsson, M., Olsson, J. and Olsson, O. (2011). Mutagenesis as a tool in plant genetics, functional genomics, and breeding. *Int. J. Plant Genomics* 142–153.

17. Waltz, E. (2016). Gene-edited CRISPR mushroom escapes US regulation.(2016) *Nature.*:532(7599):293

18. Wang, Y., Cheng, X., Shan, Q., Zhang, Y., Liu, J. and Gao, C. (2014). Simultaneous editing of three homoeoalleles in hexaploid bread wheat confers heritable resistance to powdery mildew. *Nat. Biotechnol.* 32 947–951

19. Yue, M., Yan, W., Huiqian, C., Zhong, S. S., and Xing, D. J. (2016) Recent Progress in CRISPR/Cas9 Technology. *J. Genetics and Genomics* 43: 63-75.

Chapter 14

Uncertainty Over Medicinal Marijuana: History, Pharmacodynamics and Current Drug in Market

Rajvi K. Patel

e-mai: rj.rajvi.05@gmail.com

ABSTRACT

Cannabis has a long history of medicinal use in the Middle East and Asia. Cannabis cultivation and trade for medicinal purpose are partially restricted in India. While its cultivation for industrial purposes is allowed. Overall, its use and legality come under the concern of the department of finance ministry's revenue and are governed by the Narcotic Drugs and Psychotropic Substances Act, 1985. Control over marijuana is still illegal in most countries, but many have decriminalized it and many others could be next to legalize marijuana. The purpose of this article is to acknowledge the acceptance and medicinal use of marijuana, pharmacodynamics inside the body, pharmacology and spread an awareness on the significance role of the psychoactive compounds present in marijuana.

Keywords: *marijuana, Cannabis, narco drugs, medicinal plants*

Introduction

Scientists are looking into the benefits of various indigenous plant species and their extracts for use in medicines, among which the universally demanding national attention since decades, namely cannabis (marijuana) belongs to a small family of flowering plants, Cannabaceae[1]. Marijuana is currently recognized by the U.S. Drug Enforcement Agency's (DEA's) Comprehensive Drug Abuse Prevention and Control Act (Controlled Substances Act) of 1970 as a Schedule I drug, defined as illegal drug having a high abuse potential, no medical use in treatment in the United States, and a lack of accepted safety data for use in treatment under medical supervision[2]. Despite all this, Marijuana is being legalised in some part of the world for medicinal and/or recreational purpose. Recreational use has always been subjected to criminalization, but recently popular opinion has shifted toward legalizing its use.

According to researchers, the two main psychoactive chemicals present in Marijuana for medicinal application are cannabidiol (CBD) - which seems to impact the brain without a high- and tetrahydrocannabinol (THC) - which has pain relieving properties, present in the resin produced by the leaves and buds of the female cannabis plant. CBD may be useful in reducing pain and inflammation, controlling epileptic seizures, and possibly even treating mental illness and addictions.

The two species of cannabis plant are *Cannabis sativa* and *Cannabis indica*. *Cannabis sativa*, is widely used for recreational purpose, medicinal, and religious purposes and for industrial purpose in the making of products derived from hemp (the soft fibre from the stalk). The main difference between the two is their tetrahydrocannabinol, or THC content. THC is what determines cannabis's mind-altering properties. On average, Cannabis *indica* has higher levels of THC compared to CBD, whereas Cannabis sativa has lower levels of THC to CBD[4].

The purpose of this article is to acknowledge the acceptance and medicinal use of marijuana, pharmacodynamics inside the body, pharmacology and spread an awareness on the significance role of the psychoactive compounds present in marijuana.

Historical Significance and Accpetance of Cannabis (Marijuana)

Cannabis has a long history of medicinal use in the Middle East and Asia. It was introduced in Western Europe as a medicine in the early 19th century to treat epilepsy, tetanus, rheumatism, migraine, asthma, trigeminal neuralgia, fatigue, and insomnia[5,6]. According to the World Health Organization (WHO), marijuana consumption has an annual prevalence rate of approximately 147 million individuals or 2.5 per cent of the global population[7]. In 2014, approximately 22.2 million Americans 12 years of age or older reported current cannabis use[8]. Cannabis is also one of the oldest sources of food and textile fibre. Between 1000 and 2000 BCE hemp was grown for fibre in Western Asia and Egypt and subsequently in Europe. Cultivation of hemp in Europe became widespread after 500 CE. The crop was first brought to South America (Chile) in 1545, and to North America (Port Royal, Acadia) in 1606[9].

In the U.S., cannabis was widely utilized as a patent medicine during the 19th and early 20th centuries, described in the United States Pharmacopoeia for the first time in 1850. Federal restriction of cannabis uses and cannabis sale first occurred in 1937 with the passage of the Marihuana Tax Act.[10,11] Subsequently, cannabis was dropped from the United States Pharmacopoeia in 1942, with legal penalties for possession increasing in 1951 and 1956 with the enactment of the Boggs and Narcotic Control Acts, respectively, and prohibition under federal law occurring with the Controlled Substances Act of 1970[12,13,14].

General cannabis use, both for recreational and medicinal purposes, has garnered increasing acceptance across the United States by actions like legislative actions, ballot measures, and public opinion polls; in October 2016, Gallup poll on American's views on legalizing cannabis indicated that 60 per cent of the surveyed population believed that Cannabis should be legalized[15]. In the United States, cannabis is approved for medicinal use in 28 states, the District of Columbia, Guam, and Puerto Rico as of January 2017[16].

Cannabis cultivation and trade for medicinal purpose are partially restricted in India. While its cultivation for industrial purposes is allowed. Overall, its use and legality come under the concern of the department of finance ministry's revenue and are governed by the Narcotic Drugs and Psychotropic Substances Act, 1985[17]. In February 2018 India's leading ayurvedic product manufacturer, Patanjali's chief executive Balkrishna, weighed the legalisation and importance of cannabis plant for medicinal purpose[18]. Although control over marijuana is still illegal in most countries, but many have decriminalized it and many others could be next to legalize marijuana.

Psychoactive Chemical Present in Marijuana

Cannabis is a quite complex substance. Isolation and extraction of the active ingredient present in the Cannabis is difficult even today. These active ingredients are quite unique among the various psychoactive plant substances, it contains no nitrogen and thus is not an alkaloid. Cannabis plant contains over 600 chemicals of which more than 60 compounds possess psychoactive property, these compounds are called cannabinoids. Out of these 60 cannabinoids, two major cannabinoids are delta-9-tetrahydrocannabinol (d-9-THC) and cannabidiol (CBD) (Figure 14.1 shows the chemical structure of THC and CBD respectively). The chemical structure of both the compounds is quite similar however the pharmacological property is very different. In plants, these cannabinoids are synthesized and accumulated as cannabinoid acids, but when the herbal product is dried, stored and heated, the acids decarboxylize gradually into CBD or d-9-THC[19].

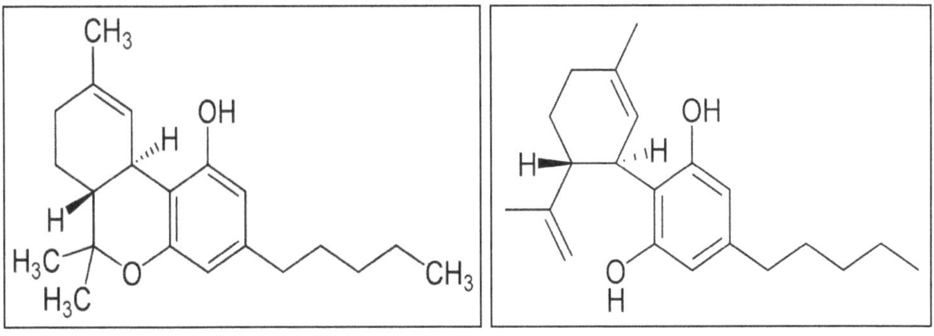

Delta-9-tetrahydrocannabinol (d-9-THC) **Cannabidiol (CBD)**

Figure 14.1: Structure of Two Main Psychoactive Compound found in Cannabis[45].

Out the two-main subspecies, *Cannabis indica* and *Cannabis sativa*, *Indica* have higher cannabidiol (CBD) content and in the *sativa* plants THC content is higher. As d-9-THC is the main ingredient which causes the desired 'stoned' effect, users prefer *sativa* strain of the plant.

Along with the discovery of these cannabinoids, further research led to the discovery of an important neurotransmitter system called the endocannabinoid system. This system is responsible for various significant functions and are present in the brain and in the body.

How is Marijuana Smoked?

Marijuana is currently used as an 'illicit' drug for recreational purpose. It is widely used among young generation. It is smoked in many ways. It is smoked in a hand-rolled cigarette or using water pipes known as bong. It is also used in vaporized form to avoid inhaling the smoke, in which the main active ingredient is separated and collected in the vaporized form in the storage unit and the vapour is then inhaled instead of the smoke. Besides this, marijuana is also used in food like brownie, candy and/or cookies or its extract is used in tea also.[20] A newly popular method of use is smoking or eating different forms of THC-rich resins.[20] Every time someone smokes a marijuana cigarette or ingests marijuana in some other form, THC (delta-9-tetrahydrocannabinol) and other chemicals enter the user's body from the plant and/or its extract. These chemicals make their way through the bloodstream to the brain and then to the rest of the body. The THC from marijuana goes directly to the lungs where millions of alveoli (the tiny air sacs where gas exchange occurs, having an enormous surface area) are present. The lungs absorb the smoke immediately after inhalation. Hence the person begins to experience effects almost immediately. If marijuana is consumed in foods or beverages, these effects are somewhat delayed usually appearing after 30 minutes to 1 hour because the absorption of THC occurs through the digestive system which is much slower than the lungs. Eating or drinking marijuana delivers significantly less THC into the bloodstream than smoking an equivalent amount[20].

Pharmacodynamics: Mechanism of Marijuana Inside the Body

Studying the dynamic nature of the by-products of marijuana helps us in understanding it's medicinal property. Among the several neurotransmitters, endocannabinoid neurotransmitter system (eCBs) (or endogenous cannabinoids) is present throughout the body: nervous system, internal organs, connective tissues, glands, and immune cells that are responsible for physiological processes like appetite, pain-sensation, mood, and memory[21,22]. The naturally occurring endocannabinoid ligands include anandamide (AEA), 2-arachidonoyl glycerol(2-AG), N-arachidonoyl-dopamine, and virohamine. The chemical structure of THC is similar to one of the endocannabinoid called anandamide(AEA). Because of structural similarity, the body recognize THC (when consumed) instead of AEA and alters normal brain communication[20] (Figure 14.2)

The eCB system consists of receptors, endogenous ligands, and ligand metabolic enzymes called cannabinoid receptor. A variety of physiological processes occur

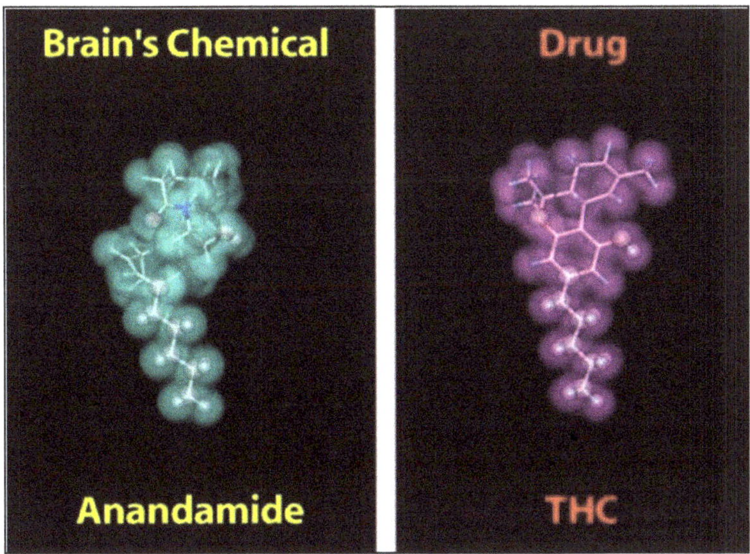

Figure 14.2: Structure of Anandamide and THC[20].

when cannabinoid receptors are stimulated. Cannabinoid receptors belong to G-protein coupled receptor[23]. Cannabinoid receptors are activated by either of the three major groups of endocannabinoid ligands that are produced by (1) the body, (2) plant cannabinoids (such as cannabidiol, produced by the cannabis plant); and (3) synthetic cannabinoids (such as HU-210). All the endocannabinoids and plant cannabinoids are lipophilic, such as fat-soluble compounds. Due to high lipid solubility of cannabinoids, it is possible that THC or CBD persist in the body for a longer period particularly in the lipid membrane of neurons.

There are currently two known subtypes of cannabinoid receptors, termed CB1 and CB2[24]:

1. CB1 receptors: are mainly found in high densities in the neuron terminals of the basal ganglia (affecting motor activity), cerebellum (motor coordination), hippocampus (short-term memory), neocortex (thinking), and hypothalamus and limbic cortex (appetite and sedation)[25].
2. CB2 receptors: are mostly expressed in immune cells, spleen and the gastrointestinal system, and to some extent in the brain and peripheral nervous system[26].

The THC attaches to these naturally occurring cannabinoid receptors in the brain. However, when the receptors pair with THC, the neurotransmitters do not function with the same efficiency and are thus unable to provide the correct information to the different parts of the brain as a result the body to doesn't respond in a normal manner and the natural regulating mechanisms becomes blocked. *E.g.*, When cannabis is used, d-9-THC as a partial agonist binds to CB1R (due to structural similarity with anandamide) and inhibiting the release of neurotransmitters that are

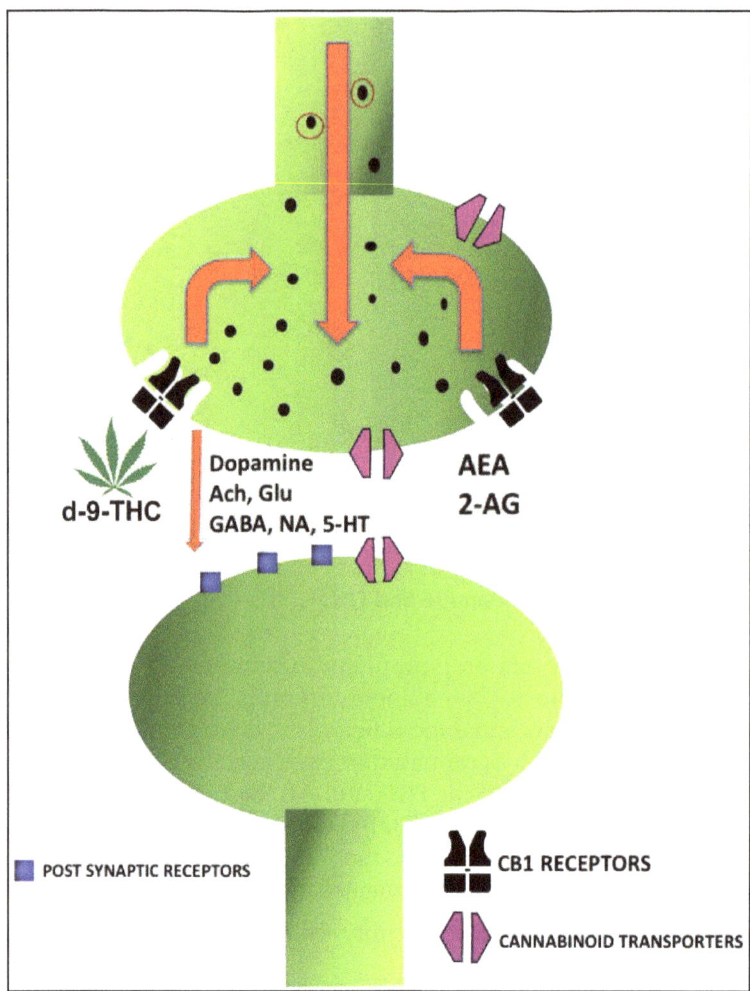

Figure 14.3: CB1 Receptors: Effects of Endocannabinoids and d-9-THC Release of Anandamide (AEA) and 2- arachidonoylglycerol (2-AG) to inhibit glutamate (Glu), Gamma-aminobutyric acid (GABA), acetylcholine (Ach), dopamine, noradrenaline (NA) and serotonin (5-HT)[27].

normally modulated by endocannabinoids such as AEA and 2-AG. It is considered that it may also increase the release of dopamine, glutamate and acetylcholine in certain brain regions, by inhibiting the release of an inhibitory neurotransmitter like GABA onto dopamine, glutamate or acetylcholine-releasing neurons[27] (Figure 14.3)

Pharmacology and Therapeutic Use of Marijuana Plant

According to researcher, marijuana medications is to be consumed in purified chemicals that are derived directly from or based on those in the marijuana plant, to be more promising therapeutically rather than using the whole marijuana plant or its crude extracts[20]. Some of the therapeutic uses of marijuana is shown below[28]:

Clinical Conditions with Symptoms that may be Relieved by Treatment with Marijuana or Other Cannabinoids[28]

Glaucoma

Early evidence of the benefits of marijuana in patients with glaucoma (a disease associated with increased pressure in the eye) may be consistent with its ability to affect a transient decrease in intraocular pressure[29,30], but other, standard treatments are currently more effective. THC, cannabinol, and nabilone (a synthetic cannabinoid like THC), but not cannabidiol, were shown to lower intraocular pressure in rabbits[31,32]. More research is needed to establish whether molecules that modulate the endocannabinoid system may not only reduce intraocular pressure but also provide a neuroprotective benefit in patients with glaucoma[33].

Nausea

Treatment of the nausea and vomiting associated with chemotherapy was one of the first medical uses of THC and other cannabinoids[34]. THC is an effective antiemetic agent in patients undergoing chemotherapy,[35] but patients often state that marijuana is more effective in suppressing nausea. Other, unidentified compounds in marijuana may enhance the effect of THC (as appears to be the case with THC and cannabidiol, which operate through different antiemetic mechanisms)[36]. Paradoxically, increased vomiting (hyperemesis) has been reported with repeated marijuana use.

AIDS-Associated Anorexia and Wasting Syndrome

Reports have indicated that smoked or ingested cannabis improves appetite and leads to weight gain and improved mood and quality of life among patients with AIDS[37]. However, there is no long-term or rigorous evidence of a sustained effect of cannabis on AIDS-related morbidity and mortality, with an acceptable safety profile, that would justify its incorporation into current clinical practice for patients who are receiving effective antiretroviral therapy[38]. Data from the few studies that have explored the potential therapeutic value of cannabinoids for this patient population are inconclusive[38].

Chronic Pain

Marijuana has been used to relieve pain for centuries. Studies have shown that cannabinoids acting through central CB1 receptors, and possibly peripheral CB1 and CB2 receptors[39], play important roles in modelling nociceptive responses in various models of pain. These findings are consistent with reports that marijuana may be effective in ameliorating neuropathic pain[40,41], even at very low levels of THC (1.29 per cent)[42]. Both marijuana and dronabinol, a pharmaceutical formulation of THC, decrease pain, but dronabinol may lead to longer-lasting reductions in pain sensitivity and lower ratings of rewarding effects[43].

Inflammation

Cannabinoids (*e.g.*, THC and cannabidiol) have substantial anti-inflammatory effects because of their ability to induce apoptosis, inhibit cell proliferation, and suppress cytokine production.[44] Cannabidiol has attracted particular interest as an anti-inflammatory agent because of its lack of psychoactive effects.[34] Animal models have shown that cannabidiol is a promising candidate for the treatment of rheumatoid arthritis[34] and for inflammatory diseases of the gastrointestinal tract (*e.g.*, ulcerative colitis and Crohn's disease) [45].

Multiple Sclerosis

Nabiximols (Sativex, GW Pharmaceuticals), an oromucosal spray that delivers a mix of THC and cannabidiol, appears to be an effective treatment for neuropathic pain, disturbed sleep, and spasticity in patients with multiple sclerosis. Sativex is available in the United Kingdom, Canada, and several other countries,[46,47] and is currently being reviewed in phase 3 trials in the United States to gain approval from the Food and Drug Administration.

Epilepsy

In a recent small survey of parents who use marijuana with a high cannabidiol content to treat epileptic seizures in their children[48], 11 per cent (2 families out of the 19 that met the inclusion criteria) reported complete freedom from seizures, 42 per cent (8 families) reported a reduction of more than 80 per cent in seizure frequency, and 32 per cent (6 families) reported a reduction of 25 to 60 per cent in seizure frequency. Although such reports are promising, insufficient safety and efficacy data are available on the use of cannabis botanicals for the treatment of epilepsy. [49] However, there is increasing evidence of the role of cannabidiol as an antiepileptic agent in animal models[50].

Pharmaceutical Drugs with Chemicals from Marijuana Plant

Many controversies have been revolving surrounding issues like legal, ethical, and social implications associated with use; safety administration, packaging and dispensing; adverse health consequences and deaths attributed to marijuana intoxication and therapeutic efficiency based on limited clinical data shows complexities in transitioning marijuana from a vilified substance to a therapeutic one.

Cannabis, or marijuana, was first used for medicinal purposes in 2737 B.C[51,52]. In 1851, it was initially classified as legitimate medical compound[53]. However, after criminalization in the United States in 1940-1942 by American Medical Association and bearing the schedule I drug status, patients have continued to consume botanical cannabis for medical purposes through state-wide programs and cannabis dispensaries, which are facilities or locations where medical cannabis is made available for qualified patients. Several types of cannabinoid medicines are available in the United States and Canada. Two types of cannabinoid medicines are used in North America:[54,55]

1. Cannabis-derived pharmaceutical: which include dronabinol (schedule III), nabilone (schedule II), and nabiximols (not approved by the U.S. Food and Drug Administration [FDA]) [54,55]
2. Phytocannabinoid-dense botanicals (*i.e.*, medical cannabis or marijuana): which include the schedule I medicinal plants *Cannabis sativa* or *Cannabis indica*[54,55]

Some of the medicines containing compounds from the Cannabis or compounds similar to that are listed below along with their worldwide acceptance figure:

I. Dronabinol: [54,55,56]

Manufacturer: Unimed Pharmaceuticals, a subsidiary of Solvay Pharmaceuticals

Medicinal use: treatment of nausea and vomiting associated with cancer chemotherapy in patients who have failed to respond adequately to conventional antiemetic therapy; treatment of anorexia associated with weight loss in patients with acquired immune deficiency syndrome[54,55]; analgesic to ease neuropathic pain in multiple sclerosis patients.[56]

Approval status: FDA approved in United States as Schedule I drug for appetite stimulation (1992) and for nausea (1985); moved to Schedule III effective July 2, 1999. Approved in Denmark for multiple sclerosis (Sep. 2003). Approved in Canada for AIDS-related anorexia (Apr. 2000) and for nausea and vomiting associated with cancer chemotherapy (1988)

II. Nabilone: [54,55,56]

Manufacturer: Valeant Pharmaceuticals International (VRX on NASDAQ)

Medicinal use: Treatment of nausea and vomiting in patients undergoing cancer treatment. In 2006, nabilone is formulated from two strains of *Cannabis sativa* into an oromucosal spray for three indications such as symptomatic relief of spasticity in adults with multiple sclerosis who have not responded adequately to other therapy and who demonstrate meaningful improvement during an initial trial of therapy, symptomatic relief of neuropathic pain in patients with multiple sclerosis, intractable cancer pain

Approval status: Originally approved by the FDA for use in the US in 1985, but removed from the market until re-approved by the FDA on May 15, 2006 and made available in US pharmacies on Aug. 17, 2006. Also approved in United Kingdom and Australia (1982), Canada (1981), and Mexico (2007)

III. Sativex: [54,55,56]

Manufacturer: GW Pharmaceuticals (GWPH on NASDAQ)

Medicinal use: Treatment of neuropathic pain and spasticity in patients with Multiple Sclerosis (MS); Analgesic treatment in adult patients with advanced cancer who experience moderate to severe pain

Approval status: Approved and launched in the UK on June 21, 2010, making it the first cannabis-based prescription medicine in the world (rescheduled from UK Schedule 1 to Schedule 4 on Apr. 10, 2013). Licensed to Bayer in the UK and to Almirall in Europe. Approved to treat spasticity caused by multiple sclerosis in Spain (July 28, 2010), Canada (Aug. 31, 2010), Czech Republic (Apr. 15, 2011), Denmark (June 8, 2011), Germany (July 4, 2011), Sweden (Dec. 22, 2011), Austria (Feb. 7, 2012), Italy (May 7, 2013), and Switzerland (Nov. 27, 2013). Also approved in Finland, Israel, Norway, and Poland[56].

Several other drugs such as dexanabinol, CT-3 (ajulemic acid), Cannabinor (formerly PRS-211,375), HU 308, HU 331, Rimonabant/Acomplia, Taranabant/ MK-0364 have been manufactured but are not approved for use outside research laboratory[56]. Developing drugs from botanical plants possess much greater difficulties as they contain various unknown active chemicals and it is difficult to decide accurate dosage of a newly developed medicine/product.

Adverse Effect of Consuming Marijuana

When consumed Cannabis has psychoactive and physiological effects[20]. The effects from consuming marijuana include relaxation and stoned, a general alteration of conscious perception, increased awareness of sensation, increased libido[57] and distortions in the perception of time and space. General effect from both long term and short term are listed below:

Effects of Short-term Use

1. Include reddening of eye, increased heart rate, increased appetite. These effects usually abate after six hours however in heavy smoker the symptoms may remain till six days[28,59]
2. Impaired short-term memory, making it difficult to learn and to retain information. Impaired motor coordination, interfering with driving skills and increasing the risk of injuries[28]
3. Altered judgment, increasing the risk of sexual behaviours that facilitate the transmission of sexually transmitted diseases[28]

Effects of Long-term or Heavy Use

1. Addiction (in about 9 per cent of users overall, 17 per cent of those who begin use in adolescence, and 25 to 50 per cent of those who are daily users)[28]
2. Effects can include altered body image, auditory and/or visual illusions, pseudo hallucinations and ataxia from selective impairment of polysynaptic reflexes. In some cases, cannabis can lead to dissociative states such as depersonalization[58] and derealization
3. In adolescence, altered brain development, poor educational outcome, with increased likelihood of dropping out of school, cognitive impairment, with lower IQ among those who were frequent users during adolescence, diminished life satisfaction and achievement[28]
4. Long term exposure to marijuana may have biologically-based physical, mental behavioural and social health consequences and may be associated with diseases of the liver (particularly hepatitis C), lungs, heart, and vasculature[59]
5. Symptoms of chronic bronchitis: Increased risk of chronic psychosis disorders (including schizophrenia) in persons with a predisposition to such disorders

However, medicinal cannabis may similarly pose health risks associated with its use, including psychoactive, intoxicating, and impairing effects, which have not been completely elucidated through clinical trials. Nevertheless, a growing number of states have legalized dispensing of marijuana or its extracts to people with a range of medical conditions.

Conclusion

The literature suggest that Cannabis may have several medicinal uses. Regardless of such literature studies published worldwide, there is still uncertainty about the promising nature of the plant because of limited clinical research based on long term usage of subjects. No proper universal conclusion has been derived till date as major potential of the psychoactive compounds (THC and CBD) present in these plants are yet undiscovered. The main barrier for this is, Cannabis is defined as a schedule 1 drug. Hence restricting this factor an open and safe research in depth should be carried on with the various active compounds present in the Cannabis (especially THC and CBD). The biochemical and therapeutic property of the two-main psychoactive compound should be studies and researched properly before coming to any conclusion. If obtained with positive and accurate results, the Cannabis plant should be considered in medicinal use.

References

1. phytochemical and biological research of cannabis pharmaceutical resources. Da Cheng Hao, Pei Gen Xiao, in Medicinal Plants, 2015
2. Drug Enforcement Administration Office of Diversion Control. Schedules of controlled substances. (b) Placement on schedules; findings required. (1) Schedule I. Springfield, Virginia: U.S. Department of Justice; 1970. Title 21 United States Code (USC) Controlled Substances Act. Subchapter I–Control and enforcement Part B–Authority to control; standards of controlled substances §812. [also known as Controlled Substances Act, 21 United States Code § 812(b) (1), 1970].
3. World Health Organization. Management of substance abuse: cannabis. 2016. [Accessed February 15, 2018]. Available at: www.who.int/substance_abuse/facts/cannabis/en.2016.
4. *Karl W. Hillig; Paul G. Mahlberg (2004). "A chemotaxonomic analysis of cannabinoid variation in Cannabis (Cannabaceae)"*. American Journal of Botany. *91 (6): 966–975.* doi:10.3732/ajb.91.6.966. PMID 21653452.
5. 5. Zuardi AW. History of cannabis as a medicine: A review. Rev Bras Psiquiatr. 2006; 28 (2):153-157
6. 4. Doyle E, Spence AA. Cannabis as a medicine? Br J Anaesth. 1995;74(4):359-361.
7. World Health Organization. Management of substance abuse: cannabis. 2016. [. [Accessed February 15, 2018]. Available at: www.who.int/substance_abuse/facts/cannabis/en

8. Office of National Drug Control Policy. Answers to frequently asked questions about marijuana. [Accessed February 15, 2018]. Available at: https://obamawhitehouse.archives.gov/ondcp/frequently-asked-questions-and-facts-about-marijuana

9. *Small E, Marcus D. Hemp: a new crop with new uses for North America. In: Janick J, Whipkey A, eds. Trends in New Crops and New Uses. Alexandria, VA: ASHS Press; 2002:284-326*

10. Malmo-Levine D. Recent history. In: Holland J, editor. The Pot Book: A Complete Guide to Cannabis. Rochester, Vermont: Park Street Press; 2010.

11. The Marihuana Tax Act of 1937. Musto DF, Arch Gen Psychiatry. 1972 Feb; 26(2):101-8.

12. Giancaspro GI, Kim N-C, Venema J, *et al.*, The advisability and feasibility of developing USP standards for medical cannabis. U.S. Pharmacopeial Convention; [Accessed February 16, 2018]. Available at: http://flboardofmedicine.gov/forms/usp-standards-cannabis.pdf

13. Cameron JM, Dillinger RJ. Narcotic Control Act. In: Kleiman MAR, Hawdon JE, editors. Encyclopedia of Drug Policy. Thousand Oaks, California: SAGE Publications, Inc; 2011. pp. 543–545.

14. Drug Enforcement Administration Office of Diversion Control. Schedules of controlled substances. (b) Placement on schedules; findings required. (1) Schedule I. Springfield, Virginia: U.S. Department of Justice; 1970. [Accessed February 16, 2018]. Title 21 United States Code (USC) Controlled Substances Act. Subchapter I–Control and enforcement Part B–Authority to control; standards of controlled substances §812. [also known as Controlled Substances Act, 21 United States Code § 812(b)(1), 1970]. Available at: https://www.deadiversion.usdoj.gov/21cfr/21usc/812

15. Swift A. Support for legal marijuana use up to 60 per cent in U.S. Oct 19, 2016. [Accessed February 16, 2018]. Available at: www.gallup.com/poll/196550/support-legalmarijuana.aspx

16. National Conference of State Legislatures. State medical marijuana laws. Nov 9, 2016. [Accessed February 17, 2018]. Available at: ncsl.org/research/health/state-medical-marijuana-laws.aspx

17. *India's cannabis economy has a new hope—Patanjali. [Accessed February 17, 2018] Available at:* https://qz.com/1191203/patanjali-the-indian-cannabis-economys-new-hope/

18. *Weed Energy: Baba Ramdev's Patanjali Wants Marijuana Legal in India! [Accessed February 17, 2018] Available at:* https://www.indiatimes.com/news/india/weed-energy-baba-ramdev-s-patanjali-wants-marijuana-legal-in-india-339252.html

19. The inheritance of chemical phenotype in Cannabis sativa L. (Cannabinoid pharmacology. Dewey WL, Pharmacol Rev. 1986 Jun; 38(2):151-78.) de Meijer EP, Bagatta M, Carboni A, Crucitti P, Moliterni VM, Ranalli P, Mandolino G. Genetics. 2003 Jan; 163(1):335-46)

20. *How does marijuana produce its effect? National institute of drug abuse. [Accessed February 17, 2018] Available at:* https://www.drugabuse.gov/publications/research-reports/marijuana/how-does-marijuana-produce-its-effects

21. Emmanuel S Onaivi; Takayuki Sugiura; Vincenzo Di Marzo (2005). Endocannabinoids: The Brain and Body's Marijuana and Beyond. Taylor and Francis. p. 58. ISBN 978-0-415-30008-7. Gordon AJ, Conley JW, Gordon JM. "Medical consequences of marijuana use: a review of current literature". Curr Psychiatry Rep. 15 (12): 419. doi:10.1007/s11920-013-0419-7. PMID 24234874.

22. McPartland JM, Duncan M, Di Marzo V, *et al.*, Are cannabidiol and Δ9-tetrahydrocannabivarin negative modulators of the endocannabinoid system? A systematic review. Br J Pharmacol. 2014; 172:737–753.

23. Graham ES, Ashton JC, Glass M (2009). "Cannabinoid receptors: a brief history and "what's hot"". Front. Biosci. 14 (14): 944–57. doi:10.2741/3288. PMID 19273110.]

24. Mackie K (May 2008). "Cannabinoid receptors: where they are and what they do". J. Neuroendocrinol. 20 Suppl 1: 10–4. doi:10.1111/j.1365-2826.2008. 01671.x. PMID 18426493

25. Matsuda LA, Lolait SJ, Brownstein MJ, Young AC, Bonner TI (1990). "Structure of a cannabinoid receptor and functional expression of the cloned cDNA". Nature. 346 (6284): 561–4. doi:10.1038/346561a0. PMID 2165569

26. A tale of two cannabinoids: the therapeutic rationale for combining tetrahydrocannabinol and cannabidiol. Russo E, Guy GWMed Hypotheses. 2006; 66(2):234-46

27. The pharmacology of cannabinoid receptors and their ligands: an overview. Pertwee RG Int J Obes (Lond). 2006 Apr; 30 Suppl 1(): S13-8

28. Nora D. Volkow, M.D., Ruben D. Baler, Ph.D., Wilson M. Compton, M.D., and Susan R.B. Weiss, Ph.D. Adverse Health Effects of Marijuana Use. N Engl J Med. 2014 Jun 5; 370(23): 2219–2227. doi: 10.1056/NEJMra1402309

29. Merritt JC, Crawford WJ, Alexander PC, Anduze AL, Gelbart SS. Effect of marihuana on intraocular and blood pressure in glaucoma. Ophthalmology 1980; 87:2228.

30. Hepler RS, Frank IR. Marihuana smoking and intraocular pressure. JAMA 1971; 217:1392

31. Chen J, Macias J, Dinh T, *et al.*, Finding of endocannabinoids in human eye tissues: implications for glaucoma. Biochem Biophys Res Commun 2005; 330:1062-7

32. Song ZH, Slowey CA. Involvement of cannabinoid receptors in the intraocular pressure-lowering effects ofWIN55212,,2. J Pharmacol Exp Ther 2009; 292:136-9

33. Nucci C, Bari M, Spanö A, *et al.*, Potential roles of (endo) cannabinoids in the treatment of glaucoma: from intraocular pressure control to neuroprotection. Prog Brain Res 2008:17

34. Zuardi AW. Cannabidiol: from an inactive cannabinoid to a drug with wide spectrum of action. Rev Bras Psiquiatr 2008; 30:271-80

35. Sallan SE, Zinberg NE, Frei E Ill. Antiemetic effect of delta-^{C}D-tetrahydrocannabinol in patients receiving cancer chemotherapy. N Engl J Med 1975; 293:795-7

36. Parker LA, Kwiatkowska M, Burton P, Mechoulam R. Effect of cannabinoids on lithium-induced vomiting in the Suncus murinus (house musk shrew). Psychopharmacology (Berl) 2004; 171:156-61

37. D'Souza G, Matson PA, Grady CD, *et al.*, Medicinal and recreational marijuana use among HIV-infected women in the Women's Interagency HIV Study (W IHS) cohort, J Acquir Immune Defic syndr

38. Lutge IEE, Gray A, Siegfried N. The medical use of cannabis fijr reducing morbiclity and mortality in patients with HIV/AIDS. Cochrane Database Syst Rev 2013; 4:CD005175

39. Chiou LC, Hu SS, Ho YC. Targeting the cannabinoid systern for pain relief? Acta Anaesthcsiof Taiwan 2013; 51:161-70

40. Wilsey B, Marcotte T, Tsodikov A, *et al.*, A randomized, placebo-controlled, crossover trial of cannabis cigarettes in neuropathic pain. J Pain 2008; 9:506-21. 65

41. Wallace M, Schulteis G, Atkinson JH, *et al.*, Dose-dependent effects of smoked cannabis on capsaicin-induced pain and hyperalgesia in healthy volunteers. Anesthesiology

42. Wilsey B, Marcotte T, Deutsch R, Gouaux B, Sakai S, Donaghe H. Low-dose vaporized cannabis significantly improves neuropathic pain. J Pain 2013; 14:136-48. 67

43. Cooper ZD, Comer SD, Haney M. Comparison of the analgesic effects of dronabinol and smoked marijuana in daily marijuana smokers. Neuropsychopharmacology 2013;38

44. Nagarkatti P, Pandey R, Rieder SA, Hegde V L, Nagarkae-i 1M. Cannabinoids as novel anti-inflammatory drugs. Future Med Chem 2009; 1:1333-49

45. Esposito G, Filippis DD, Cirilio C, *et al.*, Cannabidiol in inflammatory bowel diseases: a brief overview. Phytother Res

46. Collin C, Davies P, Mutibol<0 1K, Rat^{e}cliffe S. Randomized controlled trial of cannabis-based medicine in spasticity caused by multiple sclerosis. Eur J 2007; 14:290-6.

47. Centonze D, Mori F, Koch G, *et al.*, Lack of effect of cannabis-based treatment on clinical and laboratory measures in multiple sclerosis. Neurol Sci 2009:30

48. Porter BE, Jacobson C. Report of a parent survey of cannabidiol-enriched cannabis use in pediatric treatment-resistant epilepsy. Epilepsy Behav 2013; 29:574-7

49. Rogan NM, Mechoulam R. Cannabinoids in health and disease. Dialogues Clin Neurosci 2007; 9:413-30

50. Hill TD, Cascio MG, Romano B, al. Cannabidivarin-rich cannabis extracts are anticonvulsant in mouse and rat via a CBI receptor-independent mechanism. Br J Pharmacol2013:17

51. Hi HL. An archaeological and historical account of cannabis in China. Econ Bot 1974; 28:437–48

52. Aggarwal SK, Carter GT, Sullivan MD, ZumBrunnen C, Morrill R, Mayer JD. Medicinal use of cannabis in the United States: historical perspectives, current trends, and future directions. J Opioid Manag 2009; 5:153–68

53. Extractum cannabis. In: The pharmacopoeia of the United States of America, 3rd ed. Philadelphia: Lippincott, Grambo and Co., 1851

54. Cesamet (nabilone) package insert. Meda Pharmaceuticals, 2009. [Accessed march 20, 2018] Available from https://www.cesamet.com/pdf/Cesamet_PI_50_count.pdf

55. Marinol (dronabinol): package insert. Unimed Pharmaceuticals, Inc., September 2004. [Accessed February 20,2018] Available at: https://www.accessdata.fda.gov/drugsatfda_docs/label/2005/018651s021lbl.pdf

56. 10 Pharmaceutical Drugs Based on Cannabis. [Accessed march 20, 2018] Available at https://medicalmarijuana.procon.org/view.resource.php?resourceID=000883

57. Emmanuel S Onaivi; Takayuki Sugiura; Vincenzo Di Marzo (2005). Endocannabinoids: The Brain and Body's Marijuana and Beyond. Taylor and Francis. p. 58. ISBN 978-0-415-30008-7

58. Short term effects of cannabis. Available at http://www.self.gutenberg.org/articles/Short-term_effects_of_cannabis [Accessed march 20, 2018]

59. hufman, E; Lerner, A; Witztum, E (2005). "Depersonalization after withdrawal from cannabis usage" (PDF). Harefuah (in Hebrew). 144 (4): 249–51, 303. PMID 15889607.

60. Graham ES, Ashton JC, Glass M (2009). "Cannabinoid receptors: a brief history and "what's hot"". Front. Biosci. 14 (14): 944–57. doi:10.2741/3288. PMID 19273110.]

61. Mackie K (May 2008). "Cannabinoid receptors: where they are and what they do". J. Neuroendocrinol. 20 Suppl 1: 10–4. doi:10.1111/j.1365-2826.2008. 01671.x. PMID 18426493

62. Matsuda LA, Lolait SJ, Brownstein MJ, Young AC, Bonner TI (1990). "Structure of a cannabinoid receptor and functional expression of the cloned cDNA". Nature. 346 (6284): 561–4. doi:10.1038/346561a0. PMID 2165569

63. A tale of two cannabinoids: the therapeutic rationale for combining tetrahydrocannabinol and cannabidiol. Russo E, Guy GWMed Hypotheses. 2006; 66(2):234-46

64. The pharmacology of cannabinoid receptors and their ligands: an overview. Pertwee RG Int J Obes (Lond). 2006 Apr; 30 Suppl 1(): S13-8

65. Hi HL. An archaeological and historical account of cannabis in China. Econ Bot 1974;28:437–48

66. Aggarwal SK, Carter GT, Sullivan MD, ZumBrunnen C, Morrill R, Mayer JD. Medicinal use of cannabis in the United States: historical perspectives, current trends, and future directions. J Opioid Manag 2009;5:153–68

67. Extractum cannabis. In: The pharmacopoeia of the United States of America, 3rd ed. Philadelphia: Lippincott, Grambo and Co., 1851

68. Imaging the neural effects of cannabinoids: current status and future opportunities for psychopharmacology. Bhattacharyya S, Crippa JA, Martin-Santos R, Winton-Brown T, Fusar-Poli P, Curr Pharm Des. 2009; 15(22):2603-14.

69. Kriese U, Schumann E, Weber WE, Beyer M, Brühl L, Matthäus B. Oil content, tocopherol composition and fatty acid patterns of the seeds of 51 Cannabis sativa L. genotypes. Euphytica. 2004;137(3):339-351

70. Small E, Marcus D. Hemp: a new crop with new uses for North America. In: Janick J, Whipkey A, eds. Trends in New Crops and New Uses. Alexandria, VA: ASHS Press; 2002:284-326

71. Ranalli P, Di Candilo M, Mandolino G, Grassi G, Carboni A. Hemp for sustainable agricultural systems. Agro Food Ind Hi Tech. 1999;10(2):33-38.

72. Kalant H. Medicinal use of cannabis: history and current status. Pain Res Manag. 2001 Summer; 6(2):80-91

73. Baron EP. Headache. Comprehensive Review of Medicinal Marijuana, Cannabinoids, and Therapeutic Implications in Medicine and Headache: What a Long Strange Trip It's Been 2015 Jun;55(6):885-916. doi: 10.1111/head.12570. Epub 2015 May 25

74. Grotenhermen F. Pharmacokinetics and pharmacodynamics of cannabinoids. Clin Pharmacokinet. 2003;42(4):327-60

75. Ther Adv Psychopharmacol. 2012 Dec; 2(6): 241–254. Cannabis, a complex plant: different compounds and different effects on individuals. Zerrin Atakan

76. Nora D. Volkow, M.D., Ruben D. Baler, Ph.D., Wilson M. Compton, M.D., and Susan R.B. Weiss, Ph.D. Adverse Health Effects of Marijuana Use. N Engl J Med. 2014 Jun 5; 370(23): 2219–2227. doi: 10.1056/NEJMra1402309

Chapter 15

An Efficient Protocol for Increased Fosmid Transformation in Preparation of Metagenomic Gene Bank

Verruchi Gupta, Sonam Nain, Shafaq Rasool, V. Verma

[1]School of Biotechnology, Shri Mata Vaishno Devi University, Katra (J&K), India
[2]Microbial Biotechnology and Genomics Unit, CSIR-Institute of Genomics and Integrative Biology, Mathura Road, New Delhi, India
e-mail: verma211@gmail.com

ABSTRACT

Objective: To increase transformation efficiency of recombinant Fosmid by using it as a cloning vector for the preparation of Metagenomic gene banks.

Results: Metagenomic DNA was isolated from the soil collected from Glacier of Northern Western Himalayas of J and K state and Metagenomic gene bank was constructed by modifying the standard protocol using pCC2FOS as a vector. Restriction digestion of the recombinant Fosmid showed an average insert size of ~45kb. The transformation efficiency was calculated to be 10^{11} cfu/ml using 1 µg of metagenomic DNA. Besides, the protocol was helpful in saving processing time up to 48 hours compared to earlier reported methods.

Conclusions: This paper describes an efficient protocol for obtaining increased transformation efficiency for construction of Fosmid metagenomic gene bank.

***Keywords**: Fosmid vector, Cloning, Metagenomics, Transformation.*

Introduction

Fosmid libraries have demonstrated their utility for a number of applications which include filling gaps between BACs and small insert libraries in detecting insertions, deletions, and rearrangements in structural variation studies (Tuzun *et al.*, 2005). A Fosmid cloning system employs a low-copy number cosmid vector based on the *Escherichia coli* (*E.coli*) F-factor replicon and provides a method for preparing genomic bank with an average insert size of 40 kb with high efficiency (Kim *et al.*, 1995). The Fosmid vector offers many advantages over other genomic library systems, including ease of handling and propagation of clones, stability of the insert DNA, and unbiased cloning (Liu *et al.*, 2016). The Fosmid system offers advantages over other genomic libraries and has been widely used in metagenomic research (Lee *et al.*, 2014; Lu *et al.*, 2014), genome sequencing (Li *et al.*, 2013; Oshiki *et al.*, 2015), and other applications.

It is now widely accepted that as much as 95 per cent of the microorganisms present in nature are not cultivable by the standard techniques but the exploitation of this genetic reservoir has now been made possible by advances in our ability to recover significantly more genetic information from environmental samples in a culture- independent manner called metagenomics (Handelsman 2004). Metagenomics is defined by revolutionary approaches in the modern microbial ecology to the genomic analysis of microbial communities that are present in samples taken from the environment (Handelsman 2004). Total community DNA extraction technology is giving researchers access to the genomes of previously "unculturable" microorganisms, the result of which is insight into microbial ecology and greater access to potentially novel genes through the adaptation of classical molecular biology techniques on a metagenomic DNA scale (Handelsman 2004).

In the present communication we report a modified protocol for construction of metagenomic Fosmid library by modifying the method of Copycontrol ™ HTP Fosmid Library Production kit (Epicenter, Madison, Wisconsin) protocol using soil samples collected from the Glacier of Northern Western Himalayas of J and K state. The manufacturer's protocol has been modified and optimised for the construction of Fosmid metagenomic library with high transformation frequency. This Fosmid metagenomic gene bank is being used for harnessing novel genes encoding enzymes of industrial/pharmaceutical importance. As these environmental samples harbour non-culturable microorganisms cloning of these genes is of great importance.

Material and Methods

Sample Collection

The soil sample was collected from Glacier of Northern Western Himalayas of J and K state, India. The temperature of the glacier was -20°C. The height of the glacier is 4,700 metres above sea level. The longitude and latitude of the Glacier is 34° 92 493 N, 75° 192 493 Ehttps://tools.wmflabs.org/geohack/geohack.php?pagename=Apharwat_Peak and params=33.9995402_N_74.325517_E_type:mountain_scale:100000_. The soil is moist and collected in sterile bags. The sample was carried in sterile bags to the institute.

Preparation of Soil Metagenome

Total soil DNA was extracted using ultrapure ultraclean Megaprep., soil DNA kit (Mobio Laboratory U.S.A) as per the manufacturer's instructions and then precipitated overnight with 5M NaCl and ethanol at -20°C. The sample was centrifuged at 13,500×g for 30 min. The pellet was washed with 70 per cent ethanol twice by centrifuging at 13,500×g for 10 min. The pellet was air dried, dissolved in

1× TE and analysed on 0.8 per cent agarose gel.

Construction of Soil Metagenomic Library with the Modified Protocol

Copycontrol ™ HTP Fosmid Library Production kit (Epicenter, Madison, Wisconsin) was used for the construction of metagenomic library using manufacturer's instructions with some modifications in the described protocol. The different steps involved in the modified protocol for the preparation includes purification of DNA using β- agarase method, end-repairing, ligation of the blunt-ended DNA, and pCC2FOS™ vector, *in vitro* packaging and infection of EPI300™-T1R. Transformants were grown for 12hr at 37°C on LB agar plates containing 12.5μg/ml chloroamphenicol. The transformants were subsequently checked for the quality of library by looking for the vector and insert DNA.

The detailed modified protocol for the construction of Fosmid metagenomic library using Copycontrol ™ HTP Fosmid Library Production kit (Epicenter, Madison, Wisconsin) is described below.

After the metagenomic DNA was isolated, it was purified using β-agarase method in which the isolated metagenomic DNA was checked on 0.8 per cent agarose gel against a molecular weight ladder for the concentration of DNA. The metagenomic DNA was run on 1 per cent Low Melting Point (LMP) agarose gel (Merck) without EtBr overnight at 35 V/cm. The DNA fragments from 30-40 kb were excised from the gel with the help of a scalpel. The agarose gel containing DNA fragments was incubated at 70°C till the gel completely dissolves in water bath (Dry bath). β-agarase enzyme (NEB 10 U/μl) was added to the eppendorff and incubated at 42° C for 2 hours. The sample was centrifuged at 13,500×g for 10 min. An aliquot of 5 M ammonium acetate; (pH 7) was added to make a final concentration of 2.5 M and the contents were incubated in ice for 10 min. The sample was centrifuged at 13,500×g for 10 min and the supernatant was recovered with the help of a pipette. 0.1 volume of 3 M sodium acetate and double the volume of chilled ethanol were added for DNA precipitation. The mixture was incubated at -20°C overnight. The sample was centrifuged at 13,500×g for 20 min. and the pellet was washed twice with 70 per cent ethanol. The air dried pellet was dissolved in an appropriate amount of 1× TE (Tris- EDTA). The eluted DNA was checked on 0.8 per cent agarose gel along with lambda DNA *Hind*III digested marker and the Fosmid control DNA. The insert DNA was then End–repaired to generate blunt ended, 5′-phosphorylated DNA following the steps by mixing the reagents in the sequence and complete reaction of 200 μl AMQ water, 10 × End repair buffer, 2.5 mM dNTP's, 10 mM ATPs, Genomic DNA, and End-repair Enzyme mix. The tubes were incubated at room temperature for 45 min and in order to inactivate the End repair enzyme mix the reaction was subsequently incubated at 70°C for 10 min.

The sample along with Green view DNA dye (Agilent) and Fosmid control DNA and lambda DNA mix was then run for size selection of End- repaired insert DNA on 1 per cent LMP Agarose and the gel was run overnight at 30-35 V/cm. The fragments of required size were excised from LMP agarose gel and purified using β-agarase method (as described in purification of DNA step). DNA was then eluted in 40 μl 1× TE buffer. The ligation reaction includes insert DNA (250 ng), pCC2FOS vector, AMQ water, 10 mM ATP, Ligase Buffer, and Fast DNA ligase enzyme and a total reaction of 10 µl. First, insert DNA and pCC2FOS vector was added and the mixture was incubated at 42°C for 2 min and kept it on ice for 2 min. Later, ATP, Ligase buffer, enzyme were added. The reaction was carried out at 16°C for overnight.

Preparation of Competent Cells

E.coli EPI300 cells were streaked on an LB agar plate without any antibiotic and incubated at 37°C overnight incubation. A single colony of *E.coli* EPI300 cells was inoculated into 5 ml LB broth and incubated at 37°C overnight. Next,50 ml LB broth with 0.2 per cent maltose and 10 mM $MgSO_4$ was inoculated with 0.5 ml of *E.coli* EPI300 cells grown overnight for the growth to reach A_{600} of 0.8 -1.0(approx. 2.5 hrs).

Packaging of Ligated DNA in Fosmid Cloning Vector pCC2FOS

One tube of Max Plax Lambda packaging extract was thawed on ice and 10 µl of ligation reaction was added into 25 µl of the packaging extract. The extract was mixed by gentle pipetting and was incubated at 30°C for 2 hours. The remaining 25 µl packaging extract was then added and incubated at 30° C for 2 hours. 1 ml of phage dilution buffer was added to the above prepared reaction and mixed gently. 25 µl of chloroform was added and mixed. The mix was stored at 4°C until further use.

Titration of the Fosmid Packaging Reaction

Serial dilutions of the packaged reaction were prepared as 1:10^1 dilution: - 20 µl undiluted phage with 180 µl PDB (Phage dilution Buffer) (10 mM Tris HCl (pH 8.3), 100 mM NaCl, 10 mM $MgCl_2$). 1:10^2 dilution: - 20 µl of 1:10^1 dilution with 180 µl PDB.1:10^3 dilution: - 20 µl of 1:10^2 dilution with 180 µl of PDB. 10 µl of each dilution was added into 100 µl of EPI300 cells which was stored at 4°C and incubated at 37°C for 1 hour. The culture was spread on LB agar plates with antibiotic. The colonies were counted and calculated for the titre of packaged phage.

Calculation

$$x = \frac{\text{No. of colonies} \times \text{dilution factor} \times 1000\mu\frac{1}{\text{ml}}}{\text{Volume of phage plated } (\mu\text{l})}$$

Where "*x*" denotes the titer of the fosmid library (cfu mL–1).

Results and Discussion

The construction of the metagenomic Fosmid library using this vector gives very high transformation rate of approx. 10^{11} cfu/ml by modifying the manufacturer's protocol. The maximum transformation efficiency reported using manufacturer's protocol is 10^5 cfu/ml (Kim *et al.*, 2003). The given protocol in the manufacturer's protocol starts with the shearing of the DNA, End repairing, Size selection, ligation and *invitro* packaging but in the modified protocol the genomic DNA is purified using β-agarase method for the selection of the correct size of DNA of 30-40kb fragment for further experimental procedures with changes in the given protocol.

The modified protocol gives increased transformation rate of Fosmid gene bank vis-a-vis existing protocols. The present strategy was designed to increase the transformation rate for the construction of metagenomic gene bank to harness the unknown genes in *E. Coli*. The recombinant Fosmid DNA was isolated from random clones and checked for the insert size which was found to be at an average of 45kb.

Survey of literature shows that earlier protocols reported for Fosmid metagenomic gene banks construction have reported maximum of 10^5 cfu/ml as maximum titration (Kim *et al.*, 2003). Magrini generated a Fosmid library representing 10-fold coverage of the *Histoplasma capsulatum* G217B genome (Magrini *et al.*, 2004). A Fosmid library for Chinese cabbage consisting of 97,536 clones with an average insert size of approximately 40 kb, corresponding to seven genome equivalents was reported (Park *et al.*, 2011). Fosmid library of Vg1 consisted of 574,000 clones with an average insert size of 36.4 kb, representing 7.9-fold coverage of the maize genome (Liu *et al.*, 2016). A gorilla Fosmid library of 261,120 independent clones was constructed and characterized for Hox A gene cluster of the gorilla genome (Kim *et al.*, 2003).

The above Fosmid metagenomic gene bank has been screened for the presence of genes encoding novel cold active enzymes like lipases, cellulases, amylases and asparaginases, and, 6 bioactivities like antimicrobial activity for *Staphylococcus aureus, Bacillus subtilis, Candida albicans*. These libraries are also being screened for anti-diabetic and anticancer activities. Cloning of these genes encoding above activities are in the process of subcloning and hyperexpression.

Conclusion

We report here construction of as many as 10^{11} cfu/ml using 1μg of metagenomic DNA isolated from Glacier soil of Northern Western Himalayas of J and K state. Looking into the literature this is the highest reported transformation using recombinant Fosmid DNA so far. Besides, it saves time up to 48 hours of processing in the protocol as compared to the published protocols. 20,000 Fosmid clones were screened for lipases, cellulases, amylases and asparaginase activities. 6 clones have been found to positive for lipase, 3 clones for cellulases, 2 clones for amylase and 2 clones for asparaginase activities. Besides, 10,000 Fosmid clones were screened for antimicrobial activity in which 11 clones show activity against *Staphylococcus aureus*, 3 show activity against *Bacillus subtilis* and 2 clones show activity against *Candida albicans*. Sequencing of the positive clones is underway to identify the desired genes and their sub-cloning and hyper-expression.

References

Handelsman J (2004) Metagenomics: application of genomics to uncultured microorganisms Microbiol Mol Biol Rev 68:669-685 doi:10.1128/mmbr.68.4.669-685.2004

Kim CG, Fujiyama A, Saitou N (2003) Construction of a gorilla fosmid library and its PCR screening system Genomics 82:571-574

Kim UJ, Shizuya H, Sainz J, Garnes J, Pulst SM, de Jong P, Simon MI (1995) Construction and utility of a human chromosome 22-specific Fosmid library Genet Anal 12:81-84

Lee CM *et al.* (2014) Screening and characterization of a novel cellulase gene from the gut microflora of Hermetia illucens using metagenomic library J Microbiol Biotechnol 24:1196-1206

Li S, Liu G, Chen Z, Wang Y, Li P, Hua J (2013) Construction and initial analysis of five Fosmid libraries of mitochondrial genomes of cotton (Gossypium) Chinese Science Bulletin 58:4608-4615 doi:10.1007/s11434-013-5962-4

Liu C, Liu X, Lei L, Guan H, Cai Y (2016) Fosmid library construction and screening for the maize mutant gene Vestigial glume 1 The Crop Journal 4:55-60 doi:http://dx.doi.org/10.1016/j.cj.2015.09.003

Lu J, Du L, Pang H, Ma G, Wei Y, Huang R (2014) Construction of a metagenomic library from hot spring soil and cloning of pullulanase gene Journal of Southern Agriculture 45:725-730

Magrini V, Warren WC, Wallis J, Goldman WE, Xu J, Mardis ER, McPherson JD (2004) Fosmid-based physical mapping of the Histoplasma capsulatum genome Genome Res 14:1603-1609 doi:10.1101/gr.2361404

Oshiki M, Shinyako-Hata K, Satoh H, Okabe S (2015) Draft Genome Sequence of an Anaerobic Ammonium-Oxidizing Bacterium, "Candidatus Brocadia sinica" Genome Announcements 3:e00267-00215 doi:10.1128/genomeA.00267-15

Park TH, Park BS, Kim JA, Hong JK, Jin M, Seol YJ, Mun JH (2011) Construction of random sheared fosmid library from Chinese cabbage and its use for Brassica rapa genome sequencing project J Genet Genomics 38:47-53 doi:10.1016/j.jcg.2010.12.002

Tuzun E *et al.* (2005) Fine-scale structural variation of the human genome Nat Genet 37:727-732 doi:10.1038/ng1562

Chapter 16

Molecular Mechanism of Drought Resistance in Plant

Abhinandan S. Patil[1], *Viralkumar B. Mandaliya*[2], *Kirankumar G. Patel*[3] *and S.A. Patil*[4]

[1]*Plant Sciences Institute, Agricultural Research Organization, Rishon Lezion, Israel*
[2]*Gujarat National Law University, Gandhinagar, Gujarat, India*
[3]*P. D. Patel Institutes of Applied Sciences, Charotar University of Science and Technology, Anand, Gujarat, India*
[4]*Deptt. of Zoology, Smt. Kasturbai Walchand College, Sangli, Maharashtra, India*
e-mail: agrilstar25@gmail.com

ABSTRACT

Despite the many genes that have been identified in association with drought stress, much of the data is descriptive, with the functions of only a few of the encoded proteins established. The production of mutants using an antisense- RNA approach is a powerful technique that should continue to elucidate certain aspects of stress tolerance, but it has been most successful only with well-characterized areas of plant metabolism. It is also difficult to devise screening procedures for useful dehydration-tolerance mutants, because of the array of processes simultaneously affected by drought. Another valuable approach may be to identify those metabolic steps that are most sensitive to drought stress (a technique used to genetically dissect salt stress in yeast). Little progress has been made with the cloning and analysis of drought-related transcription factors, although a biochemical approach and use of the recently established yeast one- and two-hybrid systems should produce new insights. The complexity of drought tolerance apparent throughout this review points to control by multiple genes, and thus the identification of quantitative-trait loci (QTLs) for drought resistance may well be an effective analytical tool. The approach has just begun to be applied to the environmental-stress responses of plants and is particularly promising considering that saturated DNA–marker maps are now available for both genetic model plants and crop plants. The use of novel approaches combining genetic, biochemical, and molecular techniques should provide exciting results in the near future.

Keywords: *Draught, Drought-related transcription factors, Resistance, Genetics and Drought biochemical.*

Introduction

Drought stress is the most common adverse environmental condition that can seriously reduce crop productivity. This is especially important in countries where crop agriculture is essentially rain-fed. Biotechnology offers a promising array of tools that may be useful in achieving drought tolerance in plants. A new approach to crop production by which crops are modified to suit the environment in which they are growing, rather than modifying the environment to meet the needs of the crop. This approach is advantageous in areas where water supplementation by irrigation is either difficult or unaffordable. Increasing crop resistance to drought stress would be the most economical approach to improve agricultural productivity and to reduce agricultural use of freshwater resources. The biological basis for drought tolerance is still largely unknown and few drought tolerance determinants have been identified (Araus *et al.*, 2002; Bruce *et al.*, 2002). Physiological and molecular biological studies have documented several plant responses to drought stress (Schroeder *et al.*, 2001). In the last decade, molecular and biochemical studies have identified many of these ABA and stress-responsive genes and increased biosynthesis of these hormone as well as the induction of drought and ABA-responsive genes and a few of the transcription factors responsible for their induction in model plants as well as crop plants (Yu and Setter, 2003; Poroyko *et al.*, 2005). Most of their gene products may function in stress response and tolerance at the cellular level. To overcome these limitations and improve crop yield under stress conditions, it is important to improve stress tolerance in crops. The responses of plants to various abiotic stresses have been important subjects of physiological studies (Levitt, 1980) and, more recently, of molecular and transgenic studies (Zhang *et al.*, 2000). The identification of novel genes, determination of their expression patterns in response to the stresses, and an improved understanding of their functions in stress adaptation will provide us the basis of effective engineering strategies to improve stress tolerance (Cushman and Bohnert 2000). A number of genes have been reported to be induced by drought and their products are thought to function in stress tolerance and response (Shinozaki and Yamaguchi- Shinozaki, 2000). An assortment of genes with diverse functions is induced or repressed by these stresses (Bartels and Sunkar, 2005; Yamaguchi-Shinozaki and Shinozaki 2005).Significantly, the introduction of many stress-inducible genes via gene transfer resulted in improved plant stress tolerance (Umezawa *et al.*, 2006). Now, analyzing the functions of these genes is critical to further our understanding of the molecular mechanisms governing plant stress response and tolerance, ultimately leading to enhancement of stress tolerance in crops through genetic manipulation. Several drought-inducible genes are induced by exogenous ABA treatment. Their gene products are thought to function in stress tolerance and response. Stress-inducible genes have been used to improve stress tolerance of plants by gene transfer. It is important to analyze functions of stress-inducible genes not only for the further understanding of molecular mechanisms of stress tolerance and response of higher plants but also for improvement of stress tolerance of crops by gene manipulation. Molecular studies of drought stress in plant use a variety of strategies for this a large number of genes with a potential role in drought tolerance have been discovered its a major part in the molecular biology. Control of Gene expression and understand the gene function is the main factor of this area.

Drought Reistance

It causes minimum loss of yield in a draught environment relative to the maximum yield in a constraint-free.

Type of drought resistance: draught escape, dehydration avoidance, and dehydration tolerance.

Drought Escape

Drought Escape is the situation in which drought susceptible variety performs well in a drought environment condition simply avoiding the period of drought by early maturity such type of plant has lower leaf index, lower total evaporation type features to cope of with such condition.

Dehydration Avoidance

Dehydration Avoidance is the ability of a plant to retain a relatively higher level of hydration under the condition of soil or atmosphere water stress. This can be archived either by reducing transpiration (water saver) by stomata sensitivity, osmotic adjustment, cuticular wax, ABA acid Proline, leaf rolling or increased water uptake (water spender) by the deep root system, root length density, root hydraulic resistance.

Dehydration Tolerance

Dehydration tolerance is the ability of a plant to live without water.

Genetics of Drought Resistance

The genetic control of these traits ranges from oligogenic to polygenic. Generally, leaf characters like waxy bloom, 'glossy' traits, glaucousness, glabrous leaves are under oligogenic character, ABA accumulation while in polygenic both additive and dominance gene effect involved (Table 16.1).

Gene with Up-regulated and Expressed in Response to Dehydration

Table 16.1: Genes Up-regulated by Drought Stress and Encoding Polypeptides of known Function

cDNA	*Source*	*Encoded Polypeptide*
GapC-Crat	*Caterostigma plantagineum*	*Cytosolic glyceraldehyde 3-phosphate dehydrogenase*
pSPS1	*C. plantagineum*	*Sucrose-phosphate synthase*
pSS1; pSS2	*C. plantagineum*	*Sucrose synthases 36*
pPPC1	*Mesembryanthemum crystallinum*	*Phosphoenolpyruvate carboxylase*
pBAD	*Hordeum vulgare* (barley)	Betaine aldehyde dehydrogenase
cAtP5CS	*Arabidopsis thaliana*	*d1-pyrroline-5-carboxylate synthetase*

cDNA	Source	Encoded Polypeptide
RD28	*A. thaliana*	*Water channel*
SAM1; SAM3	*Lycopersicon esculentum*	*S-adenosyl-L-methionine synthetases*
rd19A; rd21A	*A. thaliana*	*Cysteine proteases*
UBQ1	*A. thaliana*	*Ubiquitin extension protein*
pMBM1	*Triticum aestivum*	*L-isoaspartyl methyltransferase*
SC514	*Glycine max* (soybean)	*Lipoxygenase 10*
cATCDPK1; cATCDPK2	*A. thaliana*	*Ca2+-dependent, calmodulin-independent protein kinases*
PKABA1	*T. aestivum*	*Protein kinase 4*
cAtPLC1	*A. thaliana*	*Phosphatidylinositol- specific phospholipase C*
Apx1 gene	*Pisum sativum* (pea)	*Cytosolicascorbate peroxidase*
Sod 2 gene	*P. sativum*	*Cytosolic copper/zinc superoxide dismutase*
P31	*L. esculentum*	*Cytosolic copper/zinc superoxide dismutase*
pcht28	*L. chilense*	*Acidic endochitinase*
Atmyb2	*A. thaliana*	*MYB-protein-related transcription factor*
ERD11; ERD13	*A. thaliana*	*Glutathione S- transferases*
cAtsEH	*A. thaliana*	*Soluble epoxide hydrolase*

Metabolisms

Changes in primary metabolism are a general response to stress in plants some enzyme shows increased expression during drought and upon ABA treatment. Proteases may also be an important feature of stress metabolism, dispensing with redundant proteins and depolymerizing vacuolar storage polypeptides, thereby releasing amino acids for the massive synthesis of new proteins. Enzymes of sugar metabolism also play important role in tolerance there are certain sugars may be central to the protection of organisms against drought. Enzymes involved in the synthesis of other compounds that can act as compatible solutes—and whose transcript levels are clearly upregulated during drought—include dD1-pyrroline 5carboxylate synthetase (proline biosynthesis) and betaine aldehyde dehydrogenase (glycine betaine biosynthesis). The induction of the mRNA encoding phosphoenolpyruvate carboxylase in *Mesembryanthemum crystallinum* highlights the importance of Crassulacean acid metabolism in enabling carbon fixation with minimal water loss. Such metabolism is a major response in a wide variety of plants to grow in dry conditions.

Osmotic Adjustments

Total water potential can be maintained during mild drought by osmotic adjustment, which involves utilizing sugars or other compatible solutes.Both ion and water channels are likely to be important in regulating water flux, and the relevance of these channels to drought-stress has been supported by the isolation of channel protein genes expressed in response to water deficit. The 7a cDNA from pea (*Pisum sativum*) encodes a polypeptide with characteristic features of ion channels, while the RD28 cDNA (*A. thaliana*) and probably also the H2-5 cDNA (*C. plantagineum*) (J-B Mariaux and D Bartels, unpublished data) encode putative water-channel proteins.

Structural Adjustments

Drought stress has been shown to cause alterations in the chemical composition and physical properties of the cell wall (*e.g.* wall extensibility), and such changes may involve the genes encoding *S*-adenosylmethionine synthetase. Under non-stressful conditions, increased expression of *S-adenosyl- L-methionine synthetase* genes correlates with areas where lignification is occurring. Thus, the increased expression in drought-stressed tissue could thus also be due to lignification in the cell wall. Cell elongation stops under prolonged drought stress, and then lignification processes seem to begin. Fungal elicitors cause the coinduction of *S*-adenosyl-L-methionine synthetase transcript with those of other enzymes, *e.g.* *S*-adenosyl-L-homocysteine hydrolase or a methyltransferase, required for cell wall formation. The *C. plantagineum pcC37-31* cDNA encodes the dsp-protein, whose mRNA levels increase in response to various stresses. The cDNA shows significant homology to early light-inducible protein (ELIP) genes. Light is involved in the regulation of the gene expression, and the encoded dsp-22 protein is chloroplastic. ELIPs may play a role in the assembly of the photosystem (1a). During desiccation, *C. plantagineum* chloroplasts undergo morphological changes, and thus the dsp-22 protein could bind pigments or help maintain assembled photosynthetic structures essential for resuming active photosynthesis during resurrection.

Degradations and Repairs

Proteases degrade proteins irreparably damaged by the effects of drought. During an early drought in *A. thaliana,* there is an increase in levels of mRNA encoding ubiquitin extension protein, a fusion protein from which active ubiquitin is derived by proteolytic processing. This increase may be significant in terms of protein degradation because ubiquitin has a role in tagging proteins for destruction. During drought stress, protein residues may be modified by chemical processes such as deamination, isomerization, or oxidation, and it is thus likely that enzymes with functions in protein repair are upregulated in response to drought. L-isoaspartyl methyltransferases may convert modified-isoaspartyl residues in damaged proteins back to L-aspartyl residues it's a repair process. Such repair mechanisms could be particularly important during desiccation when protein turnover rates are low. The products of two drought-induced genes isolated by differential screening have sequence similarity to heat-shock proteins. These encoded proteins are probably chaperonins, involved in protein repair by helping other proteins to recover their native conformation after denaturation or misfolding during water stress. The low-molecular-weight heat-shock proteins may also be chaperonins.

Removal of Toxics

Enzymes concerned with removing toxic intermediates produced during oxygenic metabolisms, such as glutathione reductase and superoxide dismutase, increase in response to drought stress and are probably very important intolerance. Decreasing leaf water content and consequent stomatal closure result in reduced

CO_2 availability and the production of active oxygen species such as superoxide radicals. Increased photorespiratory activity during drought is also accompanied by elevated levels of glycolate-oxidase activity, resulting in H_2O_2 production. This could explain why genes encoding enzymes that detoxify active oxygen species such as ascorbate peroxidase and superoxide dismutase have been found upregulated in response to drought.

Late-Embryogenesis-Abundant Proteins

The genes encoding late-embryogenesis-abundant (LEA) proteins are consistently represented in differential screens for transcripts with increased levels during drought. LEA proteins were first described from research into genes abundantly expressed during the final desiccation stage of seed development. Circumstantial evidence for their involvement in dehydration tolerance is strong: The genes are similar to many of those expressed in vegetative tissues of drought-stressed plants, and desiccation treatments can often induce precocious expression in seeds. ABA can also induce the *lea* genes in seeds and vegetative tissues. LEA proteins appear to be located in many cell types and at variable concentrations and within the cell, they appear to be predominantly but not exclusively cytosolic. The concentrations in the cell are characteristically very high. A general structural feature of the LEA proteins is their based amino acid composition, which results in highly hydrophilic polypeptides, with just a few residues providing 20–30 per cent of their total complement.

Roles

LEA proteins can protect specific cellular structures or ameliorate the effects of drought stress, they are highly hydrophilic, proteins could help maintain the minimum cellular water requirement. A major problem under severe dehydration is that the loss of water leads to crystallization of cellular components, which in consequence damages cellular structures. This may be counteracted by LEA proteins, and some of the LEA proteins could essentially be considered compatible solutes, which supports the likely role of sugars in maintaining the structure of the cytoplasm in the absence of water

Sugars

The involvement of soluble sugars in desiccation tolerance in plants is very important for surviving. Trehalose is the most effective osmoprotectant sugar in terms of minimum concentration required. Sugar accumulation is not the only way in which plants deal with desiccation, it is considered important factor intolerance. Total water potential can be maintained during mild drought by osmotic adjustment. Sugars may serve as compatible solutes permitting such osmotic adjustment, although many other compounds usually associated with salt stress are also active, such as proline, glycine betaine, and pinitol. Increasing sucrose synthesis and sucrose-phosphate synthase activity is not only a drought-response of desiccation-tolerant plants such as *C. plantagineum* but also of plants that cannot withstand extreme drying, such as spinach.Phosphofructokinase is a tetrameric enzyme that usually dissociates irreversibly into inactive dimers during dehydration.

Regulation of Gene Expression during Drought

Expression of drought-stress genes conforms the cellular model, with a complex signal transduction cascade that can be divided into the following basic steps: (*a*) perception of stimulus; (*b*) processing, including amplification and integration of the signal; and (*c*) a response reaction in the form of de novo gene expression. No molecular data are available on the perception of drought stress, although turgor change has been suggested as a possible physical signal. An attractive model for the activation of a transduction pathway by a stress signal has been derived from studying the heat-shock response in yeast. Heat-induced activation of a particular pathway is in response to increased drought tolerance drought-activated signal transmission process has begun to be dissected at the molecular level, mostly on the basis of studies of isolated drought-responsive genes. Endogenous ABA levels have been reported to increase as a result of water deficit in many physiological studies, and therefore ABA is thought to be involved in the signal transduction. Many of the drought-related genes can be induced by exogenous ABA.

Promoter Studies

Table 16.2: *cis*-acting Promoter Elements Relevant to ABA or Drought Genes

Genes	*Elements*	*Sequences*
Rab16A (*Oryza sativa*)	ABRE (Motif I)	GT*ACGT*GGCGC
EM(*Triticum aestivum*)	Em1A	GGAC*ACGT*GGC
Hex3 (synthetic tetramer) (derived from *Nicotiana tabacum*)		GGTGACGTGGC
rab28 (*Zea mays*)	ABRE	CC*ACGT*GG
Cat (*Hordeum vulgare*)	ABRE3 and CE1	GCC*ACGT*ACA and TGCCACCGG

Treatment with ABA can also induce these changes. The best-characterized *cis*-element in the context of drought stress is the ABA-responsive element (ABRE), which contains the palindromic motif CACGTG with the G-box ACGT core element ACGT elements have been observed in a multitude of plant genes regulated by diverse environmental and physiological factors. Systematic DNA-binding studies have shown that nucleotides flanking the ACGT core specify the DNA-protein interactions and subsequent gene activation. G-box-related ABREs have been observed in many ABA-responsive genes, although their functions have not always been proven experimentally. The best-studied examples of these ABRE promoter elements are Em1a from wheat and Motif I from the rice *rab 16A* gene. Multiple copies of the elements fused to a minimal 35S promoter confer an ABA response to a reporter gene, which supports the hypothesis that ABREs are critical for the ABA induction of relevant genes.

The ABA effect on transcription was orientation independent elements, which suggests that they function as enhancer elements in their native genes. A different class of potential transcription factors with relevance to drought stress is represented by the *A. thaliana* gene *Atmyb2*. This gene encodes an MYB-related protein and is induced by dehydration or salt stress and by ABA. Plant *Atmyb2*-related genes comprise a large family that may play various roles in gene regulation. The ATMYB2 protein expressed in *E. coli* has been shown to bind the MYB-recognition sequence, PyAACTG, which supports its role as a DNA-binding protein. Another *A. thaliana* drought stress-induced gene, *rd22*, has a promoter with no ABRE but with two recognition sites for the transcription factors MYC and MYB. Binding of the ATMYB2 protein appears likely but has not been proven experimentally.

Table 16.3: Characterization of Promoters in Transgenic Plants

Gene	*Native Gene Activity*	*Reporter Gene Activity*
Rab 16B	Embryos of *Oryza sativa*	*Nicotiana tabacum* embryos
Em	Embryos of *Triticum aestivum*	*Nicotiana tabacum* embryos
Rab 17	Embryos of *Zea mays*	The embryos and endosperm of *Arabidopsis thaliana*
Hex3 (synthetic tetramer)	(derived from *Nicotiana tabacum*)	Mature seeds of *N. tabacum;* inducible in seedlings by desiccation, salt, and ABA
Rd 22	Dehydrated *A. thaliana* plants	Constitutive in flowers and stems of *A. thaliana;* inducible in *N. tabacum* by ABA or dehydration
Rd 29A	Dehydrated *A. thaliana* plants	Inducible by dehydration in most vegetative parts of *A. thaliana;* inducible in *N. tabacum* by cold, ABA, and salt
CDeT27-45	*C. plantagineum* dehydrated or ABA-treated vegetative tissues	In embryos and mature pollen of both *A. thaliana* and *N. tabacum*
CDeT6-19	*C. plantagineum* dehydrated or ABA-treated vegetative	In developing embryos and mature pollen of both *A. thaliana* and *N. tabacum* also inducible in their leaves and guard cells tissues
CDeT11-24	*C. plantagineum* dehydrated or ABA-treated vegetative tissues	Embryos of both *A. thaliana* and *N. tabacum;* inducible in *A. thaliana* leaves by dehydration
DC8	Embryos of *Daucus carota*	*D. carota* seed tissues
DC3	Embryos of *Daucus carota*	*N. tabacum* seedlings; also inducible in the leaves by either drying or ABA treatment

Assessments of Promoters in Transgenic Plants

Promoter analysis using transient expression assays has resulted in the characterization of several distinct *cis*-acting elements and the cloning of related transcription factors. However, tests with a range of promoters derived from drought- or ABA-inducible structural genes in transgenic plants have shown that the promoter activities defined in transient assays are not always correlated with the expression patterns of their corresponding structural genes. A problem with the approach could be the use of heterologous plant expression systems. Although the genes are always active in seeds, expression in vegetative tissues is not always induced upon drought or ABA treatment, which points to an incomplete activation of the transcriptional machinery. It is interesting to note that ectopic expression of the otherwise seed-specific *abi-3* gene product allows the ABA-mediated activation of *Lea* genes in vegetative tissues of *A. thaliana*. Similarly, the *CDeT27–45* promoters from *C. plantagineum* were only fully responsive to ABA in *A. thaliana* in the presence of the ABI3 product.

Role of PYR1 Protein

The structure of PYR1 (colored ribbons) (Figure 16.1) in its open, unbound state (light green loops) and how it folds around ABA (white rods) when it binds to this hormone (turquoise and purple loops). Credit: Marquez/EMBL. Under normal conditions, proteins called PP2Cs inhibit the ABA pathway, but when a plant is subjected to drought, the concentration of ABA in its cells increases.

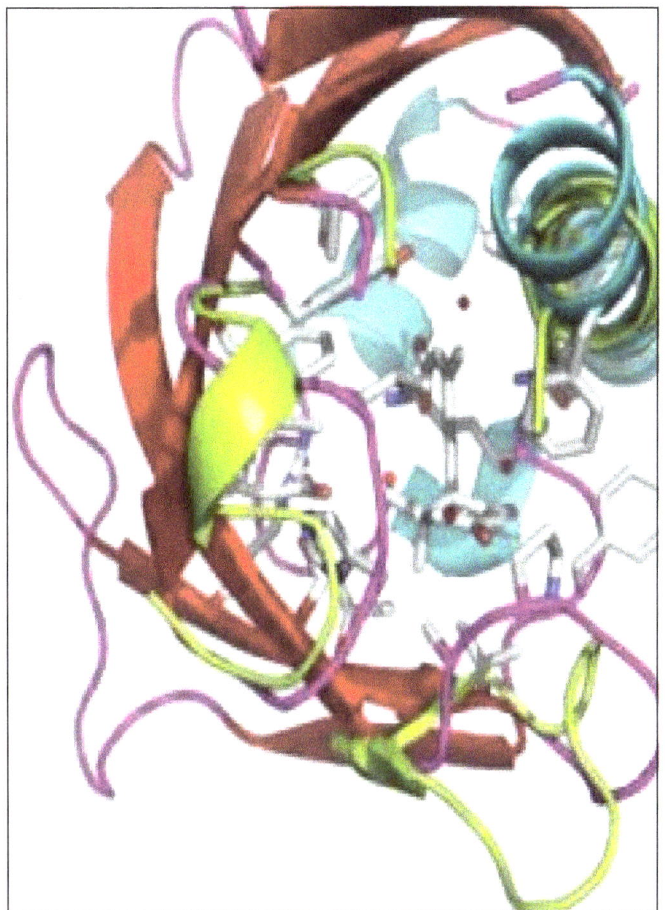

Figure 16.1: Structure of PYR1 Protein.

This removes the break from the pathway, allowing the signal for drought response to be carried through the plant's cells. This turns specific genes on or off, triggering mechanisms for increasing water uptake and storage, and decreasing water loss. But ABA does not interact directly with PP2Cs, so how does it cause them to be inhibited? Recent studies had indicated that the members of a family of

14 proteins might each act as middle-men, but how those proteins detected ABA and inhibited PP2Cs remained a mystery - until now. A group of scientists headed by José Antonio Márquez from EMBL Grenoble and Pedro Luis Rodriguez from CSIC looked at one member of this family, a protein called PYR1. When they used X-ray crystallography to determine its 3-dimensional structure, the scientists found that the protein looks like a hand. In the absence of ABA, the hand remains open, but when ABA is present it nestles in the palm of the PYR1 hand, which closes over the hormone as if holding a ball, thereby enabling a PP2C molecule to sit on top of the folded fingers. As these features seem to be conserved across most members of this protein family, these findings confirm the family as the main ABA receptors. Moreover, they elucidate how the whole process of stress response starts: by binding to PYR1, ABA causes it to hijack PP2C molecules, which are therefore not available to block the stress response.

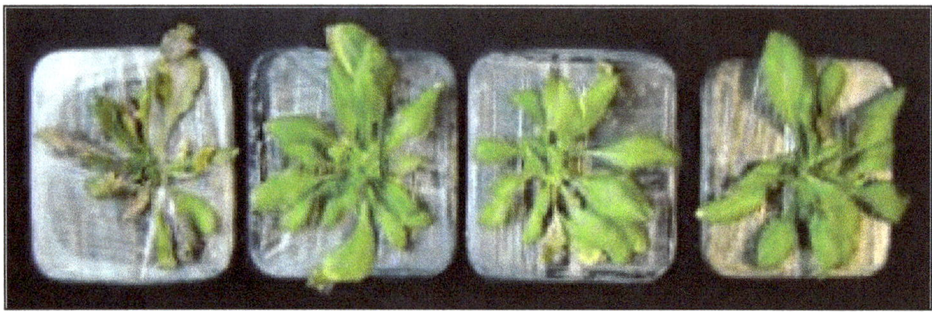

Figure 16.2: Condition of the Plant (Source: Rodriguez *et al.*, 1998).

After being subjected to drought for 15 days, an *Arabidopsis thaliana* plant will normally be withered and dry (far left), but plants from the same species that were genetically engineered to enhance their response to the plant hormone ABA (center left, center right and right) were more resistant to drought. Treat plants with ABA before a drought occurs, they take all their water-saving measures before the drought actually hits, so they are more prepared, and more likely to survive that water shortage they become more tolerant to drought", Rodriguez explains. "The problem so far", Márquez adds, "has been that ABA is very difficult - and expensive - to produce. But thanks to this structural biology approach, we now know what ABA interacts with and how, and this can help to find other molecules with the same effect but which can be feasibly produced and applied." To determine the structure of PYR1, the scientists made use of the infrastructure of the Partnership for Structural Biology, including EMBL Grenoble's high-throughput crystallization facilities and the beamlines at the European Synchrotron Radiation Facility, located on the same campus as EMBL Grenoble.

Functions of Drought-Inducible Genes

Several stress-inducible genes encode key enzymes regulating biosynthesis of compatible solutes such as amino acids (*e.g.* proline), quaternary and other amines (*e.g.* glycinebetaine and polyamines), and a variety of sugars and sugar alcohols (*e.g.* mannitol, trehalose, galactinol, and raffinose). Genes encoding LEA proteins, galactinol synthase (GolS) and heat shock proteins have also been used to improve drought tolerance in transgenic plants. Transcription factors have also proven quite useful in improving stress tolerance in transgenic plants. Other regulatory factors, such as protein kinases and enzymes involved in ABA biosynthesis, are also useful for improving stress tolerance.

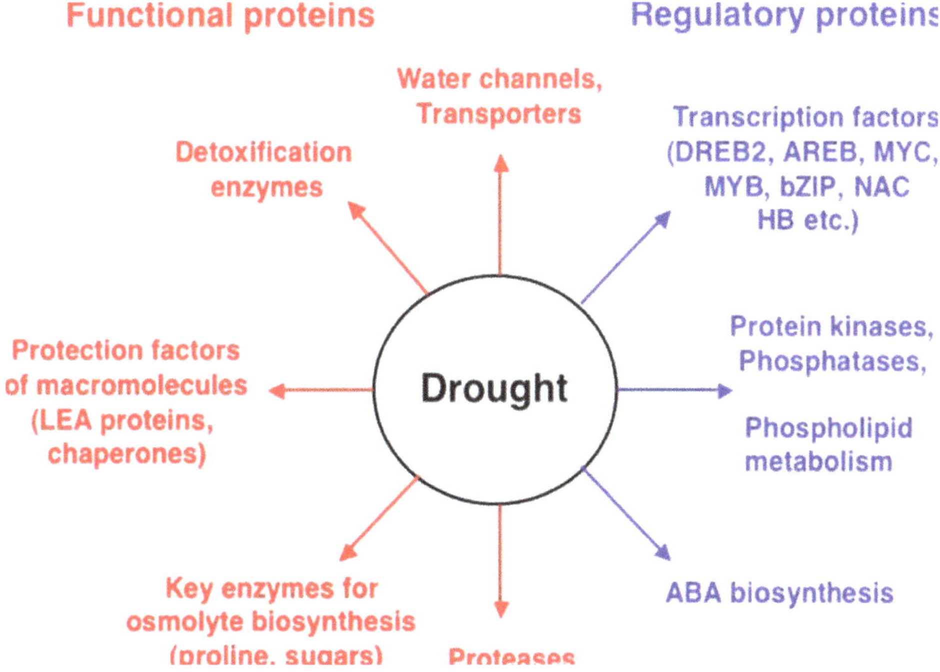

Figure 16.3: Functions of Drought Stress-Inducible Genes in Stress Tolerance and Response. Gene products are classified into two groups. The first group includes proteins that probably function in stress tolerance(functional proteins), and the second group contains protein factors involved in further regulation of signal transduction and gene expression that probably function in stress response (regulatory proteins).

At least six signal transduction pathways exist in drought: three are ABA-dependent and three are ABA-independent. In the ABA-dependent pathway, ABRE functions as a major ABA-responsive element. AREB/ABFs are AP2 transcription factors involved in this process. MYB2 and MYC2 function in ABA-inducible gene expression of the RD22 gene. MYC2 also functions in JA-inducible gene expression. The RD26 NAC transcription factor is involved in ABA- and JA-responsive gene expression in stress responses. These MYC2 and NAC transcription factors may function in cross-talk during abiotic-stress and wound-stress responses. In one of the ABA-independent pathways, DRE is mainly involved in the regulation of genes not only by drought and salt but also by cold stress. DREB1/CBFs are involved in cold-responsive gene expression.

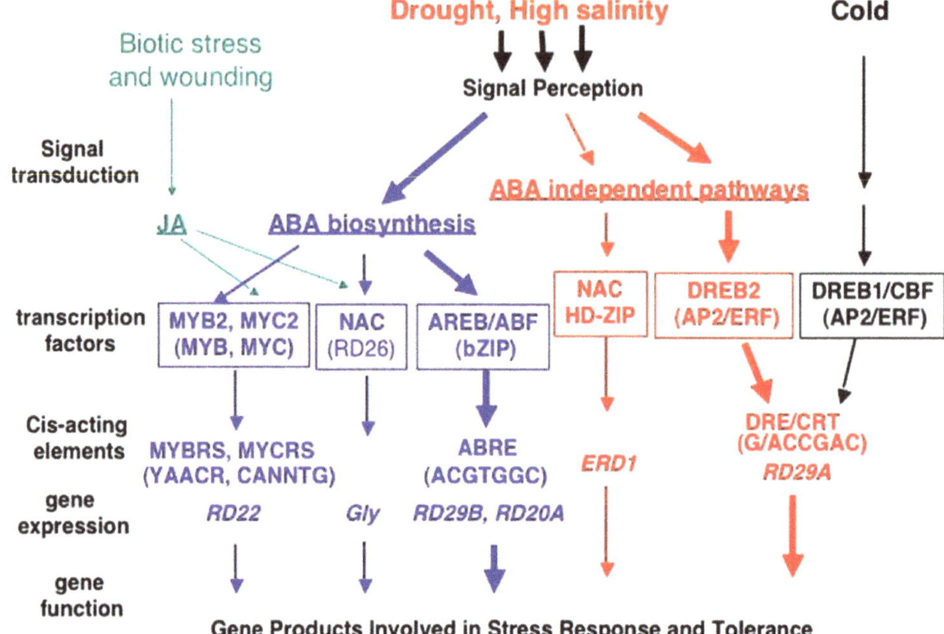

Figure 16.4: Transcriptional Regulatory Networks of Abiotic Stress Signals and Gene Expression.

DREB2s are important transcription factors in dehydration and high salinity stress-responsive gene expression. Another ABA-independent pathway is controlled by drought and salt, but not by the cold. The NAC and HD-ZIP transcription factors are involved in ERD1 gene expression.

Proline Pathways during Drought

In plants, proline is preferentially produced from ornithine under normal conditions. However, under stress, it is made directly from glutamate, the first two reactions of the pathway being catalyzed by a single enzyme δ^1-pyrroline 5-carboxylate synthetase (P5CS). The gene encoding P5CS has been isolated from soybean and moth bean and cloned. The moth bean P5CS gene has been transferred and overexpressed in tobacco. The transgenic plants produced 10- to 18-fold more proline than the control plants. The leaves of transgenic plants retained a higher osmotic potential and showed a greater root biomass under water stress than did the control plants. These findings indicate that overexpression of P5CS in plants enhances their tolerance to osmotic stress.

The primary function of the accumulation of proline and other solutes, *e.g.*, glycine betaine appears to be the regulation of intracellular water activity; under water stress, they may induce the formation of strong H-bonded water around proteins, thereby preserving the native state of cell biopolymers. Proline levels are very high at every period of water stress. Our results depicting proline accumulation are in agreement with other reports (Singh *et al.*, 1973). The greater accumulation

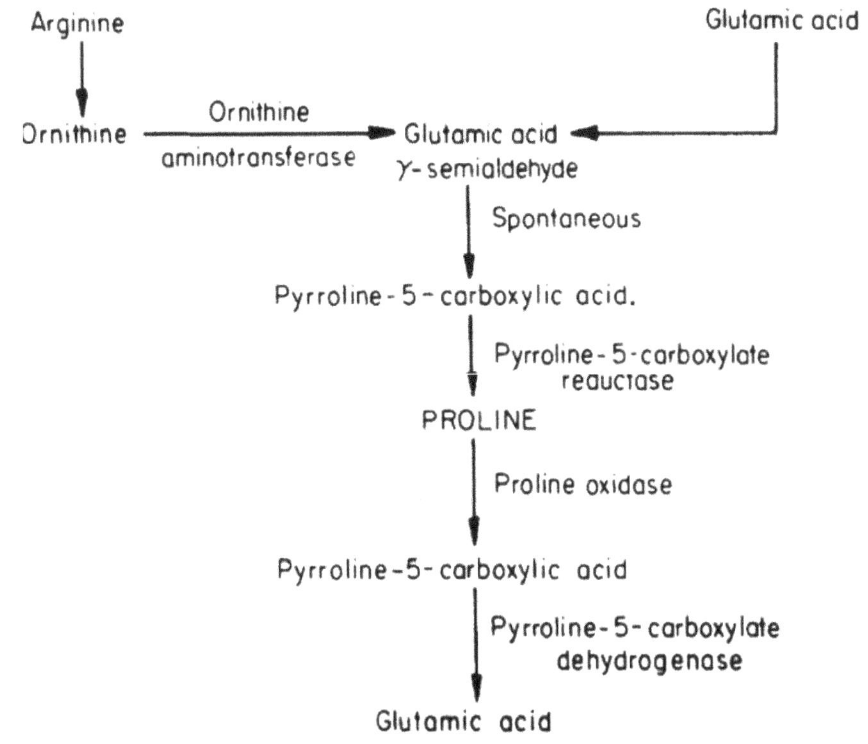

Figure 16.5: Pathway for Proline Metabolism.

of proline in these genotypes, presumably, render them drought tolerant. This hypothesis is being tested at the present time. An increase in soluble proteins during water stress and the dramatic increase in the proline levels compared to other amino acids in the free amino acid pool clearly suggest that the contribution of proteolysis may not be the major factor responsible for this phenomenon. A possible reason for these increased levels of proline during water stress could be an alteration in the activities of the enzymes involved in the biosynthesis and degradation of proline.

ROS

Central to signal transduction pathways (Figure 16.6) related to drought and other stresses are reactive oxygen species (ROS), which are molecules, formed by the incomplete one-electron reduction of oxygen. Under stress, ROS formation is usually exacerbated. Drought stress leads to the disruption of electron transport systems; therefore, under water deficit conditions, the main sites of ROS production in the plant cell are organelles with highly oxidizing metabolic activities or with sustained electron flows: chloroplasts, mitochondria, and micro-bodies.

ROS are generally damaging to essential cellular components, and plants have evolved various ROS scavenging mechanisms. These include the enzymes

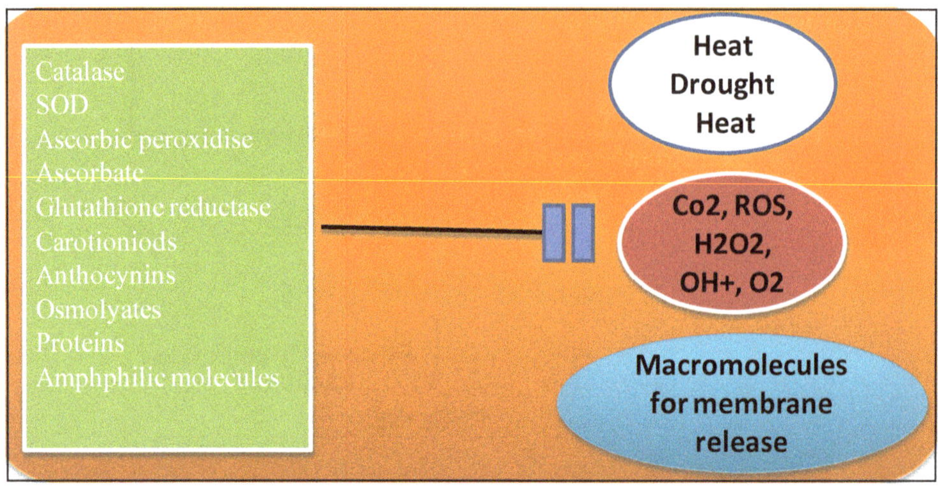

Figure 16.6: Reactive Oxygen Species Pathway.

superoxide dismutase (SOD), catalase, and peroxidases, as well as oxidized and reduced glutathione. Figure 16.6 shows the relationship between ROS-scavenging mechanisms, stress, and the damage to cellular membranes and macromolecules. Researchers have focused on expressing genes for enzymes involved in ROS scavenging to enhance plant protection against oxidative stress. Transgenic alfalfa (*Medicago sativa*) expressing Mn-superoxide dismutase cDNA tended to have reduced injury from water-deficit stress, and this improvement was also seen in field trials in yield and survival.

Secrets of Resurrection

Resurrection plants can tolerate almost complete water loss in their vegetative parts. At the University of Cape Town in South Africa, researchers are trying to unlock the secrets of the resurrection plant *Xerophyta viscosa* in an attempt to achieve drought tolerance in crops. These plants can be a source of drought tolerance genes for transgenic crop improvement. To withstand periods of drought, resurrection plants practically "die" (by losing all their vegetative parts) and then "rise again" when water becomes available. Their vegetative tissues lose all free water and then rehydrate once water becomes available again. Resurrection plants minimize ROS formation and also upregulate various antioxidant protectants during drying and rehydration. The group has identified a novel stress-inducible antioxidant enzyme, *XvPer1*, by differential screening of a cDNA library of *X. viscose*.

Osmoprotectants

Osmolytes are involved in signaling/regulating plant responses to multiple stresses, including reduced growth that may be part of the plant's adaptation to stress. In plants, the common osmolytes are proline, trehalose, fructan, mannitol, and glycine betaine. The protection mechanisms are not yet fully understood, but they are thought to work via osmotic adjustment, stabilizing macromolecules, and scavenging ROS. One proposed transgenic strategy has been to overproduce osmolytes. However, transgenic plants overproducing osmolytes often exhibit impaired growth. Trehalose, a non-reducing disaccharide, protects biological molecules in response to different stress conditions in many microorganisms. Plant biologists are interested in channeling trehalose metabolism to enhance stress tolerance in plants. Trehalose is made from UDP-glucose and glucose-6-phosphate via a two-step process. The conversion of UDP-glucose and glucose-6-phosphate to trehalose-6-phosphate is catalyzed by trehalose-6-phosphate synthase, encoded by the bacterial otsA gene. In the second step, glucose-6-phosphate is converted to trehalose by a phosphatase encoded by the bacterial otsB gene (Figure 16.7). Tobacco plants transformed with bacterial otsA have a greater ability to retain water and a greater ability to photosynthesize under water stress.

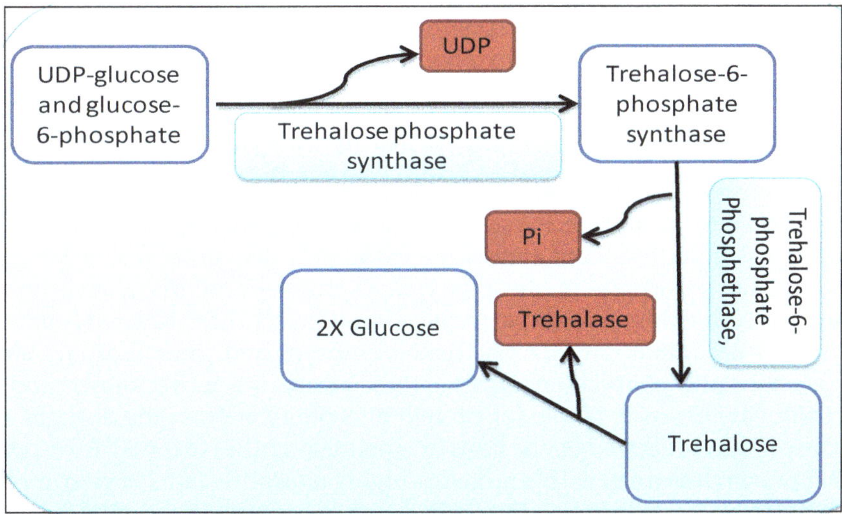

Figure 16.7: Synthesis and Metabolism of Trehalose.

Root Responses to Drought and Osmotic Stress

To develop novel methods to study drought tolerance mechanisms, we began a few years ago to search for new phenotypes that are conferred by drought stress. In this study, we found that the inhibition of lateral root development is a typical adaptive response of roots to drought stress. Significant progress has been made in understanding root growth under drought stress (Sharp *et al.*, 2004). Root response to drought stress and identified the inhibition of lateral root elongation as a reliable response to the stress and ABA.

Protect only when Needed

Genes imparting protection from drought stress can be expressed in plants in two ways: they can be expressed all the time, whether or not the plant is under stress; or they can be engineered to express only when there is drought stress. The second method is more favored, as it limits the side effects of the manipulations.

One of the challenges biologists face in trying to engineer for drought tolerance is that drought tolerance and/or resistance traits are often negatively correlated with productivity. To achieve protection only when needed, scientists use promoters that are stress-inducible, typically abscisic acid (ABA) inducible promoters.

Gene Involved in Drought Stress Response and Tolerance

Drought stress induces a range of physiological and biochemical responses in plants. These responses include stomatal closure, repression of cell growth and photosynthesis, and activation of respiration. Plants also respond and adapt to water deficit at both the cellular and molecular levels, for instance by the accumulation of osmolytes and proteins specifically involved in stress tolerance. An assortment of genes with diverse functions is induced or repressed by these stresses (Bartels and Sunkar, 2005; Yamaguchi-Shinozaki and Shinozaki, 2005). Most of their gene products may function in stress response and tolerance at the cellular level. Drought triggers the production of the phytohormone abscisic acid (ABA), which in turn causes stomatal closure and induces expression of stress-related genes.

Second Messengers and Signaling Molecules

Protein phosphorylation and dephosphorylation (*via* kinases and phosphorylases, respectively) are major mechanisms of signal integration in plant cells. Genes encoding calcium-dependent kinases are induced by dehydration, which suggests that they may participate in phosphorylation processes occurring in response to drought. A serine-threonine- type protein kinase has also been isolated from wheat and shows accumulation in ABA-treated embryos and in dehydrated shoots. However, the phosphorylation targets of these kinases are not yet known, and their exact roles are obscure. A role for protein phosphorylation in the drought-stress response is also suggested on the basis of functional studies of the ABA-responsive RAB17 protein from maize. This protein is highly phosphorylated in vivo, probably via catalysis by casein kinase 2. The RAB17 protein has been found to be distributed between the cytoplasm and the nucleus of maize embryos, in different states of phosphorylation. Biochemical studies showed that RAB17 binds peptides with nuclear localization signals and that the binding is dependent on phosphorylation. It has been suggested that RAB17 mediates the transport of specific nuclear-targeted proteins during stress. Cytoplasmic calcium acts as a second messenger in many cellular processes and may also be involved in the signaling pathways mediating the expression of drought-related genes. Stomatal closure is an early plant response to drought, and increases in the cytosolic concentration of free calcium, together with pH changes, are considered to be primary events in the ABA-mediated reduction of stomatal turgor. However, it is likely that calcium, together with phosphorylation processes, plays a more general role in the mechanisms associated with drought-stress perception. For example, the *A. thaliana ABI1* gene product is thought to be a calcium-activated phosphoprotein phosphatase. Furthermore, a transcript encoding a phosphatidylinositol-specific phospholipase C, an enzyme involved in catalyzing the synthesis of inositol 1,4,5-triphosphate, increases during dehydration, inositol triphosphate stimulates the release of Ca2+ from intracellular stores.

Drought Stress Signaling Pathways

In nature, for a plant to sacrifice a part of its structure constitutes an adaptive strategy to survive a stress episode. For adaptive or presumed adaptive responses, it may be helpful to conceptually group them into three aspects: (*a*) homeostasis that includes ion homeostasis, which is mainly relevant to salt stress, and osmotic homeostasis or osmotic adjustment; (*b*) stress damage control and repair, or detoxification; and (*c*) growth control. Accordingly, salt and drought stress signaling can be divided into three functional categories: anionic and osmotic stress signaling for the reestablishment of cellular homeostasis under stress conditions, detoxification signaling to control and repair stress damages, and signaling to coordinate cell division and expansion to levels suitable for the particular stress conditions. Homeostasis signaling negatively regulates detoxification responses because, once cellular homeostasis is reestablished, stress injury would be reduced, and failure to reestablish homeostasis would aggravate stress injury. Homeostasis and detoxification signaling lead to stress tolerance and are expected to negatively regulate the growth inhibition response, *i.e.*, to relieve growth inhibition.

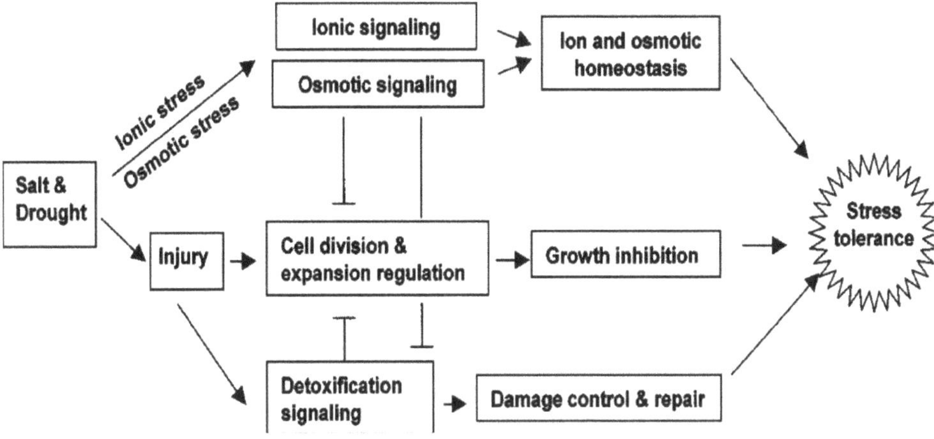

Figure 16.8: Functional Demarcations of Salt and Drought Stress Signaling Pathways. The inputs for ionic and osmotic signaling pathways are ionic (excess NaCl) and osmotic (*e.g.*, turgor) changes. The output of ionic and osmotic signaling is cellular and plant homeostasis. Direct input signals for detoxification signaling are derived stresses (*i.e.*, injury), and the signaling output is damage control and repair (*e.g.*, activation of dehydration tolerance genes). Interactions between the homeostasis, growth regulation and detoxification pathways are indicated.

Osmotic signaling pathways include gene expression and/or activation of osmolyte biosynthesis enzymes as well as water and osmolyte transport systems. Most of the other changes induced by drought stress can be considered as part of detoxification signaling. These include (*a*) phospholipid hydrolysis; (*b*) changes in the expression of LEA/dehydrin-type genes, molecular chaperones, and proteinases that remove denatured proteins; and (*c*) activation of enzymes involved in the generation and removal of reactive oxygen species and other detoxification proteins. The input signal(s) for the detoxification pathways is most likely not anionic or osmotic change, but a product of stress injury, *e.g.*, reactive oxygen species or protein denaturation. Water stress generally inhibits plant growth; they act the signal for cell division and expansion machinery. Slower cell division under water stress is probably a result of reduced cyclin-dependent kinase (CDK) activity. Reduced CDK activity may be a result of combined effects of transcription suppression of cyclins and CDKs and induction of CDK inhibitors. The direct input signal(s) for the CDK regulation is unclear but can be a product of stress injury or any of the primary or intermediary signals involved in the homeostasis and detoxification pathways (Figure 16.8).

Post-transcriptional Controls

To understand gene regulation during drought has been devoted to transcriptional mechanisms, including mRNA processing, transcript stability, translation efficiency, and protein modification or turnover. These mechanisms also play a role during stress responses. In drought stress induces some proteins that are synthesized in a light-dependent manner; for some of these proteins, the levels of the mRNA do not parallel those of the proteins, which suggest posttranscriptional regulation. A second major control point appears to be the posttranslational modification of proteins, in which phosphorylation is a key mechanism. For example, phosphorylation is involved in the modification of the fructose-1,6-bisphosphatase in drought-stressed leaves of sugar beet (Beta vulgaris). Some of the proteases induced by drought stress may also have a function in posttranslational modification. This mechanism could also operate during drought stress. Protease inhibitors induced during drought have a role in controlling the activity of endogenous proteases.

Down-regulation of Gene

Genes are up-regulated during drought stress and as well as involves the down-regulation of several genes. There are several examples which revealed that transcripts encoding proteins relevant to photosynthesis are down-regulated during the dehydration process and thus possibly reduce photo-oxidative stress. Promoter regions of storage protein genes contain the information for their downregulation during seed desiccation. Furthermore, it has recently been reported that histone H1 transcripts accumulate in response to drought stress in vegetative tissues of tomato, and it was suggested that H1 histones are implicated in the repression of gene expression.

Mutants as Tools to Understand Cellular and Molecular Drought Tolerance Mechanisms

The use of mutants: a most promising way to detect genes involved in the development or in response to environmental stress. The model species *Arabidopsis,* particularly amenable to dissect the genetics and molecular mechanisms underlying physiological responses, also offers the advantage of a wide variety of mutants. As far as drought tolerance is concerned, hormonal mutants, impaired in hormone biosynthesis deficient mutants or in the signal transduction pathway responsive mutants provide a valuable tool to analyze the role of phytohormone interaction in the plant drought behavior as well as to differentiate the mutant phenotypes with new criteria. These two categories of mutants (in particular the abscisic acid, ABA, mutants) were shown to be affected in developmental processes during seed maturation-in the desiccation phase- and/or in response to environmental stress (drought,.) in vegetative tissues. The present report will focus on this last aspect: alterations in drought responses in vegetative tissues (adaptive strategies and drought tolerance mechanisms) essentially in *Arabidopsis* hormonal mutants (ABA-deficient and ABA-insensitive, GA-deficient, auxin, and ethylene-insensitive). Some of the results are discussed with regard to the predicted functions of genes affected by the mutations. Mutant can be altered in a developmental programme or in response to environmental stress has made an important contribution to our understanding of molecular mechanism underlying physiological processes.the use of mutant to improve plant molecular genetic studies has been widely extended to all field of development, embryogenesis and germination, morphogenesis, flowering, metabolic pathway, hormone perception and action. Most of the development mutant revealed defect in a transcription factor or in specific signal transduction processes. Mutant affected in response to environmental stress also appeared as a promising way to detect genes involved in normal and stressed plant behavior, inducing signal transduction and resulting modification of cellular and developmental programme. As far as response to water stress are concerned, two approaches have been an attempted-the selection of mutant lines, adapted to increasing osmotic stress and the use of hormonal mutant, altered in hormone biosynthesis or in the signal transduction pathway. Mutant cell lines, modified in their response to environmental stress (salt, low temperature, heavy metal) have been widely developed. They may provide valuable tools for fundamental studies on the molecular and cellular basis of stress tolerance as a well as selection in the breeding programme.

Transgenic Plants Assessing Gene Function

Transgenic plants allow the targeted expression of drought-related genes in vivo and are therefore an excellent system to assess the function and tolerance conferred by the encoded proteins. With an ectopic expression of genes involved in controlling ABA biosynthesis, it should also be possible to alter the hormonal balance in vivo and thus to clarify the role of ABA in the drought response. Another purpose of using transgenic plants is to improve drought tolerance in agronomically valuable plants. A reason for this is that stress tolerance is likely to involve the expression of gene products from several pathways. The accumulation of low molecular weight metabolites that act as osmoprotectants is a widespread adaptation to dry, saline, and low-temperature conditions in many organisms. In engineering plants that synthesize protective osmolytes, microorganisms appear to be useful sources for genes. Transgenic tobacco plants that synthesize and accumulate the sugar alcohol mannitol have been obtained by introducing a bacterial gene that encodes mannitol 1-phosphate dehydrogenase. Plants producing mannitol showed increased salt tolerance. Tobacco plants that accumulate the poly fructose molecule fructan have been engineered using microbial (*Bacillus subtilis* or *Streptococcus mutans*) fucosyltransferase genes. These plants showed improved growth under polyethylene-mediated drought stress, with a positive correlation observed between the level of accumulated fructans and degree of tolerance. One consequence of drought and many other stresses is the production of activated oxygen molecules that cause cellular injury, and therefore plants with increased concentrations of oxygen scavengers should show improved performances under nonlethal stress conditions. Although *Lea*-related genes are upregulated abundantly in most plants during all types of osmotic stress, separate ectopic expression of three different representatives in tobacco did not yield an obvious drought-tolerant phenotype.

Conclusion and Future Perspectives

Despite the many genes that have been identified in association with drought stress, much of the data is descriptive, with the functions of only a few of the encoded proteins established. The production of mutants using an antisense- RNA approach is a powerful technique that should continue to elucidate certain aspects of stress tolerance, but it has been most successful only with well-characterized areas of plant metabolism. It is also difficult to devise screening procedures for useful dehydration-tolerance mutants, because of the array of processes simultaneously affected by drought. Resurrection plants would be an excellent source for mutants with decreased tolerance ought stress have been with ABA-related mutations, and the power of the approach is shown in the cloning of drought gene, which has provided new perspectives. Another valuable approach may be to identify those metabolic steps that are most sensitive to drought stress (a technique used to genetically dissect salt stress in yeast). Such an approach can at least begin to elucidate which gene products are of primary importance. The plant hormone ABA regulates different aspects of the drought-stress response, and thus the synthesis of pure active ABA analogs may help in the development of probes for ABA-binding proteins, which could then shed some light on primary signals. In contrast with the situation with signal perception, some information is available on *cis*- and *trans*-regulatory factors. Several elements in a promoter need to cooperate with multiple DNA-binding proteins to mediate gene expression. The recently described coupling elements are probably only a beginning in resolving the regulatory network. Little progress has been made with the cloning and analysis of drought-related transcription factors, although a biochemical approach and use of the recently established yeast one- and two-hybrid systems should produce new insights. Regulation at stages beyond transcription must also be further considered because this could make a major contribution to the final gene expression pattern. The complexity of drought tolerance apparent throughout this review points to control by multiple genes, and thus the identification of quantitative-trait loci (QTLs) for drought resistance may well be an effective analytical tool. The approach has just begun to be applied to the environmental-stress responses of plants and is particularly promising considering that saturated DNA–marker maps are now available for both genetic model plants and crop plants. The molecular analysis of the drought response has arrived at a stage where research can build upon a large collection of characterized genes. The use of novel approaches combining genetic, biochemical, and molecular techniques should provide exciting results in the near future.

References

Araus JL, Slafer GA, Reynolds MP, Royo C. (2002). Plant breeding and drought in C3 cereals: what should we breed for?. Annals of botany, 89(7): 925-40.

Bartels D, Sunkar R. (2005). Drought and salt tolerance in plants. Critical reviews in plant sciences, 23-24(1): 23-58.

Cushman JC, Bohnert HJ. (2000). Genomic approaches to plant stress tolerance. Current opinion in plant biology, 1-3(2): 117-24.

Levitt J. (1980). Responses of Plants to Environmental Stress, Volume 1: Chilling, Freezing and High Temperature Stresses, Academic Press.

Poroyko V, Hejlek LG, Spollen WG, Springer GK, Nguyen HT, Sharp RE, Bohnert HJ. (2005). The maize root transcriptome by serial analysis of gene expression. Plant Physiology, 1:138(3): 1700-10.

Rodriguez PL, Benning G, Grill E. (1998). ABI2, a second protein phosphatase 2C involved in abscisic acid signal transduction in Arabidopsis. FEBS letters, 421(3): 185-90.

Schroeder JI, Allen GJ, Hugouvieux V, Kwak JM, Waner D. (2001). Guard cell signal transduction. Annual review of plant biology, 52(1): 627-58.

Sharp RE, Poroyko V, Hejlek LG, Spollen WG, Springer GK, Bohnert HJ, Nguyen HT. (2004). Root growth maintenance during water deficits: physiology to functional genomics. Journal of experimental botany, 55(407): 2343-51.

Shinozaki K, Yamaguchi-Shinozaki K. (2000). Molecular responses to dehydration and low temperature: differences and cross-talk between two stress signaling pathways. Current opinion in plant biology, 3(3): 217-23.

Singh TN, Paleg IG, Aspinall D. (1973). Stress metabolism III. Variations in response to water deficit in the barley plant. Australian Journal of Biological Sciences, 26(1): 65-76.

Umezawa T, Fujita M, Fujita Y, Yamaguchi-Shinozaki K, Shinozaki K. (2006). Engineering drought tolerance in plants: discovering and tailoring genes to unlock the future. Current opinion in biotechnology, 17(2): 113-22.

Yamaguchi-Shinozaki K, Shinozaki K. (2005). Organization of cis-acting regulatory elements in osmotic-and cold-stress-responsive promoters. Trends in plant science, 10(2): 88-94.

Yu LX, Setter TL. (2003).Comparative transcriptional profiling of placenta and endosperm in developing maize kernels in response to water deficit. Plant Physiology,131(2): 568-82.

Zhang J, Klueva NY, Wang Z, Wu R, Ho TH, Nguyen HT. (2000). Genetic engineering for abiotic stress resistance in crop plants. In Vitro Cellular and Developmental Biology-Plant, 36(2): 108-14.

Chapter 17

Wickedness to Heal: Climate Change

Rajendra Parikh

Faculty of Law, The Maharaja Sayajirao University of Baroda,
Vadodara, Gujarat - 390 002
e-mail: rajendraiparikh@gmail.com

ABSTRACT

Many living thing are depend on environment. Environment is the biggest gift of the nature to the living beings. But human beings considering it as their legacy used it for development. Environment and development are related with each other. In last few decades or so we are experiencing various environmental challenges such as various kinds of pollution, deforestation, tsunami, heat waves, *etc.* 'Climate change' refers to a change of climate which is attributed directly or indirectly to human economic activity that alters the composition of the global atmosphere. It is in addition to natural climate variability observed over a comparable time periods. Climate change is also one of the evil effects of environmental degradation. We are facing the problem of greenhouse effect, ozone layer depletion as a result of climate change. In this chapter researcher has tried to find out various international as well as national response taken to curb the evil of climate change. Despite of various initiatives taken by international as well as national level issue regarding climate change has not been solved yet. Experts are of the opinion that if things will continue in the same pace then we are going to suffer evil effects of climate change in future to come. It generates very complex and multidimensional global issues in the context of its implications for the global environment and human beings. Many pollution problems give rise to impact on different social systems-social groups, countries, or regions-and on different natural ecosystems. What distinguishes climate change is the nature and potential seriousness of its human impacts, which transform the issue from a purely environmental problem into an environment and development-related one.

Keywords: *Climate change, Greenhouse effect, Greenhouse gas, Ozone, Carbon dioxide.*

Introduction

Climate Change is a serious global environmental concern. It is primarily caused by the building up of Green House Gases (GHG) in the atmosphere. The global increases in carbon dioxide concentration are primarily due to fossil fuel use and land use change, while those of methane and nitrous oxide are primarily due to agriculture. Global Warming is a specific example of the broader term "Climate Change" and refers to the observed increase in the average temperature of the air near earth's surface and oceans in recent decades. Its effect particularly on developing countries is adverse as their capacity and resources to deal with the challenge is limited.[1]

The Intergovernmental Panel on Climate Change (IPCC), set up in cooperation by the world Meteorological Organization and United Nations Environment Programme released its Fourth Assessment Report (AR4) in 2007. The Report first brought to light that climate change is a real and a very grave problem and that it is mostly man-made. From the direct observations of changes in temperature, sea level and snow cover in the northern hemisphere during 1850 to 2007. The AR4 concluded that the earth's climate system is slowly but steadily changing. According to experts, increase in atmospheric concentration of greenhouse gases and aerosols, solar radiation and ozone depletion lead to global warming, which in turn, affect the energy balance of the climate system, thereby causing climate change.[2]

Meaning: Climate Change

"Changes in the earth's weather, including changes in temperature, wind patterns and rainfall, especially the increase in the temperature of the earth's atmosphere that is caused by the increase of particular gases, especially carbon dioxide". – *Oxford Dictionary*

The United Nations Framework Convention on Climate Change defines this subject as "a change of climate which is attributed directly or indirectly to human activity that alters the composition of the global atmosphere and which is in addition to natural climate variability Observed over comparable time periods." Global warming and climate change refer to an increase in average global temperatures. Natural measures and human activities are believed to be causative to an increase in average global temperatures. This is caused primarily by increases in "greenhouse" gases such as Carbon Dioxide (CO_2).[3]

Effects of Climate Change

Green House Effect

A Green House Gas (GAG) is a gas in the atmosphere that is transparent to incoming short-wave solar radiation but can absorb and trap long-wave radiation

---

1 http://164.100.47.134/intranet/CLIMATE_CHANGE-INDIA's_PERSPECTIVE.pdf

2 Newell, Petter, climate for change, Cambridge University Press (2006).

3 http://www.globalissues.org/article/233/climate-change-and-global-warming-introduction.

emitted by the earth's surface. Green House Gases include carbon dioxide, methane, nitrous oxide, hydrofluorocarbons, perfluorocarbons and sulphur hexafluoride. It was reported by IPCC in AR4 that most of the observed increase in global average temperature since the mid -20th century was due to anthropogenic greenhouse effect, with an increase of 70 per cent between 1970 and 2004.[4]

Industrial Revolution has been one of the biggest contributors towards the increased amounts of greenhouse gases in the atmosphere. The concentration of carbon dioxide and methane have increased by 36 per cent and 148 per cent respectively since 1750. Fossil fuel burning amounts to about 3/4th of anthropogenic increase inn carbon dioxide over the past 20 years. The rest of this increase is mostly by change in land-use, especially deforestation.[5]

AR4 predicted that unless the emissions pattern change, there would be a likely increase in global mean temperature of about 1 degree C above present value by 2025 and 3 degree C before the end of the century, with negative impacts on agriculture, air, water, forestry, coastal zones *etc.*[6]

Ozone Depletion

Global warming and ozone depletion are two separate but related threats. Global warming and green house effect refer to the warming of the lower part of the atmosphere due to increasing concentrations of heat trapping gases. Converse to this, the ozone hole refers to the loss of ozone in upper part of the atmosphere. This is of serious concern because stratospheric ozone blocks incoming ultraviolet radiation from the sun, some of which is harmful to plants, animals and humans.

The ozone coat traps heat, so if it gets destroyed, the upper atmosphere actually cools, thereby offsetting part of the warming effect of other heat trapping gases. But the cooling of upper layers of the atmosphere can produce changes in the climate that affect weather patterns in the higher latitudes. Trapping heat in the lower part of the atmosphere allows less heat to escape into space and leads to cooling of the upper part of the atmosphere.[7]

Impact of Climate Change

The key environmental challenges in India have been sharper in the past two decades. Climate change is impacting the natural ecosystems and is expected to have substantial adverse effects in India, mainly on agriculture on which 58 per cent of the population still depends for livelihood, water storage in the Himalayan glaciers which are the source of major rivers and groundwater recharge, sea-level

---

4 The AR4 summary for policymakers at p.5

5 Gupta, Purmina, G-8 Summit: global warming, Yojana (2005), Vol. 49, No. 9

6 Goudie Andrew S, encyclopaedia of environmental change and human society, Oxford University Press (2001).

7 Eblen, Ruth and William eds., the environment encyclopaedia, Vol 5, Houghton Mifflin Company (1994).

rise, and threats to a long coastline and habitations. Climate change will also cause increased frequency of extreme events such as floods, and droughts. These in turn will impact India's food security problems and water security.[8]

Climate Change-International Response

Vienna Convention and Montreal Protocol[9]

The protection of the ozone layer from the destructive elements of GHGs is the subject of a complex legal regime comprising the 1985 Vienna Convention for the Protection of the Ozone layer and the 1987 Montreal Protocol. The Convention was negotiated for over five years under the auspices of United Nations Environment Programme (UNEP) and was the first treaty to address a global atmospheric issue. It did not set targets or timeframe for action but was a comprehensive approach towards the identification of the problem.

The only protocol to the Vienna Convention is the Montreal Protocol, 1987, which provided for new regulatory techniques and adoption of innovative financial mechanisms. It set forth specific limitations and reductions on the level of consumption and production of certain ozone-depleting substances. The Protocol lists a number of substances, which are to be controlled strictly in their consumption. A multilateral Fund has been set up in order to implement the objectives of the Protocol where the developed countries are required to contribute from time to time, which will financially assist the developing countries in achieving the control on the ozone depleting substances.

The United Nations' Framework Convention on Climate Change (UNFCCC)

The UNFCCC, 1992 was signed by 195 States and reflected some kind of compromise between the nations, which wanted specific emission reduction schemes and those States who advocated only for a basis for future controls.[10]

The 1992 Convention, for the first time, amidst surrounding scientific uncertainties, recognised that climate change was a problem, which would surely escalate in the near future if immediate steps were not taken. Its ultimate objective is to stabilize GHG concentration "at a level that would prevent dangerous human induced interference with the climate system."[11]

One of the preliminary responsibilities placed by the UNFCCC was for signatory nations to establish National Greenhouse Gas Inventories of GHG emission and removals which were used to create the benchmark levels decided by the 1990 Ministerial Declaration of the Second World Climate Conference. The

---

8 India, Ministry of Finance, Economic Survey, 2012-13, pp. 256-57.

9 http://legal.un.org/avl/pdf/ha/vcpol/vcpol_e.pdf

10 Hayes, Peter and Smith, Kirk, eds, the Global Green House Regime: Who Pays? Science, Economics and North-South Politics in the Climate Change Convention, UN University Press (1993).

11 http://unfccc.int/essential_background/convention/background/items/1353.php

Convention mandates that updated inventories must be regularly submitted as it is the responsibilities of the Annex I countries to reduce the 1990 benchmark levels of omission. The responsibilities of the Annex I countries are to provide financial assistance to the developing countries to help them to meet their obligations under the Convention, by assisting in transfer of technology and knowhow, sponsoring projects *etc.*[12]

The Kyoto Protocol[13]

The Kyoto Protocol is an global agreement linked to the United Nations Framework Convention on Climate Change, which entrust its Parties by setting background internationally binding emission reduction targets. Distinguish that developed countries are principally responsible for the current high levels of GHG emissions in the atmosphere as a result of more than 150 years of industrial activity; the Protocol chairs a heavier burden on developed nations under the principle of "common but differentiated responsibilities."

Under the Protocol, countries must meet their targets primarily through national measures. However, the Protocol also offers them an additional means to meet their targets by way of three market-based mechanisms:

- International Emissions Trading (IET);
- Clean Development Mechanism (CDM); and
- Joint Implementation (JI).

The Kyoto Protocol is criticised mainly on two grounds. First, the targets are set at much lower than required. Secondly, it violates the 'Polluter Pays Principle.'

The Bali Road Map

The Bali Road Map was adopted at the Thirteenth Conference of the Parties and the Third Meeting of the Parties in December 2007 in Bali. Is forward looking result that symbolizes the work that wishes to be finished under various negotiating "tracks" that is important to reaching a secure climate future? The Bali Road Map includes the Bali Action Plan, which charts the course for a new negotiating process designed to tackle Climate Change. The Bali Action Plan is a wide-ranging procedure to allow the complete, efficient and constant implementation of the Convention through long-term cooperative action, now, up to and beyond 2012, in order to reach an agreed outcome and adopt a decision.

The Copenhagen Accord

The 15th meeting of the Conference of the Parties to the UNFCCC and the 5th assembly of the Conference of the Parties helping as the Meeting of the Parties to the Kyoto Protocol took position in Copenhagen, Denmark in 2009. It produced

---

12 Divan, Shyam and Rosencranz, Armin, Environment Law Policy 2nd edition., Oxford University Press, New Delhi,(2002).

13 http://unfccc.int/kyoto_protocol/items/2830.php

the Copenhagen Accord. The Copenhagen Accord contained several key elements on which there was strong convergence of the views of the Governments. This incorporated the long term objective of limiting the maximum global average temperature increase to no more than 2 degrees Celsius above pre-industrial levels, subject to a review in 2015. It also included a reference to consider limiting the temperature increase to below 1.5 degrees - a key demand made by vulnerable developing countries.[14]

The Cancun Agreements

The Cancun Agreements achieved on December 11 in Cancun, Mexico, at the 2010 United Nations Climate Change Conference, stand for key steps forward in capturing plans to reduce Green House Gas emissions, and to help developing nations protect themselves from climate impacts and build their own sustainable futures. The main objectives include: Mitigation; Transparency of actions; Technology; Adaptation; Forests; Capacity building; and Finance. The objectives also include setting up the Green Climate Fund to disburse $100 billion per year by 2020 to developing countries to assist them in mitigating Climate Change and adapting to its impacts.[15]

The Durban Agreement

The United Nations Climate Change Conference at Durban in 2011 delivered a penetrate on the international community's answer to Climate Change. The Durban outcomes looked to address these challenges in a more connected way by embodying a road map for implementation. On this plan, four main areas of synchronized and corresponding action and implementation, designed also to build and conserve trust among countries, were agreed *viz.* (i) Second commitment period of the Kyoto Protocol; (ii) The launch of a new platform of negotiations under the Convention to deliver a new and universal Green House Gas reduction protocol, legal instrument or other outcome with legal force by 2015 for the period beyond 2020; (iii) Conclusion in 2012 of existing broad-based stream of negotiations; and (iv) To scope out and then conduct a fresh global Review of the emerging climate challenge, based on the best available science and data.[16]

The Doha Climate Gateway

At the 2012 UN Climate Change Conference in Doha, Qatar (COP18/CMP8), and Governments merged the profit of the last three years of international Climate Change negotiations and opened a entry to needed greater aim and action on all levels.[17]

---

14 http://unfccc.int/meetings/copenhagen_dec_2009/items/5262.php

15 http://unfccc.int/key_steps/cancun_agreements/items/6132.php

16 http://unfccc.int/key_steps/durban_outcomes/items/6825.php

17 http://unfccc.int/key_steps/doha_climate_gateway/items/7389.php

The Warsaw Outcomes

At the UN Climate Change Conference in Warsaw, administration acquired additional vital decisions to continue on track towards securing a universal climate change agreement in 2015. The idea of the 2015 agreement is dual: initial, to bind nations jointly into an efficient global effort to reduce emissions rapidly enough to plan humanity's longer term path out of the danger zone of climate change, while building adaptation capacity. Later to motivate quicker and broader action now.[18]

Climate Change–India's Response

Ozone Issue

The Ministry of Environment and Forest has formulated the Ozone Depleting Substances (Regulation and Control) Rules,2000 which regulates the sale, stock, distribution, or exhibit for sale of ozone depleting substances without proper registration with the enumerated authority, and their export and import from specified countries. Prohibition is also on established or expansion of any manufacturing facility for production of any ozone depleting substance.[19]

National Environment Policy

National Environment Policy, 2006 sketches vital elements of India's answer to Climate Change. These include adherence to principle of common but differentiated responsibility and respective capabilities of different countries, identification of key vulnerabilities of India to Climate Change, in particular impacts on water resources, forests, coastal areas, agriculture and health, assessment of the need for adaptation to Climate Change and encouragement to the Indian Industry to participate in the Clean Development Mechanism (CDM).[20]

National Action Plan on Climate Change, 2008 (NAPCC)

The National Action Plan on Climate Change (NAPCC) coordinated by the Ministry of Environment and Forests is being implemented through the nodal Ministries in specific sectors and areas. On June 30, 2008, Prime Minister, Dr. Manmohan Singh released India's first National Action Plan on Climate Change (NAPCC) delineating active and future policies and programmes addressing climate improvement and alteration.

National Action Plan on Climate Change[21]

1. National Solar Mission
2. National Mission for Enhanced Energy Efficiency

---

18 http://unfccc.int/key_steps/warsaw_outcomes/items/8006.php

19 Toman M.A., Chakravarty U. and Gupta S., eds, India and Global Climate Change: Perspectives on Economics and Policy from a Developing Country, Oxford University Press (2004).

20 http://www.gktoday.in/national-environment-policy-2006/.

21 India's National Action Plan on Climate change, 2008.

3. National Mission on Sustainable Habitat
4. National Water Mission
5. National Mission for Sustaining the Himalayan Ecosystem
6. National Mission for a "Green India"
7. National Mission for Sustainable Agriculture
8. National Mission on Strategic knowledge for Climate Change

Carbon Trading In India

India ranks under the third category of signatories to UNFCCC. India signed and ratified the Protocol in August, 2002 and emerged as a world leader in lessening of GHGs by adopting Clean Developing Mechanisms in past few years. India's carbon market is the rapidly mounting markets in the planet and has already generated approximately 30 million carbon credits, the second highest transacted volume in the world. Nearly 850 projects with an investment of 6, 50,000 million rupees are in pipeline. India is also one of the largest beneficiaries of the total world carbon trade through the Clean Development Mechanism claiming about 31 per cent. The National Commodity and Derivative Exchange (NCDE), by a notification and with due approval from the Forward Market Commission (FMC) also launched the Carbon Credit Future Contract (CCFC) whose aim is to provide transparency to markets and help the producers to earn remuneration out of the environmental projects. Carbon credit in India is traded on the National Commodity and Derivative Exchange and Multi Commodity Exchange only as a future contract.[22]

Parliamentary Forum on Global Warming and Climate Change

The Forum was constituted for the first time in 2008 and since then has been involving parliamentarians to interact with specialists working on Global Warming and Climate Change. The Members of the Forum have been taking a lot of interest in the meetings by participating in the discussions. Presentations on various subjects relating to Climate Change like: Impact of Climate Change on Agriculture; Population, Resources and Biodiversity with reference to Climate Change; Technology and Climate Change; National Solar Mission and related initiatives under the National Action Plan on Climate Change; National Mission on Sustainable Habitat, *etc.* have taken place. These give insight into different perspective on the issue of Climate Change and mitigation methods.[23]

Climate Change Action Programme (CCAP)

Various other science initiatives are planned by the Ministry as part of the Climate Change Action Programme (CCAP). These include National Carbonaceous Aerosols Programme (NCAP), Long Term Ecological Observatories (LTEO), and Coordinated Studies on Climate Change for North East region (CSCCNE). The

---

22 MajmudarArjya B., DebosmitaNandy and Mukherjee Swayambhu; Environment and Wildlife laws in India; LexisNexis; p.169.

23 http://164.100.47.134/committee/Forum_informations

NCAP is a major activity involving multi-institutional and multi-agency study. E-Action Programme (CCAP). These include National Carbonaceous Aerosols Programme (NCAP), Long Term Ecological Observatories (LTEO), and Coordinated Studies on Climate Change for North East region (CSCCNE). The NCAP is a major activity involving multi institutional and multi-agency study launched in 2011.[24]

Indian Network for Climate Change Assessment (INCCA)

Various initiatives have been taken to increase capacity at the institutional level for conducting research into Climate Change science and making necessary assessments. The Ministry has already set up a network, namely the Indian Network for Climate Change Assessment (INCCA) comprising of 127 research institutions tasked with undertaking research on the science of Climate Change and its impacts on different sectors of economy across various regions of India. INCCA has helped the Ministry put together its GHG Emissions Inventories and in carrying out other scientific assessments at more frequent intervals.[25]

Twelfth Five-Year Plan and Climate Change

The Government has a domestic mitigation goal of reducing emissions intensity of Gross Domestic Product (GDP) by 20-25 per cent by 2020 in comparison with 2005 level. The domestic goal and the objectives of the National Action Plan on Climate Change are proposed to be achieved through a sustainable development strategy under the Twelfth Five-Year Plan. Several thrust areas have been identified in the Twelfth Five-Year Plan for this purpose and a coordinated initiative to identify Nationally Appropriate Mitigation Actions and implement them towards this end will be taken during the Plan period. At the initiative of the Ministry, Planning Commission has recognized Climate Change as a major area of environmental intervention. Climate Change Action Programme (CCAP) has been approved by the Planning Commission for implementation during the 12th Five year Plan. The scheme aims at advancing scientific research, information and assessment of the phenomenon of Climate Change, building an institutional and analytical capacity for research and studies in the area of Climate Change, and supporting domestic actions to address Climate Change through specific programmes and actions at the national and state level. The scheme comprises of eight activities, of which, three relate to scientific studies on Climate Change, two to institution and capacity building and three others to domestic and international actions.[26]

Conclusion and Suggestions

Conclusion

From the above discussion it can be concluded that various efforts in proper direction has been initiated at international as well as national level. Various

---

24 op.cit, Annual Report, p.352

25 https://en.wikipedia.org/wiki/Indian_Network_on_Climate_Change_Assessment

26 http://164.100.47.134/intranet/CLIMATE_CHANGE-INDIA's_PERSPECTIVE.pdf

Conventions, Protocols *etc.* has been incorporated amongst various nations. Developed nations are also under an obligation to help developing nations in order to combat the problem of climate change.

The Government is implementing the National Action Plan on Climate Change (NAPCC) with a view to enhance the ecological sustainability of India's development path and address Climate Change. The Government regularly reviews the progress under the National Action Plan on Climate Change (NAPCC) based on the information provided by the concerned nodal Ministry. The Government has also constituted an Executive Committee on Climate Change in January, 2013, under the chairmanship of Principal Secretary to Prime Minister to assist the Prime Minister's Council on Climate Change in evolving a coordinated response to issues relating to Climate Change at the national level and to monitor the implementation of the eight National Missions and other initiatives under the NAPCC.[27]

Suggestions

Climate change has been proved to be the biggest environmental threat ever to the comfort of mankind. To combat it, the world has taken collective vow to reduce the concentration of the harmful gases. We can also contribute for combating against climate change by following ways:

- Reduction in use of Fossil Fuel.
- Motivating use of CNG for vehicles.
- Strict regulation on carbon emission.
- Educating people.
- Use of social media.

27 ibid.

Chapter 18

Climate Change Impacts on Crop Production and Smallholder Farmer Livelihoods in Limpopo Province, Northern South Africa

Nomcebo R. Ubisi[1], Unathi Kolanisi[2] and Obert Jiri[3]

[1]School of Agricultural, Earth and Environmental Sciences, University of KwaZulu-Natal, Private Bag X01, Scottsville, Pietermaritzburg 3209, South Africa
[2]Consumer Science Deptt., Faculty of Science and Agri., Uni. of Zululand, South Africa
[3]Faculty of Agriculture, University of Zimbabwe, Harare, Zimbabwe
e-mail: nomceboubisi@gmail.com

ABSTRACT

Climate change and variability directly influences the food supply and livelihoods of billions of people, particularly smallholder farmers who depend on climate-sensitive rain-fed agriculture. This study investigated the impacts of climate change on crop production and smallholder farmer's livelihoods in Mopane and Vhembe districts, Limpopo province, South Africa. Hundred and fifty questionnaires were administered to smallholder farmers who were subsistence farmers who produced for household consumption and only seldom sold; those who were farming for both household consumption and selling the surplus; and those who were mainly selling referred to as *'food producers'* because their primary goal was to produce for the market. Eight focus group discussions were conducted for further probing. Transect walks were done with a small group of farmers to triangulate the above mentioned tools. The study findings highlighted that most smallholder farmers especially women (64 per cent), regarded crop production as a way of life. The effect of climate change among farmers have been experienced through decline of productivity compromising food security and livelihood options of farmer's as 73 per cent depend on the income generated from sales of agricultural produce. The findings also highlighted that smallholder subsistence farmers perceived prolonged droughts (56.4 per cent) as the main shock stressing crop production. They also indicated that droughts often lead to low crop yield and high crop failure (73.3 per cent). In response to the prevailing climatic conditions, smallholder farmers used their indigenous knowledge as it was regarded as accessible and available based on trust, convenience, cost effectiveness and reliability. However, there is a need to consider integration of indigenous knowledge system-based, climate-smart agricultural approaches and interventions with scientifically derived information to empower subsistence farmers with adequate adaptive capacity to better respond to climatic challenges.

Keywords: *Smallholder farmers, Climate change, Food security, Livelihood, Climate-smart.*

Introduction

In many parts of Africa, the current climate is already marginal with respect to precipitation and further warming in semi-arid areas and it's likely to be devastating to agriculture (8). Climate may change more rapidly than expected and is projected to have complex, long term effects on the environment. According to (13) climate change brings about substantial losses especially to smallholder farmers whose main source of livelihood is derived from agriculture.

Due to their socio-economic position, smallholder farmers are among the most disadvantaged and vulnerable groups affected by climate change and variability (2). Smallholder farmers in the southern African region are set to be most affected by these climate variations due to poor access to information, access to technology and dependency on climate sensitive agriculture (18, 20, and 21). Therefore, the impact of climate change and variability threatens and weakens the already vulnerable smallholder farmers whose main source of livelihood is rain fed agriculture.

According to (13) smallholder agriculture is the engine of rural economic growth and the main source of most smallholder farmers' livelihoods. (11) Estimates that there are about 500 million smallholder farms in the world; in Asia and sub-Saharan Africa smallholder farmers produce up to 80 per cent of the food consumed and support up to two billion people. However, global climate change has increased vulnerability leading to poverty and human food insecurity. According to (8) in South Africa the agricultural sector contributes 3.4 per cent to the Gross Domestic Product (GDP) and employs 30 per cent of the labour force, and for the third quarter of 2010 Primary agriculture contributed about 3 per cent to the GDP of South Africa whose nominal value was estimated at R667 billion (4). Regardless of the great contribution agriculture to the economy, it could be greatly affected by climate related disasters such as erratic rainfalls, floods and extended dry seasons.

In South Africa rural smallholder farmers are vulnerable to climate change and according to (10),(5) and (19), it is expected to increase food insecurities and worsen the poverty status among rural communities, affecting all four dimensions of food security, which are food availability, accessibility, utilization and stability, as well as livelihood assets. As indicated by (13), smallholder farmers' production systems are directly threatened by the increasing temperatures that cause heat stress on plants, reducing water availability and lowering overall productivity.

The changing climate poses a negative impact on overall productivity; soil fertility due to the very hot temperatures accompanied by dry winds leading to erosion, wilting of plants and poor production (7). The (9) highlighted that soil is very vital for the provision of nutrients for plant growth, carbon storage as well as the regulation of water cycle. The increase in temperature and changing of precipitation patterns negatively affects soil quality which results in loss of soil organic matter. This action negatively affects the soil fertility as rising of air temperatures are likely to speed-up the natural decomposition of organic matter and increase the rates of other soil processes (1). (8), also highlighted that yields could fall quite dramatically in the absence of adaptation measures. This degrades soils which are critical for crop production subsequently compromise food quantity and quality. Majority of smallholder farmers in rural areas have no or primary level education, therefore it is difficult for them access information on new technologies on soil management (6). These farmers mostly practice mono-cropping, which is disadvantageous as it degrades soils even more. Climate change has also impacted on the erratic rainfalls in South Africa and Limpopo is no different to the effects with the current drought the country is facing.

The Limpopo province in South Africa is relatively dry with an annual average rainfall of 400mm (15). The (15) highlighted that in Limpopo province, drought is a very serious problem as the province is semi-arid area with low and erratic rainfall. The impact of low rainfall in this region has resulted in loss of livestock, shortage of drinking water, low yields and shortage of seeds for subsequent cultivation. The loss of these natural assets among smallholder farmers minimize their ability to cope with the climatic changes, hence they are vulnerable to climate change. The (6) highlighted that increasing temperatures in South Africa may support expansion of the borders of vector and water borne diseases (*e.g.* malaria and cholera), and that climate change may also potentially trigger new and emerging infection epidemics and environmental toxins caused by disruptions to human well-being and to agricultural and natural ecosystems. It is for these reasons that the mitigation and adaptation to climate change should be given attention.

In various South African rural areas, smallholder farmers are generally found in remote areas, making it difficult to reach because roads are either in poor condition or non-existent. Smallholder farmers' adaptation to climate change at a local level faces poor infrastructure as part of the main challenges due to erratic rains causing floods, destroying buildings, eroding roads and bridges. As a result, there is long transportation time with high costs, due to inadequate transport infrastructure. According to(16) transportation of produce to the markets on time is one of the key constraints for smallholder farmers in rural areas. This therefore, results in loss of quality and late delivery to the markets, leading to produce being sold at lower prices or rejected, so, this means a lack of sustainable income for the smallholder farmers, which affects their livelihoods as well as their food security (3).

According to (14) the negative impacts of climate change can be significantly reduced through adaptation strategies. Therefore, there is a need for investments to improve agricultural productivity under the risk of climate change. This paper investigates the impacts of climate change on crop production and smallholder farmer's livelihoods in Mopane and Vhembe districts, Limpopo province, South Africa.

Materials and Methods

Description of the Study Area

The study was conducted in Limpopo province, Northern South Africa, within two district municipalities namely Mopani (23.31670 S, 30.71670 E) and Vhembe (22.93330 S, 30.46670E) (Figure 18.1). The Mopani District is situated in the North eastern part of the Limpopo Province covering an area of about 25 344, 13 km2 in the province, with farming as the second largest employer in the district. However, this district is characterized by low rainfall (between 400mm to 900mm per year), resulting in limited water resources causing severe water shortages and regular drought conditions particularly in the lower-lying areas of the district. Vhembe district is located in a semi-arid area that is frequently affected by dry spells, often growing into severe drought.

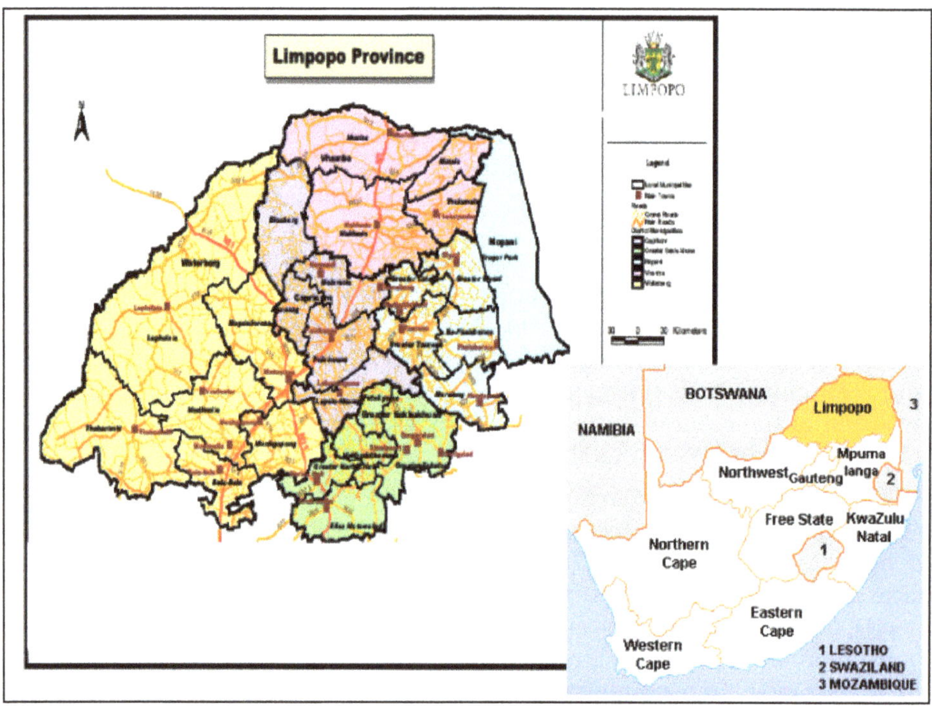

Figure 18.1: Location Map of the Study Area, Limpopo Province.

The district is the most northern district of Limpopo province with a rainfall pattern ranging between 246mm to 681mm per annum. Vhembe district covers an area of about 25 592 km2 which is predominantly rural, with a population size of about 1, 294,722 people. As reported by the (15) the two district municipalities were the most vulnerable to climate change experiencing extreme climatic risk as well as high climate variability in the province.

Data Collection

Both qualitative and quantitative methods were used to collect data in the study. The quantitative research method was used to compare responses across the participants since they were asked identical questions in the same order to allow for significant comparison of responses across participants. On the other hand, the qualitative research method was used to seek understanding of the farmer's perspective or situation by regarding the participants as experts of their situation. This methodology was found appropriate for this study because the study aimed to find meaningful answers and experiences of farmers with regards to the impacts of climate change on crop production and variability on smallholder farmer's livelihoods and food security

A representative population of 150 smallholder farmers in Mopani and Vhembe districts participated in this study. The local extension officer of each local municipality provided a list of households and the smallholder farmers were randomly selected from each local municipality. The extension worker selected every fifth household in their area for administering the questionnaire. Focus group discussions as well as transect walk participants were also selected to be representative of the youths, women, and elderly and cheer leaders in both communities.

Data Analysis

A Statistical Package for Social Sciences (SPSS) version 23.0, Microsoft excel 2010 statistical package and STATA version 8 were used for questionnaire data analysis. Focus group discussions and secondary data were analyzed through content analysis by identifying themes, concept, patterns and trends.

Results and discussions

Negative Effects of Climate Change

The study findings highlights that the majority of individuals involved in rural agriculture were women (64 per cent) and they regarded crop production as a way of life, compared to 36 per cent men. These findings confirm the stereotype denoting agriculture as an activity for women, due to their perceived roles as custodians of families while men are usually involved in other cash-based activities to secure the livelihoods. Most of the farmers had income of $100 or less per month mainly from farming 73 per cent (Table 18.1).

Farmers observed climatic and non-climatic shocks caused by climate change. According to the respondents 65 per cent of female farmers had no idea about the climate change concept. They were the most vulnerable group as they reported to have experienced very severe losses of agricultural based food over the past 10 years (54 per cent) whereas the losses for male farmers were moderately severe 46 per cent (Table 18.2).

Table 18.1: Household Source of Income

		Gender	
		Male	*Female*
Total household income Per month ($)	Below 50	19	16
	51–100	52	64
	101–200	20	11
	Above 200	9	9
Source of income	Pension	58	
	Farming	73	
	Part-time job	5	
	Remittances	1	
	Social grant	13	
Total per cent of the different gender		36	64

Table 18.2: Loss of Crop Production Due to Climate Change

		Gender	
		Male	*Female*
Have you ever heard about climate change?	Yes	56	35
	No	44	65
How severe has the crop loss been over the past 10 years?	Very Severe	52	54
	Moderately severe	46	38
	Not severe	2	7
Total per cent of the different gender		36	64

The study findings revealed that different type of farmers had experienced different climatic shocks over the past ten years. Prolonged droughts were observed to have increased (51.3 per cent) as well as very hot seasons. About 5.3 per cent of the farmers observed increase in floods, and of them majority were subsistence farmers (7.4 per cent), with only 4 per cent of the farmers stated not to have observed any climatic changes (Table 18.3).

Table 18.3: Climatic Shocks Observed by Smallholder Farmers

Type of farmers	*Floods*	*Prolonged Droughts*	*Very Hot Seasons*	*Haven't Observed Any Changes*
Subsistence	7.4 per cent	56.4 per cent	29.8 per cent	6.4 per cent
Selling and consumption	0 per cent	44 per cent	56 per cent	0 per cent
Food producers	3.2 per cent	41.9 per cent	54.8 per cent	0 per cent

The respondents also highlighted the negative effects climate change had on the socio-economic aspect, emotional status as well as their food and nutrition security status (Table 18.4).

Table 18.4: Negative Effects of Climate Change on Limpopo's Smallholder Farmers

Theme	*Concept*	*Quotes*
Socio-economic effect on crop production	Declining crop yields	"Our production yield have dropped, so we experience food insecurities"
	Water scarcity	"there is no rain, hence no water, no crops"
	New pest and disease	"We keep on losing crops due to new pests such as aphid attacks"
Emotional effect	Loss of Hope	"We keep on losing our crops"
	Fear	"If these prolonged droughts persist and there's no rain, we are afraid wedie will of hunger and food insecurity"
	Helpless	"The issue of climate change is beyond our control, there's nothing we cando"
Food and nutrition security status	Food availability and access compromised	"We have not planted because there are no rains"
		"Last year we did not plant we were waiting for rains, and we suffered"

Discussions

Household Source of Income

The study findings confirm the (15) report that agriculture in Limpopo is viewed as a cornerstone of the rural economy because most farmers generate their livelihoods from it. In this study, agriculture was the main diversification strategy used by the farmers to complement their household income. The findings indicate that agricultural income was the major stabiliser and buffer of the household economic status (Table 18.1). As a result for these agriculture dependent vulnerable groups, any exposure to risks and minor changes in climate can have disastrous impacts to their household food security status and poses imbalances in livelihoods.

Loss of Crop Production Due to Climate Change

These findings are in agreement with previous studies that indicated that, in rural Limpopo the concept of *'climate change'* was virtually unknown among farmers (17). Although the concept of *'climate change'* was unknown, the farmers had their own understanding and some observations noted on what was happening (Table 18.2). According to the farmers the so called *'climate change'* was a day-to-day weather occurrence, that was observed through prolonged droughts and a significant decline in crop production due to lack of water. Therefore, there is also a need of weather stations (rain gauges) in the fields of these smallholder farmers communities as this will help them keep track of rain received yearly.

Climatic Shocks Observed by Smallholder Farmers

Smallholder farmers in the study areas were exposed to a number of shocks and stresses that affects their livelihoods. The farmers highlighted that they have been experiencing prolonged droughts, heat waves, increased dry seasons and reduced rainfall seasons which led to frequent livestock deaths, human disease outbreaks, crop failure, reduced yield and food insecurities over the past 10 years (Table 18.3). This was also highlighted by the key informants of the local municipalities.

Subsistence farmers perceived prolonged droughts (56.4 per cent) as the main shock stressing their production whilst other farmers were of the opinion very hot seasons were the significant shock (56 per cent). To further confirm these findings, during the conduct of the research, observations were made that the subsistence farmers had not planted anything because there were no signs of rain in areas such as Tzaneen and Maruleng.

Negative Effects of Climate Change on Limpopo's Smallholder Farmers

The focus group discussions held with the respondents highlighted that the climate change effects had a negative effect on the socio-economic aspects of the smallholder agricultural production, their emotional status as well as their food and nutrition status (Table 18.4).

As mentioned by the smallholder farmers the climate change over the past few years has resulted in prolonged droughts, reduced rainfall and very high temperatures which resulted in low crop yields. The smallholder farmers stated that lack of water for irrigation was another major challenge so the negative changes in rainfall patterns affected their livelihoods, because they end up delaying their planting seasons in anticipating for rainfall until it is too late in the season to plant. These findings support the (15) that Limpopo province has been experiencing extreme droughts, heat waves and reduced rainfall. These negative climatic effects compromise the well-being of the farmers as they experience food shortages.

As the respondents experienced erratic temperature changes and unpredictable rainfall they observed new pest and disease invasions. The "aphid attacks" of cabbage was one of the troublesome pests. Similar results were highlighted by (13) that smallholder farmers' production systems are directly threatened by the increasing temperatures that cause heat stress on plants, reducing water availability, lowering overall productivity and introducing new pests and diseases. According to the report by the (12) the invasion of crops by pests and diseases were caused by the rising temperatures and changes in precipitation patterns. Therefore, the increasing temperatures result in great loss of smallholder farmers' crop production. As some farmers highlighted during the FGDs even their indigenous ways of controlling pests seemed to be less effective, subsequently the new invasions infer some economic demands and unfortunately their knowledge seems to be limited on how to manage and control the pests (aphid attacks).

The negative effects of climate change have been seen to also affect the farmers emotionally. The prolonged droughts resulted in some of the farmers losing hope since they lost almost everything the previous year and it was still hard for them to recover from the loss. The farmers highlighted that they were aware of their vulnerability status towards climate as they are highly exposed to the negative impact of climate change mainly rainfall shortages (drought). The farmers also stated that they are now more confused and living in fear, as they are not sure whether to continue farming or not, since there is less rain due to prolonged droughts. These farmers greatest fear is that the agricultural sector is the driver of their well-being, so they are bothered as unfavourable weather threatens their food security status and limits their livelihood options.

The focus group discussions revealed the smallholder farmer's willingness to progress and to adopt strategies that will mitigate the climatic stresses and threats. However they feel like the situation is beyond their control, thus feeling helpless since their indigenous knowledge which is cost-effective and most accessible seems to be outdated.

Conclusions and Recommendations

This study investigated the impacts of climate change on crop production and smallholder farmer's livelihoods in Mopane and Vhembe districts, Limpopo province, South Africa. The results of this study showed that in Mopani and Vhembe district municipalities agriculture is the back-bone and the primary source of the smallholder farmers' livelihoods. The study revealed that smallholder farmers in these municipalities were categorized in three groups: subsistence farmers who produced for household consumption and only sold seldom; then those who were farming for both household consumption and selling the surplus; and those who were referring to themselves as *'food producers'* because their primary goal was to sell to the market. However, the majority of smallholder farmers were not aware of climate change. Subsistence farmers more especially women were found to be the most vulnerable to climate change due to their high dependency on rainfall for their farming and lack of flexibility to employ different adaptation strategies.

Smallholder farmers were affected by prolonged droughts, reduced rainfall and invasion of new pests and diseases such as aphid attacks. In order to counter these effects, the majority of smallholder farmers in Mopani and parts of Vhembe relied on their indigenous knowledge for their farming practices since most of them suffered a serious lack of climate information that would help them adapt.

Therefore, there is need to bring awareness of the implications of climate change and to consider integration of indigenous knowledge system-based, climate-smart agricultural approaches and interventions with scientifically derived information to empower subsistence farmers with adequate adaptive capacity to better respond to climatic challenges.

Acknowledgements

The research team wishes to thank the National Research Foundation (NRF) for funding this research. The African Centre for Food Security staff members at the University of KwaZulu-Natal for information sharing throughout the year towards the research is also acknowledged. The LDA for approval to conduct the study in Mopani and Vhembe District Municipalities and The community members and agricultural advisors of Tzaneen, Maruleng, Mutale and Musina Local municipalities for participating in this study and for the valuable information they provided.

References

1. Altieri MA, and Koohafkan P (2008).Enduring Farm: climate change, smallholders and traditional farming communities. Third World Network, Malaysia.
2. ASFG (2013). Supporting smallholder farmers in Africa: A framework for an enabling environment.International NGOs working together with Africa's smallholder farmer, London.
3. Baloyi JK (2010). An analysis of constraints facing smallholder farmers in the agribusiness value chain. University of Pretoria, South Africa.
4. Chamuka T (2011). Possible Short to Long-Term Impacts of the January 2011 Floods to South African and Some of Her SADC Trading Partners,http://www.sangonet.org.za, accessed on 20 April 2015.
5. Clarke C (2012). Responses to the linked stressors of Climate Change and HIV/AIDS amongst vulnerable rural households in the Eastern Cape, South Africa.Unpublished Msc thesis.Department of Environmental Science, Rhodes University, Grahamstown, South Africa.
6. DEA (2010).Climate Change – A Critical Emerging Issue, http://soer.deat.gov.za/Climate_change_-_a_critical_emerging_issue__May_2010_1ZyIN.pdf.file, accessed on 18 May 2015.
7. DEDEA (2013). Limpopo green economy plan: Including provincial climate change response,https://www.environment.gov.za/sites/default/files/docs/limpopogreen_economyplan.pdf, accessed on 10 May 2015.
8. Dinar A, Hassan R, Mendelsohn R and Benhin J (2008). Climate change and agriculture in Africa: Impact assessment and adaptation strategies. Earthscan publishers, London.
9. EEA (2009). Soil and climate change, http://www.eea.europa.eu/themes/soil/climate, accessed on 2 May 2015.
10. FAO (2008). Climate change, energy and food: Climate-related transboundary pests and diseases. FAO, Rome.
11. IFAD (2010).Rural Poverty Report, http://www.ifad.org/rpr2011/, accessed on May 2015.
12. IPCC (2007). "Summary for Policymakers. In: Climate Change 2007: Impacts, Adaptation and Vulnerability". Contribution of Working Group II to the Fourth Assessment Report of the Intergovernmental Panel on Climate.Cambridge. UK. Cambridge University Press.
13. KombaC, and Muchapondwa E(2012). Adaptation to climate change by smallholder farmers in Tanzania. Economic research Southern Africa, Tanzania.

14. Kurukulasuriya P, and Mandelsohn R (2008).Crop Switching as an Adaptation Strategy to Climate Change.African Journal of Agricultural and Resource Economics, 2: 105-12.
15. LDA (2012). The Mapping of Agricultural Commodity Production in the Limpopo province, South Africa.
16. Louw A, Chikazunga D, Jordan J, and Bienade E (2007).Regoverning markets: small scale producers in modern agrifood markets, agrifood sector series: restructuring food markets in South Africa. Dynamics within the context of the tomato sub-sector, Pretoria.
17. Maponya P, and Mpandeli S (2012).Climate Change and Agricultural Production in South Africa, Impacts and Adaptation options. Journal of Agricultural Science, 4: 10.
18. Mutekwa VT (2009). Climate change impacts and adaptation in the agricultural sector: The case of smallholder farmers in Zimbabwe. Journal of Sustainable Development in Africa, 11: 237-256.
19. Mpandeli S and Maponya P (2013). The use of climate forecasts Information by farmers in Limpopo Province South Africa. Journal of Agricultural Science, 5: 2.
20. Morton J F (2007). The Impact of Climate Change on Smallholder and Subsistence Agriculture. *PNAS, 104:50.*
21. Oxfam (2007). Adapting to climate change, What's needed in poor countries, and who should pay. Oxfam Briefing Paper 104, Oxfam International.

Chapter 19

Conservation of Biodiversity in Sacred Groves and its Connection with Wild Food and Agricultural Practices

D.K. Kulkarni and D.S. Nipunage

BAIF Development Research foundation, Pune 411058.
K.M.C. College, Khopoli, Dist.- Raigad
e-mail: dilipkkulkarni@gmail.com dsnipunage@gmail.com

ABSTRACT

Western Maharashtra, has rich biodiversity conserved in 'Sacred groves or *Devrais* or *Deorahat*'. These preserved forests had been maintained by local people on religious belief. These forests are preserved to respect specific deity. Tribal communities are preserving these virgin forest patches for social, cultural, religious and even for funeral activities. These forests are sources of wild food plants, which are useful as future germplasm of plant resources.

Tribal communities from Western Maharashtra consume vegetables, flowers, fruits, tubers, seeds, mushrooms, *etc.* They also consume toxic plants with some traditional recipes during famine. Traditional wisdom of these communities in their dietary practice places a premium on nutrition. These wild food plants are nutritious and can add value to the dietary pattern of undernourished communities.

During last few decades, correlation between food consumption and various diseases has been established. Chronic diseases like obesity, diabetes, cancer and asthma are now seen to be diet related. In United states, obesity has risen to epidemic levels. Obesity is a risk factor for serious diseases like Type II diabetes and heart disease. It is also a risk factor for certain cancers. National Institute of Health reported increase in obesity. 65 per cent US adults are overweight or obese, with nearly 31 per cent adults meeting criteria for obesity. The Institute has programme for prevention and treatment of obesity through lifestyle modification by specific diet and physical activity. One of the solutions to these health problems is the Indian system of Medicine - Ayurveda. According to Ayurvedic system of medicine certain foods should be regularly consumed or certain foods should be avoided based on the constitution of an individual. Even in traditional medicine, practitioners recommend a range of diets.

Taking the clue from their traditional knowledge of various communities, utilizing modern scientific tools to evaluate functional food resources is a major area of research in coming years.

The role of ethno-biologist is well recognized for documentation of indigenous cultures and knowledge. Scientific information on the genetic wealth conserved by tribal communities is useful for selecting genotypes for resistance or tolerance to wide range of biotic and abiotic stresses. The yield of rice has been dramatically improved due to conservation of intra-specific wide varieties. Rural or tribal people have conserved biological diversity, remained poor, while those who have applied modern technology to convert biodiversity into economic wealth, have grown rich. The wild variety of genetic diversity of plants is still available in tribal areas, due to harmony with nature which is inherited in the culture and life of tribal societies. These communities collect wild food plants for their consumption from near by forest which was not preserved on religious ground. Even some agricultural operations require some instruments and some medicines for human and livestock are also collected and used. It is clear that Sacred groves and surroundings forest is key issue of biodiversity conservation.

Keywords: *Coservation of sacred groves, Wild food resources, Agricultural implements.*

Introduction

Forest preserved on religious grounds is known as Deorai or Deo rahati or Sacred grove. It is a traditional heritage of natural bioconservation in Indian culture and civilization [14]. Generally, sacred groves are classified into different forest types and they preserve climax vegetation. These sacred groves are conserved with varied degree of ecological and socio-cultural dimensions. It may be noted that even as the social changes occur, the rejuvenation of cultural heritage –one of the important ecosystem services of sacred groves, can act to support the conservation and restoration of groves. It may also be pointed out that cultural heritage and forest vegetation are complementary to each other in determining ecosystem health of community –based bio-diversity conservation institutions like sacred groves. Imbalance of these components can severely affect all other ecosystem services.[1].

The term "remnant vegetation" is broadly used to traditional conservation of native vegetation that occurs within fragmented landscapes. Remnants are generally small to medium sized patches of vegetation surrounded by highly modified land, such as cropping or grazing lands. Remnants are often thought of as patches of trees, shrubs and huge climbers 46. However, remnants may also be used to describe any fragmented native ecosystem preserved on religious aspect. The flora and fauna of these sacred groves are protected under sanctions and taboos which provide limits to over exploitation [47, 48].

The ecosystem service has been directly or indirectly responsible for regulating floods, purifying water, maintaining the temperature, botanical garden for students and plant lovers, bank of wild relatives of cultivated plants, treasure trove of wild medicinal and edible plants, shelter for birds and insects, areas of regional environmental studies, house of microbes and fungi, *etc.* Biological processes occurred in sacred groves are responsible for recycling nutrients, soil formation and providing the supporting services to the human societies. These human societies are also culturally dependent on the ecosystems for spiritual, aesthetic and recreational purposes and usages.[51, 52].

Scientific information on the genetic wealth conserved by tribal communities is useful for selecting genotypes for resistance or tolerance to wide range of biotic and abiotic stresses. The yield of rice has been dramatically improved due to conservation of intra-specific wide varieties. Rural or tribal people have conserved biological diversity, remained poor, while those who have applied modern technology to convert biodiversity into economic wealth, have grown rich. The wild variety of genetic diversity of plants is still available in tribal areas, due to harmony with nature which is inherited in the culture and life of tribal societies. These communities collect wild food plants for their consumption from near by forest which was not preserved on religious ground. Even some agricultural operations require some instruments and some medicines for human and livestock are also collected and used. It is clear that Sacred groves and surroundings forest is key issue of biodiversity conservation.[39.]

Section I: Importance of Sacred Groves as Sanctum Sanctorum

Environmental impact of sacred groves serve the vital function of preservation of plants, wild animals, fauna, *etc.* which have become very rare and extinct elsewhere [6.] Kulkarni and Nipunage [12] recorded floristic diversity and ecological studies of Dhup-Rahat from Bhor region in Pune district. It is situated near village Hirdoshi on Bhor-Mahad road. It is named after magnificent trees of Dhup *i.e. Canarium strictum* Roxb. It covers an area of 5 hectares along a gentle slope near Varandha pass, only a few km away from the origin of Nira river. The tree is very rare in Western ghats of Maharashtra and hence Dhup rahat should be preserved as a national monument.

Two sacred groves from Pune district namely Sagadara and Navaliachi rai were studied for their monotypic plants. In Sagdara sacred grove, trees of *Tectona grandis* L. are dominant while Navaliachi rai harbours *Miliusa tomentosa* (Roxb.) Sinclaee in higher numbers [18.]

Nine sacred groves from Bhudargad taluka of Kolhapur district were surveyed for rare and endemic plants. Village Patgaon has two sacred groves namely Swayambhuchi rai and Hanumantachi rai. Shivdav village has two groves namely Shivadavchi rai and Maharthak rai. Tirwade village has three groves namely Khetarpalchi rai, Tondalichi rai and Nagnatchi rai. Kadgaon village has Tambayachi rai and Pal village has Palchi rai having predominant unique tree species in the sacred grove namely *Bischofia javanica* Bl having 200 trees. From these nine sacred groves rare and endemic plants are reported as per IUCN and BSI records like *Holigarna grahamii* Kurz., *Garcinia indica* Choiss, *Ancistroclades heyneanus* Wall, *Senecio dalzellii* Clarke, *Asystasia chelonoides* Nees, *Hydnocarpus pentandra* Oken *and Cissus elongate* Roxb. [15].

Konkan area of Maharashtra was surveyed to carry out status of rare, endangered plants from preserved forests for medicine and food resources. The field visits were made in 4 talukas of Ratnagiri districts and data on 35 preserved forests have been documented for their IUCN status. The local informants were interviewed to document the medicine and food resources which are used in their daily life. The CAMP exercise was carried out by Noroji Godrej Centre for Plant Research (NGCPR) in Collaboration with Department of Botany University of Pune for threatened medicinal plants of Maharashtra in September 1998. Another Conservation Assessment and Management plan exercise was carried out by FRLHT in year 2000. These documents of species richness,rare, endangered, vulnerable, *etc.*, were evaluated as per IUCN guidelines. 15 plants were evaluated as endangered,

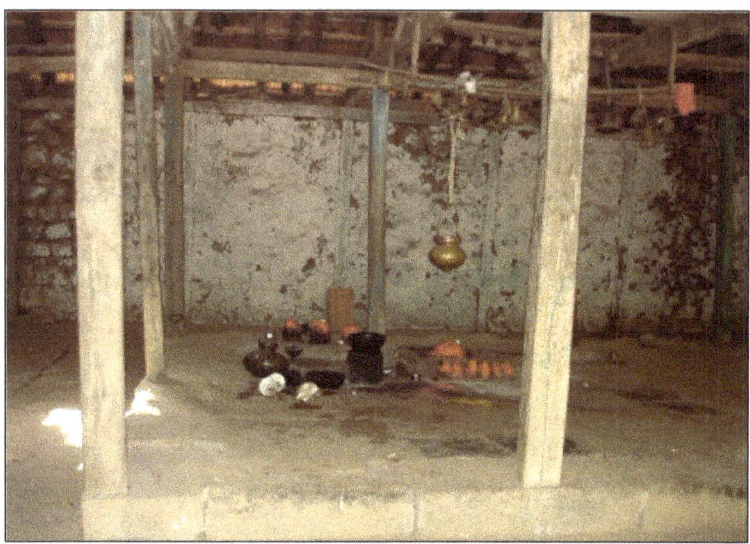

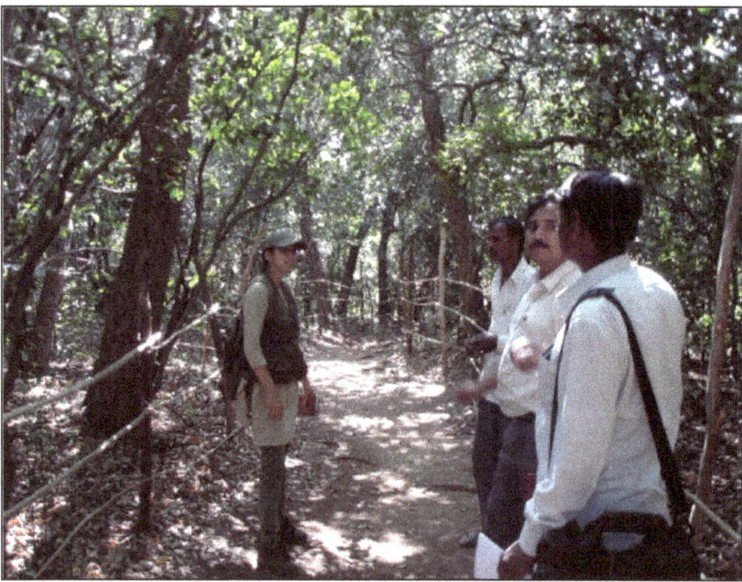

Figure 19.1: Bhiravnath Sacred grove-Ajnawale-Junnar-Photo by Author–Dr. D.K. Kulkarni.

vulnerable, least concern, threatened, critically endangered and near threatened categories [49]. In addition to rare, endemic and endangered plants available in sacred groves they are also reported from ethnobotanical point of view [53].

Phansalkar and Kulkarni [22]. conducted ecological survey in Ajnawale sacred grove in Junnar taluka of Pune district. Floristic diversity of plants was recorded in sacred grove. It includes maximum population of *Memecylon umbellatum* Burm.f.-311, *Ixora brachiata* Roxb.- 110, *Olea dioica* Roxb-55, *Canthium dicoccum* Teys and Binn.-56 and others 118. The numbering on each tree species has been made. During first shower of monsoon some ephemerals are occurring in the core zone. Maximum populations are of *Nervilia aragoana* Gaud, *Dioscorea pentaphylla* L., *Dioscorea belophylla* Haines, *Curcuma inodora* Blatt., *Zingiber purpureum* Rosc. *Zingiber nassanum* (Grah.) Ramam., *Zingiber cernuum* Dalz. *Arisaema tortuosum* Schott and Endl. and *Malaxis rheedii* Sw. This indicates that ephemeral composition is found in core zone due to habitat conservation and absence of external biotic pressure.

Balanophora abbreviata Bl. has been observed on *Memecylon umbellatum* Burm.f. plant in the core area. There are several reports of the host plant, but in Junnar area it is the first ever report on *Memecylon umbellatum.*

The sacred groves in Bhor taluka are in the range of 0.02 to 10.00 ha in area. The sacred groves with lofty trees, shrubs and giant lianas are peculiar features of natural ecosystem. Natural heritage of forest conservation in Bhor region was recorded 16. Local people from the region have maintained eight sacred groves and conserved the forest patches with religious taboos. Floristic composition of few of them is as below:

Giant climbers which are recorded in Dhamunshi sacred grove are *Entada pursaetha* DC. *Ancistrocladus heyneanus* Wall, *Gnetum ula* Brong., *Butea superba* Roxb., *Diploclisia glaucescens* Diels. It indicates that the evergreen elements are present in natural floristic wealth of sacred groves.

Baneshwar sacred grove is under control of Forest Department of Maharashtra State. This grove has been developed as garden and a good picnic spot. Water stream is flowing near the sacred grove and visitors enjoy the water fall. Big trees and some rare plants like *Tacca leontopetaloides* (L.) O. Ktze., *Acacia polyacantha* Willd. are prominent features of Baneshwar sacred grove.

Dhup rahat sacred grove harbours trees like *Terminalia bellirica* Roxb., *Syzygium cumini* (L.) Skeels., *Holigarna grahami* Hk. and *Canarium strictum* Roxb. which are prominent species of the vegetation.

Nageshwar grove has been encroached by Govt. buildings and Schools. Due to Nageshwar temple local people use it as picnic spot. Natural water source is present inside the grove. This grove harbours big trees of *Miliusa tomentosa* Roxb, *Plumeria alba* Linn, *Artocarpus heterophyllus* Lamk, *Celtis cinnamomea Lindl.* A.Juss, *Mallotus philippensis* Muell. which are remnants of past floristic wealth. Some climbers like *Vallaris solanacea* O. Ktze *Clematis gourina* Roxb. ex DC., *Acacia caesia* Willd. are well preserved. In recent years many exotic species of plants are introduced like *Parthenium hysterophorus* L., *Synedreall nodiflora* (L.) Gaertn. *Mirabilis jalapa* L. *etc.*

Andharwadachi rai–means once upon a time light was not passing through the thick vegetation on ground. Due to human activities around the sacred grove in last century like agriculture, road construction, cutting of large trees, *etc.* it has

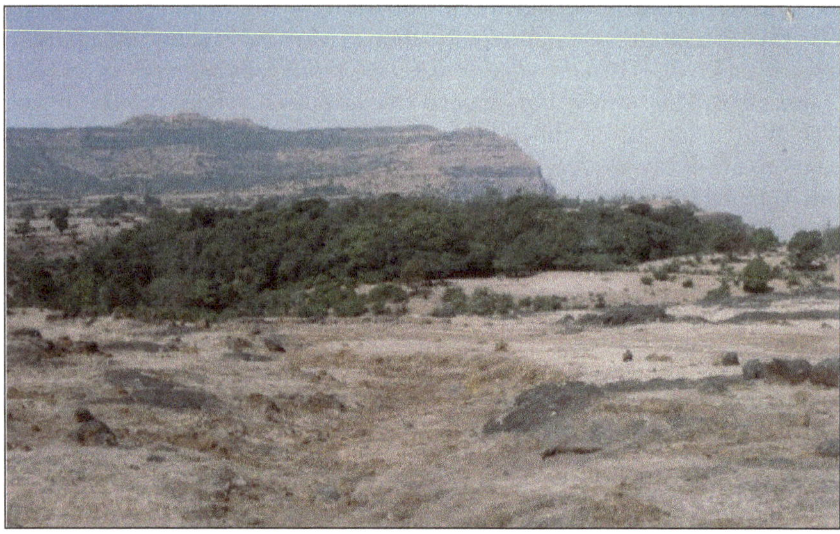

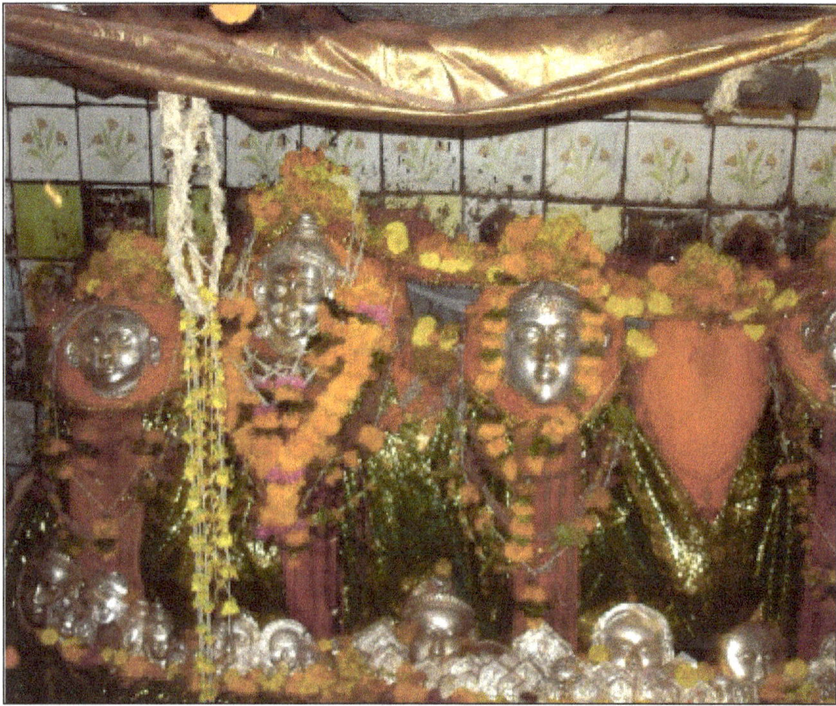

Figure 19.2: Kalubai Sacred Grove–Nanewadi-Near Malshej Ghat-Photo by Author –D.K.Kulkarni.

vanished its total plant wealth and only one tree of *Ficus benghalensis* L. is survived with *Capparis zeylanica* L. climber on it.

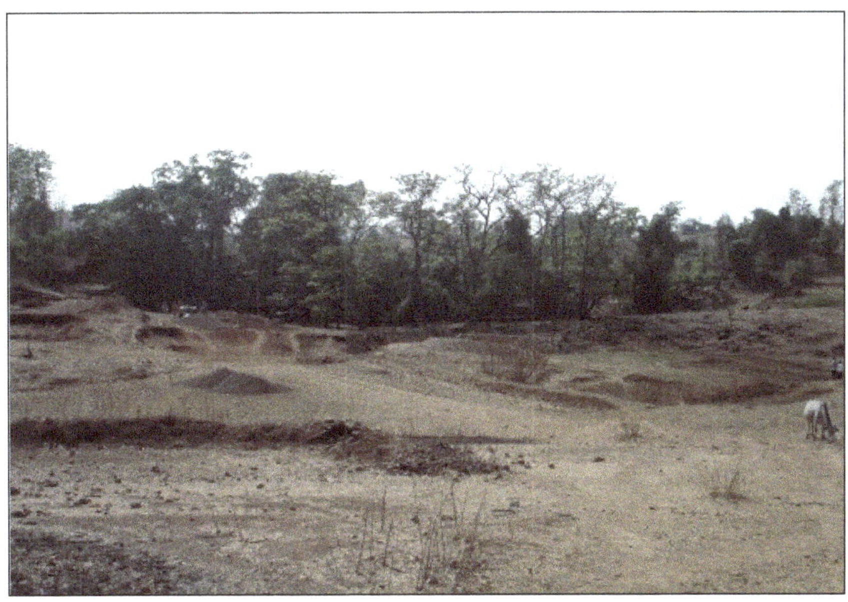

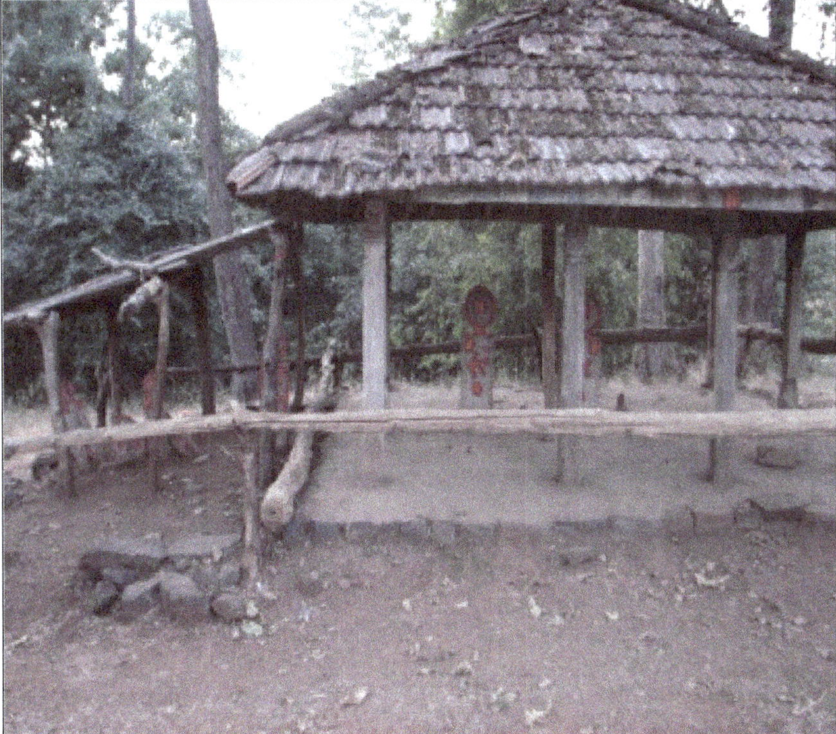

Figure 19.3: Kalamvihira Sacred and Deity Waghoba Photo by Author-Dr. D.K. Kulkarni.

In Kalubaichi rai near Nanewadi village, natural regeneration of *Memecylon* and *Zanthoxylon* is observed. Surrounding area is protected by plantations of *Eucalyptus* done by Forest Department, Maharashtra State.

In village Nandghur, there are six sacred groves protected by Mahadeokoli tribe. Some of them are located in remote places and scanty vegetation is present in Somjaichi rai. There are well protected trees like *Bombax ceiba* L., *Mangifera indica* L., *Zanthoxylum rhetsa* DC *Cassia fistula L. Heterophragma quadrilocularis* K. Schum, *Nothapodytes nimmoniana* (Grah.) Mabb. and *Dendrocalamus strictus* Nees is abundant along with shrubs and climbers.

Maulichi rai near Varvand village has thick population of trees, shrubs and climbers as well as natural regeneration of *Smilax zeylanica* L., *Teramnus labialis* (L. f.) Spreng., *Hemidesmus indicus* R. Br. *etc.*

Plant species like *Caryota urens* L., *Memecylon umbellatum* Burm. F., *Holigarna grahamii* Hook, *Terminalia bellirica* Roxb., *Bomabx ceiba* L. *Gnetum ula* Brongn., *Dalbergia horrida* Mabb., *Jasminum malabaricum* Wt., *etc.* are preserved in many sacred groves. A holy tree *Plumeria alba* L. is observed in sacred groves. It is also interesting to note that *Pongamia pinnata* Pierr., *Erythrina suberosa* Roxb., *Cassia fistula* L., *Phoenix sylvestris* Roxb., *Xantolis tomentosa* Raf. *etc.* are occasionally found in the sacred groves from Bhor region.

Quantitative floristic composition was determined by studying ten quadrats, each with an area of ten square meters chosen at random. Percentage, frequency and occurrence were documented. In this survey 8 sacred groves were visited and was recorded dominant tree species, shrubs, climbers and natural regeneration within sacred groves. Surrounding area of sacred grove was denuded or partly covered with few trees, shrubs, herbs and grasses. Hangarge *et al.*, [29] made attempt to study four sacred groves from the area and focused on plant diversity inside as well as outside the sacred groves.

Nipunage *et al.*[27]. documented 8 sacred groves from Palghar distract with natural diversity of each sacred groves. Detail survey of Waghobachi sacred groves in Kalalmvihira village in Palghar district was undertaken for anthropogenic impact by [4]. Bhusare *et al.*[24]. documented traditional knowledge associated with Kalamvihira sacred grove and cultural diversity.

Section II: Wild Food Resources

Tribal communities in Maharashtra depend upon agricultural food grains and are hardly sufficient for a few months to maintain their families. To make up for the shortage of food grains they have to depend on wild food plants to supplement their diet. 35 reported food resources from Indian aborigines. Aborigines consume a main staple diet and it is supported with supplementary wild foods. These species are consumed by various communities depending on the local availability. Various preparations of plant species are made and sold in tribal markets. Tribals and local communities have accurate knowledge of wild food resources due to their long association with nature. They also know the natural history of each species for obtaining sustained harvest of forest species by preserving forest patches and the traditional knowledge of natural ecosystems. The wide variety of tribal/local communities with their distinctive cultural practices possesses a huge reservoir of time tested information, which should be properly documented. In recent years, due to industrialization, developmental activities in tribal areas and rapid modernization, traditional knowledge of tribals is eroding faster [60.] It is high time to document ethnobotanical knowledge and wisdom of local people to find out new food/crop and horticultural resources which may be useful for modern agriculture [10]. Nene [36] reported 300 diverse plant species belonging to 90 families utilized as food resources during famine. It includes herbs, flowering stalks, leaves, seeds, kernels, fruits, tubers, *etc.* district was studied by [31].

Mahadeokoli tribe is the second largest tribal community in Maharashtra State. They utilized wild plants in their day-to-day life for food, medicine, farming practices, social and cultural aspects, *etc.* Information was gathered on wild food plants including tubers, leafy vegetables, flowers, fruits, toxic and non-toxic tuber consumption with appropriate methods/recipes. These wild food plants play an important role in the dietary pattern 33. These tribals consume 144 non-conventional food resources. They also consume hunger depressing/thirst depressing, plants during scarcity and even hunger increasing, tonic plants. Tribal people collect different types of fruits as an additional income source. Fruit of Karvanda (*Carissa* L.) is one of them and it has natural variability 34. These wild edible plants are also analysed for their chemical compositions.[2,41].

Famine or Scarcity Foods

The Indian subcontinent has natural and artificial causes of famine or scarcity of food resources. The famine conditions occurred 50 times over a period of 2300 years. States that suffered most under drought conditions were Gujarat, Rajasthan, Maharashtra, Punjab, Delhi, Uttar Pradesh, Madhya Pradesh, Bihar, Orissa and Bengal 54. During the famine people were desperate and utilized anything that was found edible. Tribals and the affected population had to find out non-conventional wild food plant species. The aim of such species is to supplement food or to depress hunger by its consumption. Unripe fruits of Arogyappacha (*Tricopus zeylanicus*) are eaten by Kani tribe to remain healthy and agile during their long trips in the high mountainous forests of Agasthyar hills in Kerala. Kani tribals claim that one can live energetically without food for longer days and perform rigorous physical work after consumption of a few fruits of this plant daily [38]. Mahadeokoli tribe from Western Maharashtra consume wild plants during scarcity and for hunger depression.

Wild plants consumed by Mahadeokoli's as thirst depression are shown in Table 19.2.

Nutritional Analysis of Wild Plants

Nutritional science was established in the 19th century by doctors, physiologists, chemists and hygienists. Food is required for the maintenance of human body. Fats and carbohydrates serve as fuel of the human machine, but proteins alone seem to be the source of muscular power. Chemical composition of food stuffs suggest the possibility of determining the value of proteins, carbohydrates, fats, ashes, moisture and specific calorific value by way of exact figures. It means higher value of a substance that exists in the food has higher quality and quantity of nutrients [57].

Table 19.1: Hunger Depressing Wild Plants Consumed by Mahadeokoli's

Name of Plant	*Local Name*	*Part Used*	*Locality*
Achyranthus aspera L.	Aghada	Seeds- hunger depression	Raigad, Thane
Bombax ceiba L.	Katesawar	Roots-used as vegetable in scarcity	Ahmadnagar
Bridelia squamosa Gehrm.	Asana	Leaf juice- drink-hunger depression	Nasik
Coix lacryma-jobi L.	Kusar gavat	Seed flour- hunger depression	Nasik.
Colocasia esculenta Schott.	Alu	Dried Leaves and shoots used in scarcity.	Raigad, Nasik
Cordia dichotoma Forst.	Bhokar	Young leaves used as vegetable in scarcity.	All area.
Dioscorea bulbifera L.	Kadkin	Tubers- scarcity	Raigad, Thane, Nasik, Pune
Dioscorea sativa L.	Goda karanda	Tubers preserved in soil -scarcity	Raigad, Thane, Pune
Ensete superbum Cheesman	Kavadar	Flowering axis and tubers- hunger depression	Raigad, Pune
Firmiana colorata R.Br.	Khavis	Mature fruits-scarcity	Raigad
Jasminum multiflorum Andr.	Naval	Fruits-vegetable-hunger depression	Nasik
Sauromatum pedatum Schott.	Badad	Dried leaves used in scarcity	Raigad

Table 19.2: Thirst Depressant Plants Consumed by Mahadeokoli's

Name of Plant	*Local Name*	*Part Used*	*Locality*
Pueraria tuberose DC.	Pithana	Tubers- Tonic	Pune
Vigna vexillata A.Rich.	Halunda	Tuber-increase hunger	Pune, Thane, Raigad, Nasik, Ahmadnagar
Solena heterophylla Lour.	Gometi	Fruits- increase hunger	Nasik
Coriandrum sativum L.	Dhana	Seed powder- thirst depressant	Raigad

Tribal communities consume wild tubers, rhizomes and corms either in raw or baked or boiled or roasted form. Tender shoots and petiole strips of Wild banana *Kauder* (*Ensete superbum*) are chewed. These are previously cooked in salt water. It is believed to suppress hunger for several days. Similarly, Halunda (*Vigna capensis*) is supposed to stimulate the hunger [37]. Efforts were also made to explore the nutritive potential of wild edible tubers, rhizomes, leafy vegetables and wild fruits which supplement several nutrients particularly calcium and carotenoids. Such unconventional wild edible plants are resources of fats, proteins and are rich sources of micro-nutrients and trace elements [11,40,56].

Table 19.3: Chemical Composition of some Wild Edible Tubers, Rhizomes and Corms (g/100 g fresh samples)

Plant Species	*Edible Portion*	*Moisture (Per cent)*	*Protein*	*Ash*	*Fat G (Per cent)*	*Reducing Sugar*
Dioscorea pentaphylla	—	84	3.6	0.95	1.3	7.2
D.esculanta	—	82	1.7	1.3	0.6	12.2
D.oppositifolia	—	86.5	2.5	0.7	1.5	4.4
D.tomentosa	85	79.9	2.1	1.1	2.1	10.3
D.bulbifera	90	76	2.8	1.0	1.2	14.0
Ensete superbum	—	73.1	1.9	—	1.4	19.6
Pueraria tuberosa	92	84.2	1.7	2.3	0.2	8.7
Vigna vexillata	82.4	88.3	1.5	1.0	1.2	7.0
Arisaema murrayi	—	83	3.7	—	—	9.03
Remusatia vivipara	—	77.2	2.1	2.3	2.6	11.6

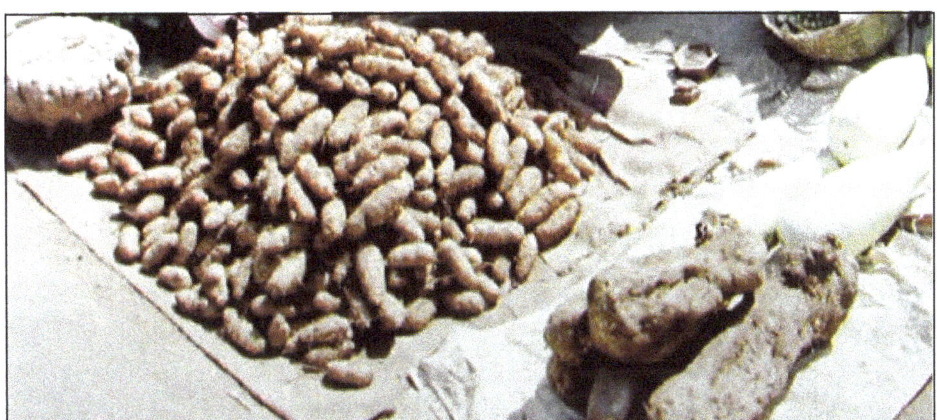

Figure 19.4: Wild Edible Tubers Consumed by Tribal Communities–Photo by Author Dr. D.K. Kulkarni.

Chemical Analysis of some Wild Edible Fruits

Fruit material collected in bulk quantity was brought in the laboratory for chemical analysis. The fruit material was cleaned, washed and chopped for further analysis in laboratory. The material was dried at 50°C for 4 days and kept in airtight containers. Results of proximate chemical analyses of the processed samples are expressed as g per 100 g dry powder (Table 19.5). Detailed procedure for moisture, fat, protein, fiber, ash, *etc.* was followed as per AOAC [58].

Table 19.4: Chemical Analysis of Leafy Vegetables (Expressed as amount per 100 gram powder)

Plant Species	*Moisture (Per cent)*	*Ash (Per cent)*	*Fat g (Per cent)*	*Protein g (Per cent)*	*Iron mg (Per cent)*	*Phosphorus mg (Per cent)*	*Carbohydrates g (Per cent)*	*Energy Kcal (Per cent)*
Ampelocissus tomentosa Planch	12.05	11.6	13.9	10.4	85.00	472.7	64.2	424
Ariopsis peltata Nimmo	67.27	10.9	7.1	18.6	32.2	380.1	63.4	392
Launaea intybacea Beauv.	84.64	9.8	17.6	18.8	87.8	270.7	53.8	449
Remusatia vivipara Kurz.	51.92	13.2	16.3	22.3	29.3	295.9	48.1	401
Spondias pinnata Kurz.	87.8	10.8	10.0	15.3	14.6	276	63.9	407
Smithia hirsuta Dalz.	78.00	1.39	1.19	4.45	--	--	14.97	88
S.bigemina Dalz.	68.60	5.90	1.44	5.58	--	--	18.48	109
S. setulosa Dalz.	57.10	5.96	1.72	7.75	--	--	27.47	156
Vigna khandalensis Sant.	80.40	1.32	0.69	4.02	--	--	13.57	77

Table 19.5: Analysis of Fruits (Expressed as g per 100 g dry powders)

Plant Species	*Moisture (Per cent)*	*Ash (Per cent)*	*Fat g (Per cent)*	*Protein g (Per cent)*	*Iron mg (Per cent)*	*Phosphorus mg (Per cent)*	*Carbohydrates g (Per cent)*	*Energy Kcal (Per cent)*
Ixora coccina L.	81	5.1	11.6	3.7	0	155.4	79.4	437
Dillenia pentagyna Roxb	78.3	2.8	1.1	1.3	0	0	16.3	810
Oxystelma secamone Karst.	79.51	6.08	29.5	16.84	6.32	199.6	47.61	523
Flacourtia montana Grah.	79.01	2.34	6.6	0.92	0.08	52.89	188.5	817
Flacourtia latifolia Cooke	76.92	2.89	10.4	1.18	0.22	68.59	144.2	675.

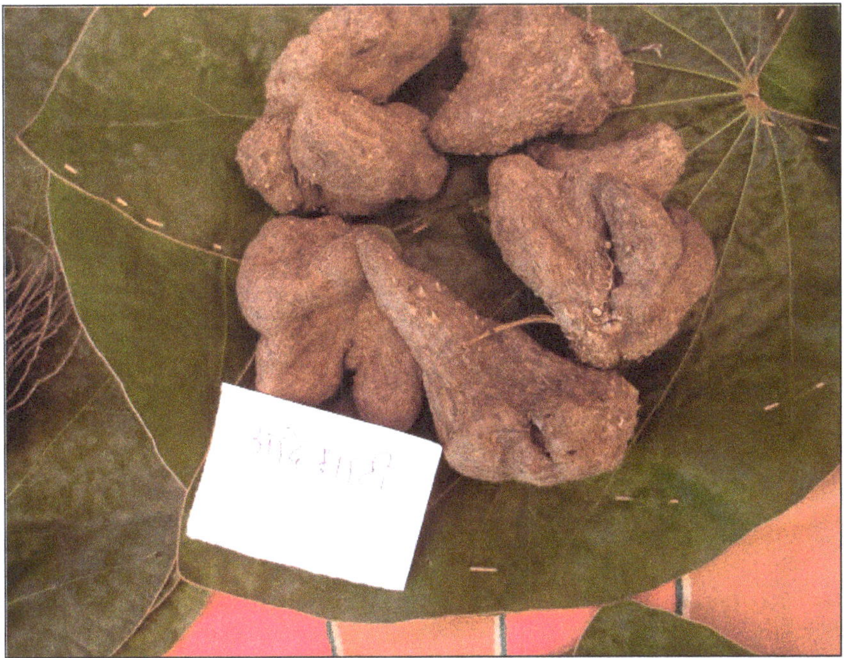

Figure 19.5: ***Vigna vexillata*** **Tubers Consumed by Tribal Communities Photo by Dr. D.K. Kulkarni.**

Wild Relatives of Fruit Crops

Traditional knowledge of plant resources and their propagation/multiplication is necessary for sustainable development of Konkan region. Kankavali Taluka, especially Deogad region is famous for Alphonso mango. They are getting higher price during the season. On the other hand, local people neglect natural potential of plant wealth which can be used for sustainable development. Therefore, it is necessary to train the teachers and students for documentation of indigenous knowledge of plant resources and their propagation techniques. Table 19.6 gives potential resources of wild fruit/seed plants.

Among wild fruits one of the economically important fruit is *Carissa* or Karanda, one of the underutilized fruit in tribal pockets. Tribal people collect fruits from surrounding forests and sell in the nearby markets. The species has been rarely studied for natural selection required for horticultural practices. In this respect, germplasm collection from different locations in eight districts of Maharashtra State was carried out. Fruit characters were mainly considered for selecting and documenting diversity. A random sampling method was followed for fruit samples. The sugar content was measured with the help of hand refractometer to correlate sweetness of the fruits in the field.

Table 19.6: Economically Important Germplasm-Wild Fruit/Seed Plants

Botanical Name	*Part Used*	*Habit*
Syzygium cumini Skeel.	Fruits	Tree
Buchanania lanzan Spreng	Seed	Tree
Carissa congesta Wt.	Fruits	Shrub
Dillenia pentagyna Roxb	Fruits	Tree
Firmiana colorata R.Br.	Seeds	Tree
Mimusops elengi L.	Fruits	Tree
Mangifera indica L.	Fruits	Tree
Trewia nudiflora L.	Fruits	Tree
Garcinia indica Choisy	Fruits	Tree
Ziziphus rugosa Lamk.	Fruits	Tree
Ziziphus mauritiana Lamk.	Fruits	Tree
Meyna laxiflora Robyns	Fruits	Shrub
Sterculia guttata Roxb.	Seeds	Tree

A total of 111 accessions from 45 locations were scanned in fruiting time during April-May from Western Maharashtra. Commercial collection of fruits were recorded from Mulshi-Maval-Velha in Pune district, Karjat- Kashele from Raigad district, Dolkhamb-Shahapur-Murbad from Thane district, Kalsubai-Ghatghar from Ahmadnagar district. Collected fruit samples were categorized in to 16 distinct types based on exomorphic characters such as shape, size, colour, pulp colour, taste, number of seeds per fruit and spines. Konkan region represents rich population of the species [8]. Variables studied in fruits are shown in Table 19.7.

Table 19.7: Range of Variation in Carissa Fruits

Fruit Characters	*Range Observed*
Fruit bunch (No. of fruits)	3-17
Size of fruit	9x9- 44x43 mm
Shape	Round –oblong
Colour	Red-purple-black-green
Taste	Sour-sweet
Pulp colour	White-pink –red
No. of seeds per fruit	1-4
TDS content	10-31 per cent

In this respect, germplasm collection of high value wild fruit species is an essential and important part of research activity [3,41]. These wild fruits are useful for processing into pickles and other bio-products. Tribal communities preserve fruits in traditional method and scientific processing training given to tribal women by [21].

Section III: Natural Resources for Agriculture Purpose

Pune district has different local communities comprising Kunabis, Konkanas, Katkari, Dhangar and Mahadev koli residing in hilly regions of Western Part. They have small holding of land in which they cultivated hill millets, rice, some pulses *etc.* required for their own consumption. They are preserving forest for their own needs like food, fodder, medicines for human and animal, shelter and also for agriculture purpose and storage of harvested agriculture produce. Forests preserved by Maharashtra Govt. and sacred forests are part and parcel of their traditional agriculture which controls soil erosion and maintains heavy precipitation during monsoon season. Traditional farming systems are based on forest cover and hence role of forest is an important part. The tribal people or local people from Bhor region use natural resources for preparing agricultural implements. They generally use special wood available in the surrounding forest. They follow different agricultural operations such as plowing, hoeing, leveling, trampling, manuring, sowing/transplanting, weeding, pest and disease control, harvesting, threshing and preservation of seeds or grains. The plow is the most sacred and essential implement in traditional agriculture and it is prepared from wood of *Acacia chundra* (Roxb.ex Rottler) Willd. (*khair*) *Albizia amara* (Roxb.) Boiv. (*kala shiras*), *Lagerstroemia lanceolata* Wall.(*nana*), *Syzygium cumini* Skeels (*jambul*), *Terminalia crenulata* Roth (*ain, sadada*) *etc.* The hoe is used to weed out the stubble from the ground, an operation that is essential in tillage of land before sowing. This implement is made from *Acacia nilotica* (L.) Willd. Ex Del.(*babul*); *Cassia fistula* L.(*bhava*); *Lannea coromandelica* (Houtt.) Merr. (*mogari*); *Randia spinosa* Poir.(*gel*), *etc.* A heavy wooden log, locally called *Maind,* is pulled by two bullocks over the soil to crush the clods. A wooden soil leveler known as *petari* is used for leveling the plowed land. These implements are prepared from woods such as *Garuga pinnata* Roxb. (*kakad*) and *Terminalia bellirica* Roxb. (*yela*). While the petari is made from *Bridelia squamosa* Gehrm. (*asana*), or *Terminalia chebula* Retz.(*hirda*), other implements like, sickle handles, yokes, and threshing poles are prepared from special wood. The produce of the farmer increases depending on the quality of the threshing pole. The threshed grain is stored in a granary locally called *kanagi,* prepared by using sticks of bamboo, *Vitex negundo* L., and *Carvia callosa* (Wall.) Bremek. [10]

The study was undertaken to identify various traditional implements used for agricultural operations by the farmers of Bhor and Mahad region of Western Maharashtra. Agricultural implements are as old as Stone Age. Traditional agricultural implements were economical in terms of labour, money and time saving. These implements were made up of locally available materials, wood, *etc.* Traditional implements are operated easily without any special skills. Information was documented by using Participatory Rural Appraisal (PRA) techniques like observation and discussion. In the study, 5 traditional agricultural implements were identified and described. [20]. These traditional implements are generally used for traditional farming system of agriculture [17].

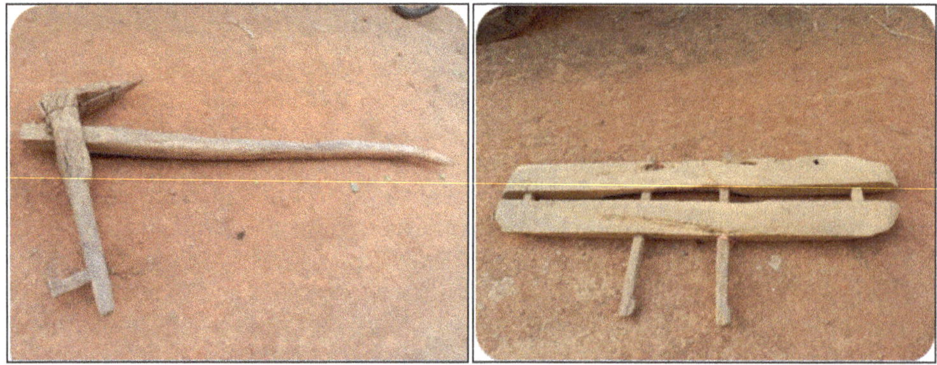

Figure 19.6: The Plow is the most Sacred Essential Implement. Petari used for crushing soil boulders-Photo by author Dr. K. Kulkarni.

Livestock Management in the Area

The tribal people control animal diseases in their livestock by using natural resources. They depend on wild plants for collection of herbs throughout the region. Majority of Mahadeokoli tribals collect plants to cure bone fractures, rinderpest, wound maggots, eye infections, dysentery, tympany, foot-and-mouth disease, prolapse of uterus, *etc.*[9]. This heritage of using herbal medicines for animal health care has a long historical background in India. Ancient non-script verbal knowledge from Bhor area regarding commonly used veterinary medicinal plants has been collected and documented. [28.]

To cure certain ailments like woud healing and maggoty wounds tribal people use different plant resources like *Annona squmosa* L. (Sitaphal), *Acorus calamus* L (Vekand) and others[19]. Other EVM (Ethnoo-veterinary-medicine) practices are also used in Vidharba region [23]. This traditional knowledge is very useful in deworming of cattle [5].

Fodder resources in rural areas are depleting day by day due to over exploitation of natural forest resources and majority of the land used for cultivation of crops is decreasing due to developmental activities. Indian people or tribals are depending on livestock for milk, meat and agricultural operations. Food stuffs are used not only to build up the body but are also used to perform work and convert into various products like milk, wool and meat. Grazing land utilized by farmers is waste land, hill sides and forest patches. This land furnishes grazing only during the monsoon season. After the monsoon season the grazing land begins to dry up and these pasture lands are not suitable for grazing. The condition of pasture land is rather poor due to over grazing followed by soil erosion. The productivity of such pastures is low and can not meet the requirement of the livestock. This shortage of palatable fodders is supported by wild fodder plant species. Generally tribal people from Bhor region prefer tree species like *Grewia tiliifolia* Vahl. (Dhaman), *Hardwickia binata* Roxb. (Anjan), *Dalbergia sissoo* Roxb. ex DC. (Sisav), *Ailanthus excels* Roxb. (Maharukh), *etc.* Tribal people from Maharashtra are also facing shortage of crop residue and they use 20 different fodder species belonging to trees, shrubs and herbs [55.]

Analysis of naturally available fodder resources is an important factor. In this connection fodder samples were collected from tribal region of Vidarbha and Akola region of Ahmadnagar district and analysed for their proximate values [30,32].

Germplasm Collection of Plant Resources for Mitigating Climatic Change

The biggest sources of biodiversity in tropical countries are threatened due to over exploitation, changing ecosystems and global warming. Department of Environment food and rural affairs warned against temperature increase of as much as 3-4°C towards the same time line in India. Further more it is speculated that an increase of only 2°C will have consequences in terms of shifting of cultivation pattern and yield reduction of rice and wheat, which are staple food for more than one third of the world population.[43]

Naturally there is variation in social and cultural practices and food resources used by tribal communities. In recent years, natural wealth is disappearing due to habitat destruction and developmental activities like roads, dams, social and cultural development in tribal areas[59].

The spread of modern landraces and hybrids which began in the mid-1960s has made an important impact on small farmers of India. The loss of crop genetic resources can be linked to the spread of modern agriculture. Uniform cultivar over wide areas has resulted in abandonment of genetically variable, indigenous varieties by subsistence farmers [44].

Millets are among the oldest cultivated crops in the world and cultivated over more than 35.8 million ha around the world as per estimates for 2007. They are referred as coarse cereals and this term is highly misleading in view of their nutritional profiles and strategic importance to the livelihood of millions of people [45]. Millets comprise two main groups of species, major millets includes Sorghum and pearl millets. Minor millets are represented by six cultivated species, Little millets, Indian barnyard millets, Kodo millet, Foxtail millets, Finger millets, Proso millet.

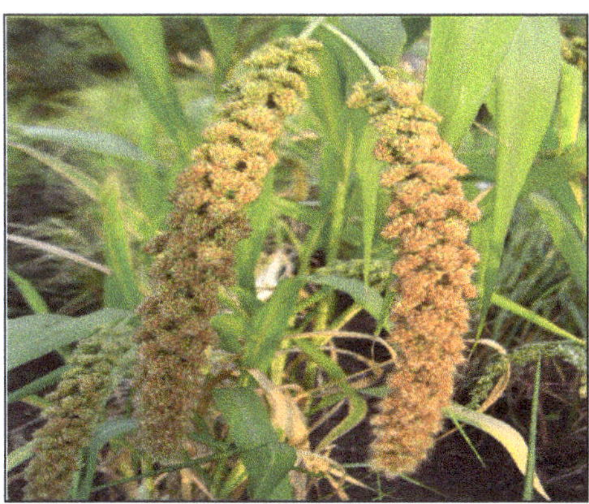

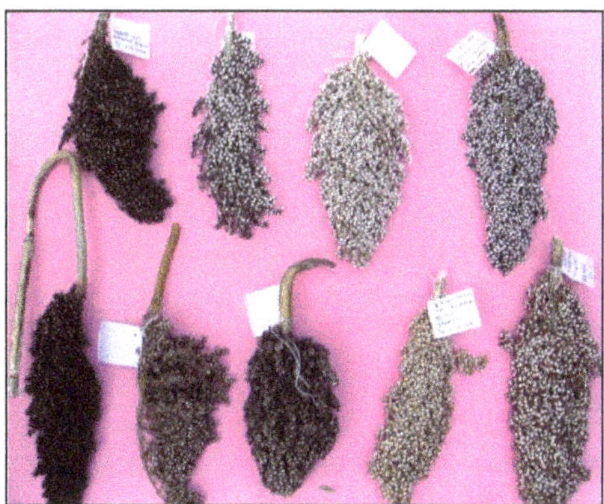

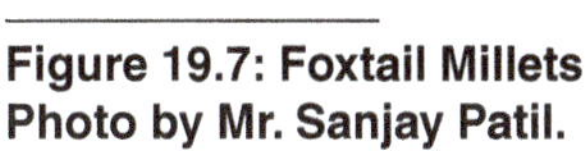

Figure 19.7: Foxtail Millets Photo by Mr. Sanjay Patil.

Sorghum Diversity

In India minor millets are cultivated mainly as rainfed crop and occupy an area of about 2.7 million ha which is about 12 per cent of the whole area under coarse cereals in the country.[42].

The area under minor millets cultivation in India has significantly decreased. The factors responsible are characterized by poor agro-ecosystem and largely inhabited by socio-economically fragile farming system which are largely from section of below poverty line. The production systems followed for their cultivation are generally marginal, based mainly on locally available seeds with minimum or no external inputs or often under default organic farming conditions. Mostly, they are grown only in one season with the main monsoon season (June –November)., they are predominantly grown as mixed or intercrop along with fodder yielding crops like maize and sorghum, high value crops such as grain legumes (Pigeon pea, Green gram or Black gram) or oil seed crops (mustard and niger)

These areas have retained the traditional crop varieties and the knowledge regarding their specific qualities. This rich heritage of crop diversity is required to be conserved for mitigating climate change [13.] These landraces are known for their specific qualities like tolerance to biotic and abiotic stress, nutritional characteristics, taste, *etc.* which are not known to the scientific community and social workers in tribal societies. Systematic and accurate data collection from tribal blocks of Dhadgaon and Akkalkuwa has been documented before it is vanished forever [26]. Ancient rice varieties are still growing in the tribal region of Western Maharashtra their documentation and collection is worth for land races conservation [7.]

Conclusion

Sacred groves in Maharashra are conserved through people's participation still now. Some of the groves are under threat due to developmental activities and few of them cover the biodiversity which plays important role in tribal life, for sustainable livelihood. Surrounding forest gives them necessary wood, food and medicinal resources which they require time to time. Even tribal people conserve wild food resources for their seasonal consumption. Wild fruit diversity and germplasm of wild relatives of cultivated plants and land races of food/grain resources are conserved *in situ*. This traditional knowledge needs to be documented and conserved before it vanishes forever and for mitigating climatic changes.

Acknowledgement

Authors are thankful to President, BAIF development research foundation, Pune and Principal, K.M.C. College, Khopoli for their encouragement.

References

1. Josh Rajeshree, Kulkarni, Shruti, Bhusare, Sampada, Phansalkar, Neha, Nipunage, Dinesh and Kulkarni Dilip. 2015. Ecosystem services of Sacred groves in Western Maharashtra through multiple facets. *Life science leaflets*: 156-172.

2. Kulkarni, D.K. 2006. Role of ethno-botany in Modern Agriculture. In Proceeding of National Conference on Bridging gap between Ancient and modern

technologies to increase agricultural productivity. Ed. S.L. Chudhary, R.C. Saxena and Y.L.Nene. Pub. Central Arid Zone Research Institute, Jodhpur, Rajasthan,India.:104-115.

3. Kulkarni, D.K. 2007. Germplasm collection of High value wild fruit species for global nutraceuticals. In Proceeding of the National Workshop on 'Under -utilised Fruit Species for Food–Nutrition Security and Enhanced Rural Livelihood' held on 14-17 September 2005 at BAIF, Development Research Foundation, Pune. (Eds. Daniel, J.N., Hegde, N.G. and Dhar S.):42-46.

4. Kulkarni Shruti and D.K. Kulkarni 2013. Anthropogenic impact on sacred grove of Kalamvihira in Jawhar Taluka, Dist. Thane. The processing of UGC sponsored National conference on Sacred groves as a repository of Ethno-medicinal plants. Held at Rajaram College, Kolhapur, Sacred groves –from Tradition to Conservation on 1-2 February, 2013: pp.79-85.

5. Deo Avinash, D.K. Kulkarni and P.B.Kamble 2013. EVM for Deworming in the ruminants for sustainable health Paper presented at International conference on Inclusive and sustainable growth conducted by Institute of Management Technology, Nagpur and BAIF Development Research Foundation, Pune on Oct. 4-6, 2012 held at BAIF campus, Pune. Online publication- 142-463.

6. Kumbhojkar, M.S. and D.K.Kulkarni 1998 Environmental impact of sacred groves in Western Ghats of Maharashtra. *Science and Culture*,64 (9-10): 205-207.

7. Kulkarni, D.K., M.S.Kumbhojkar and Rajeev Khedkar 1998. Rice germplasm collection, conservation and use:A case study in Western Maharashtra. *Ethnobotany*,10:27-31

8. Ghate, V.S., D. K. Kulkarni and A.S. Upadhye 1999. Screening of Natural diversity in Karvanda (*Carissa* L.) commercially potential wild fruit in Maharashtra. *Indian Journal of Plant Genetic Resources,* 12 (1): 10-15.

9. Kulkarni, D. K. and M.S.Kumbhojkar 2002. Ethnobotanical resources for veterinary medicinal practices by Mahadeokoli tribe from Western Maharashtra, India. *Journal of Maharashtra Agric. Univ.*,27(2):172-176.

10. Kulkarni, D. K. and M.S.Kumbhojkar. (2003) Ethno-agricultrual Study of Mahadeokolis in Maharashtra,India.*Asian Agri-History.* 7(4): 295-312.

11. Kulkarni, D.K., V. V. Agte and M.S.Kumbhojkar.(2003) Leafy vegetables consumed by Mahadeokoli tribe in Western Maharashtra with their Nutritional potential. *Ethnobotany.* 15(1 and 2):34-38.

12. Kulkarni, D. K. and D. S. Nipunage (2009) Floristic diversity and ecological evaluation of 'Dhup-Rahat' sacred grove from Pune district. Geobios 36:298-302

13. Patil, P.V., P.B. Kamble and D. K. Kulkarni. (2009) Role of traditional crops and varieties to mitigate emerging climate changes on agriculture- a case study from Bhor region, Maharashtra. *Indian Journal of Plant Genetic Resources*.22(1): 76-79.

14. Nipunage, D.S. and D. K. Kulkarni. (2010) *Deo Rahati*: ancient concept of biodiversity conservation. *J. Asian Agri-History*.14(2)185-196.

15. Nipunage D.S., A.R. Kasarkar and D.K. Kulkarni (2010) Sacred groves from Bhudargad Taluka of Kolhapur district, Maharashtra State, India. a store house of rare and endemic plants. An International Journal of Bioscience Guardian 1(1): 60-65.

16. Kulkarni, D.K., D. S. Nipunage, L.M. Hangarge and P.B. Kamble (2010) Natural heritage of forest conservation in Bhor region of Pune, India. *Asian Journal of Environmental Sci.* 5(2): 94-98.

17. Patil, P.V. and D.K. Kulkarni (2011) Traditional farming systems in hilly regions of Bhor and Mahad, Maharashtra State, India. *Bioscience Guardian* 1(2): 653-658.

18. Kulkarni, D. K., D.S. Nipunage, L.M. Hangarge and A.D. Kulkarni (2013) Quantitative Plant Diversity Evaluation of Sagadara and Navalachi rai-Monotypic Sacred Groves in Pune District of Maharashtra state, India. *Annals of Biological Research* 4(2): 234-240.

19. Kamble, P.B. A. Deo and D.K. Kulkarni (2014) Social Validation of Ethno-Veterinary Medicines for wound healing in Cattle. *Asian Agri- History*, 18(1) 63-68.

20. Patil, P.V., D.K. Kulkarni and D.S. Nipunage (2014) Wisdom of local people on selection of wood for agricultural implements from Bhor and Mahad regions of Western Maharashtra. *Indian Journal of Advances in Plant Research* (IJAPR) 1(2): 11-17.

21. Ashwini Chothe, Sanjay Patil and D. K. Kulkarni (2014) Unconventional wild fruits and processing in tribal area of Jawhar, Thane District. *Bioscience Discovery*. 5(1): 19-23.

22. Phansalkar, N.S. and D.K. Kulkarni (2014) Ecological survey of Ajnawale sacred grove from Junnar area of Pune district, Maharashtra, India. *Indian Journal of Advances in Plant Research* (IJAPR) 1(4): 10-12.

23. Sajal Kulkarni, D.K. Kulkarni, A.D. Deo, A.B. Pande and R.L. Bhagat (2014) Use of Ethno-Veterinary medicines (EVM) from Vidarbha Region (MS) India. *Bioscience Discovery*, 5(2):180-186.

24. Bhusare S., Bhosale B. and Kulkarni D. K. (2014) Traditional heritage of Kalamvihira sacred grove conservation and culture practices associated in tribal's of Jawhar, Thane district Maharashtra State,India. *Indian Journal of Advances in Plant Research* (IJAPR) 1(6): 5-9.

25. Deshpande Suwarna, Rajeshree Joshi and D.K. Kulkarni (2015) Nutritious wild food resources of Rajgond tribe, Vidarbha, Maharashtra, India. *Indian Journal of fundamental and applied life sciences* 5(1):15-25

26. Patil, Sanjay, Ketaki S. Patil, Prafulla Sawarkar and D.K. Kulkarni (2015) Germplasm conservation of Maize, Sorghum, Millets and Vegetables from Dhadgaon and Akkalkuwa tribal block of Nandurbar district, Maharashtra State. *Science Research Reporter* 5(2): 137-146

27. Nipunage D.S. Ketaki Sathe, Rajeshree Joshi and D.K. Kulkarni (2016) Natural heritage of biodiversity conservation in Palghar district,Maharashtra State, India. Indian Journal of Fundamental and Applied Life Sciences.6(1): 21-32.

28. Kamble, P B and D K Kulkarni (2016) Ethno-veterinary medicinal plant resources for wound healing and maggoty wound from Bhor region,Pune district, Maharashtra *Life science leaflets*:77: 92-101

29. Hangarge L.M.[1], D.K. Kulkarni[2], V.B. Gaikwad[3], D.M. Mahajan[4] and V.R. Gunale[3] (2016)Plant diversity in four sacred groves from Bhor region and their comparative floristic composition in relation to denuded hills *Bioscience Discovery* 7(2) 121-127.

30. Sayed M.A.I, Sajal Kulkarni, Dilip Kulkarni, Ashok Pande and Vitthal Kauthale (2017) Nutritional study of local fodder species in Ahmednagar district of western Maharashtra. Agric. Sci. Digest., 37(2) 2017: 154-156.

31. Vitthal Kauthale*, Dilip Kulkarni, Lilesh Chavan, Sanjay Patil and Anjali Nalawade (2017) Diversity of Wild Edible Plants in Dhadgaon Block of Nandurbar District in Maharashtra, India. Int. J. Curr. Res. Biosci. Plant Biol. 4(6), 62-73.

32. Sajal Kulkarni, Surekha Kale, R.L. Bhagat, A.B. Pande and D.K. Kulkarni (2016) Natural fodder species and analysis for diet pattern in breeding tract of Kathani cattle in Maharashtra. Research Journal of animal husbandry and dairy science 7(1):24-27.

33. Chitre, R.G., S. Deshpande and Naiknimbalkar, S. (1983) The process of human adaptation in malnourished population with special reference to tribals.Part –I: Food and nutritent intake of Mahadeokoli from Khireshwar. The Ind.J. Nutr, Dietet. 20:46-55.

34. Ghate V.S, D. K. Kulkarni and Upadhye, A.S. (1997) Karvanda (*Carissa* L.): an underutilized minor fruit of India. *Plant Genertic Resources Newsletter*, 109: 20-21.

35. Jain,S.K. and B.K.Sinha (1988) Ethnobotanical aspect of life support species-some emergency and supplementary foods among aboriginals in India. *Life support species: Diversity and Conservation,* (Eds. Paroda, R.S, Kapoor, P, Arora R.K. and Mal Bhag) National Bureau of Plant Genetic Resources, New Delhi,: 173-180.

36. Nene, Y.L. (2004) Plant species utilized as food during famines and their relevance today.Asian Agri-History 8(4):267-278.

37. Nilegaonkar, S., V.D.Vartak and R.G. Chitre (1985) Nutritional evaluation of some wild food plants from Pune and neighbouring districts, Maharashtra state-part-I. *J.Econ.Tax.Bot.* 6(3): 629-635.

38. Pushpangadan, P., S. Rajsekaran, P.K. Rtheshkumar, C.R. Jawahar, V. Velayudhan Nair, N. Lakshmi and L. Sarada Amma. (1988) Agogyappacha (*Trichopus zeylanicus* Gaertn) The ginseng of Kani tribes of Agastyar Hills (Kerala) for ever green health and vitality. *Ancient Science of Life* 8(1): 13-16.

39. Swaminathan, M.S.(1996) Inaugural Address at IV International Congress of Ethnobiology. In proceeding IV International Congress of Ethnobiology, *Ethnobiology in Human Welfare* (Ed. S. K. Jain) Deep publications, New Delhi.: 1-7.

40. Vartak, V.D. and Kulkarni D.K. (1987). Monsoon wild leafy vegetables from hilly regions of Pune and neighbouring districts,Maharashtra State. *J.Econ.Tax. Bot.* 11(2):331-335.

41. Vartak, V.D. and Ghate V.S. (1994) Alu-*Meyna laxiflora* Robyns a less known but promising wild fruit tree for tribal areas of Western Maharashtra. *Indian J.Forestry* 3(Addl.ser.) 99-103.

42. Seetharam A, 2006. *Millets In Handbook of Agriculture*. Director of Information and Publication of Agriculture, Indian Council of Agriculture Research, Krsihi Anusandhan Bhavan, Pusa, New Delhi-11 0012,India: **892-912**.

43. Padulosia S, Mal Bhang S, Bala Ravi J, Gowda KTK, Gowda G, Shathakumar N,Yenagi and Dutta M, 2009. Food security and climate change: Role of Plant Genetic Resources of Minor Millets. *Indian J. Plant Genet. Resour.* **22(1):**1-16.

44. Altieri MA, Merrick LC, 1987. In Situ Conservation of Crop Genetic Resources through Maintenance of Traditional Farming Systems; *Economic Botany*, **41(1):** 86-96.

45. Bala Ravi, 2004. Neglected millets that save the poor from starvation; *LEISA India*; **6(1)**: 34-36

46. Carle B. and Mike Y. 1997. Motivating people: using management agreement to conserve remnant vegetation. National Research and development program on rehabilitation, management and conservation of remnant vegetation. Research report-I. CSIRO, Division of wildlife and ecology, environment, Department of the environment and Heritage, Australia: 1-4

47. Lebbie A.R. and Guries R.P. 1995. Ethnobotanical value and conservation of sacred groves of the Kpaa Mende in Sierra Leone. *Econ Bot.* 49(3): 297-308

48. Kulkarni, D.K and Upadhye A. S. 2006. Threats to remnant vegetation and traditional ecosystem. In Ecological traditions of Maharashtra. Pub. C.P.R. Environmental Education Centre, Chennai pp.60-70.

49. Upadhye, A. S., d.K.Kulkarni and Kumbhojkar, M.S. 2004.Threatened medicinal plants from sacred groves of Pune district, Maharashtra, India. *Focus on Sacred groves and Ethnobotany* (Eds. Ghate,V.;Sane,H. and Ranade,S.S.) 2004. Published by *Prism Publications, A Division of Timely Management Consl. Servs. Pvt. Ltd.* Mumbai pp.150-154.

50. Kulkarni, D.K. and Kumbhojkar, M. S. 1999 Dams-disaster to biodiversity in sacred groves. *The Deccan Geographer*, 37: 65-72.

51. Bhusare Sampada and Kulkarni, D.K. 2013. Ecosystem services from Kalamvihira sacred grove Jawhar Taehasil, Thane District, Maharashtra. In abstract book of UGC Sponsored National Conference on Sacred groves as a repository of ethno- medicinal plants (1 and 2 Feb. 2013)

52. Gokhale Y. and Pala N.A. 2011. Ecosystem services in sacred Natural sites (SNSs) of Uttarakhand: A Preliminary Survey. J. Biodiversity 2(2): 107-115.

53. Upadhye, A. S., Rani Bhagat and Kulkarni D. K. 2010. Ethnobotany of Endemic and threatened Plants from Western Ghats of Maharashtra. *Journal of Economic Taxonomic Botany*,34 (2) 434-439.

54. Balkundi HV 1998. Famines and droughts in the Indian subcontinent during the 5th century BC to 18th Century AD. Asian Agri-History 2:305-315.

55. Kulkarni, D. K. and M.S.Kumbhojkar 1992. Ethnobotanical studies on Mahadeo koli tribe in Western Maharashtra.Part II. Fodder plants. *J.Econ. Tax. Bot.* Addl. Ser.,10: 123-128.

56. Kulkarni, D.K. and M.S.Kumbhojkar 1992. Ethnobotanical studies on Mahadeokoli tribe in Western Maharashtra. Part III. Non-conventional wild edible fruits. *J.Econ. Tax. Bot.* Addl. Ser.,10: 151-158.

57. Spiekermann, U. 1998. Food quality in a changing social environment: a historical perspective. In proceedings of the ECBA-Symposium and workshop held in February 27-March 1998in Heidelberg, Germany *Food quality,Nutrition and health*. (Eds. Grimme, L.H. and Dumontet, S.) Pub: Springer –Verlag Berlin Heidelberg New York. 37-45.

58. Annonymous (1965 and 1984) Official methods of Analysis. Association of Official Analytical Chemist, Washington, D.C.

59. Kulkarni, D.K. 2005. Dams: disaster to heritage of traditional agriculture through displacement of local people from the Sahyadri region in Maharashtra State. In Proceedings of the International Conference on Agricultural Heritage of Asia. (Ed. Y.L. Nene) Pub. Asian Agri-History Foundation, Secunderabad, Andhra Pradesh, India.:155-164.

60. Kulkarni, D.K. 2005.Threat to sacred grove conservation in tribal pockets of Pune district, Western Maharashtra State. In Proceeding of National workshop on Strategy for Conservation of Sacred groves. (Eds. Kunhikannan, c and B. Gurudev Singh) Pub. By.Direcotr, Institute of Forest Genetics and Tree Breeding Coimbatore, India, p. 141- 150.

Chapter 20

Legal Aspects of Biosafety Issues in Green Biotechnology: with Special Reference to India

Amit K Kashyap & Ayushi Gupta

Institute of Law, Nirma University, Ahmedabad, Gujarat 382481
e-mail: amit1law@gmail.com

ABSTRACT

Since 1990 the Biotechnology has grown rapidly & it is well evident that the application of biotechnology in Agriculture & Biodiversity is coupled with potential risks coupled with biotechnology. The usage and trade of living genetically modified organisms (GMOs) has caused a debate for sustainable development and use of biological resources & has thus become an issue of global relevance. Laterally Biosafety is an emerging discipline built from traditional risk assessment and risk management rationale various subjects interdisciplinary aspects of Biology. In this paper, the authors have reviewed the regulatory framework to reconcile the respective needs of trade and environmental protection with respect to a rapidly growing global biotechnology industry while addressing regulatory & policy framework in India. The authors also made an effort to address relevant challenges and the extent to which regulation fosters or constrains the development of Green Biotechnology in India.

Key Words: *Green biotechnology, biosafety, Genetically Modified Crops, GMO*

Conceptual Framework for Biosafety in Green Biotechnology

Biosafety or the prevention of potential dangers from products emerged from genetic engineering, has risen as a significant scientific and political concern all over the world. As a signatory to the Cartagena Protocol on Biosafety, India has the obligation to fulfil the criteria indicated in the provision, which includes the safe transfer, managing and utilizing GMOs, with focus on the Transboundary movement. In India, concerns and debate are connected for the most part with social-economic issues vis-à-vis agricultural biotechnology as a novel technology and biodiversity preservation. An organism whose genetic material has been altered using genetic engineering techniques, also known as recombinant DNA technology is referred to as a Genetically Modified Organism (GMO) or living modified organisms (LMOs). Insulin was approved in 1982 as a GMO in the United States. Green biotechnology can be defined as the utilization of environmentally friendly solutions instead of using conventional processes based on agriculture, horticulture, and animal breeding (Chatterjee and Ghose, 2010). An illustration is the designing of transgenic plants that are altered for enhanced flavour, for increased resistance from irritations and illnesses, or for enhanced development in adverse climatic conditions.

GMOs & Green Biotechnology

It is presently a recognized fact that the fast adoption of biotechnology in India, particularly in agriculture, has been faced with by severe scientific dangers and uncertainty. These doubts and questions raise a few difficulties for policy and governance. Though developed country calls for a major part of the investment in biotechnology, in the developing countries a large number of derived products or genetically modified organisms (GMOs) are exported and marketed. This trade between the countries has been happening notwithstanding the way that there are a few logically unsubstantiated claims about GMOs and their effect. These worries are typically looked to be managed within the domain of biosafety. Biosafety or the prevention of potential dangers from products developed from genetic engineering has risen as an essential scientific and political concern around the world. Until now, India has not traded in GMOs with other nations, yet the steady increment in the worldwide acreage of GMOs is maybe a sign of things to come. Be that as it may, lessons drawn from India's involvement with it's first commercially developed GM crop – Bt cotton – uncover few gaps in the current execution of the national biosafety regulation. The long-term financial effect of reliance on this technology may additionally require more prominent legitimate and scientific investigation. These different shortcomings question India's level of responsibility towards a comprehensive policy on agricultural biotechnology. (Lianchawii, 2005)

Biosafety Issues in Green Biotechnology

Different areas associated with biosafety include:

- **Agriculture and food system issues:** Potential harmful impacts of GE food which have caused concerns comprises of lethality, allergenicity, variation in the nutritional value and development of resistant strains of microorganisms. There is a chance that GE could inadvertently cause a lethal substance, for instance, a recently expressed protein, or raise the outflow of an endogenous harmful substance. Allergenicity includes extreme reactions of the body that may happen in sensitive people after introduction to specific substances, generally proteins. During the creation of biotech plant, unintended impact might be the bringing down of its nutritional quality when the comparison is made with its traditional equivalent. This could happen when the nutrients become unavailable or indigestible to people through the intervention of key metabolic pathways. (David P. Keetch, Diran Makinde, Cholani K. Weebadde and Karim M. Maredia)

- **Environmental Issues:** The dangers comprises of contamination of different crops genetically, transmission of poison/allergen from one living thing to another and development of some new poisons/allergens and effect on the fertility of the soil. Likewise, inappropriate discharge of hazardous substances or pathogens utilized as a part of the tests, into the surroundings might be a risk. (Prof. S.C. Bhatla)
- **Market and consumer issues:** A significant part of the resistance to GM products emerges from consumer's concern over their safety due to the fact that GM products and foods are not healthy and natural.
- Institutional issues: As a signatory to the Cartagena Protocol on Biosafety, India is determined to to make domestic biosafety controls, in consensus to the provisions of the protocol. Such type of determination needs prominent institutional and technical endeavours. Be that as it may, there is no credible system till now to oversee or identify the import of unapproved GM agricultural or plant material since there is numerous entry passage in the nation. This can turn out to be fatal. In the same manner, it has been contended that the separation, identification and traceability of GM products are difficult to actualize in India because of the restrictions in government administrative machinery. These insufficiencies would make it troublesome for the farmers to select amongst GM, non-GM and organic crops. Subsequently, consumers would likewise be denied the right to make an informed decision.
- Socio economic issues: Some of the social and economic issues include patent with respect to genes by organizations; because of the commercial significance of biotechnology products originating from them. This is a real danger as large number of people of the country is still poor and because of such patenting genes and life forms become inaccessible to these unprivileged people. Generation of biological warfare agents/weapons is likewise a worry. Moral issues related to the production of GMOs; which is regarded as 'anti-nature' by a few people. (Prof. S.C. Bhatla)
- Human Health issues: The procedure of recombinant DNA technology includes utilization of microorganisms and methods which might be a risk to the labourers if utilized rashly. Also, the finished results i.e. GM-nourishment/bolster might be poisonous or cause hypersensitivities. The selectable marker utilized for the cultivation of GM products may have some harmful effects on drug (antibiotic) resistance. The utilization of these marker genes has prompted the doubt that these genes may be transmitted to the nearby surroundings and lead to the formation of drug (antibiotic) resistance to human pathogens. (Prof. S.C. Bhatla)

International Law & Biosafety

Application of Biotechnology in Agriculture & Biodiversity has given rise to a universal open debate about its prospects and potential risks.

OECD's Ad hoc Biotechnology Statistics Group

In the year 2002, the OECD came up with two definitions of biotechnology including a single definition and the one containing a list of various kinds of biotechnology techniques. The one containing the list was amended in 2005. The OECD prescribes that statistical agencies give both of these definitions to survey respondents when gathering data on biotechnology-related activities. The single definition characterizes biotechnology as:

"The application of science and technology to living organisms, as well as parts, products and models thereof, to alter living or non-living materials for the production of knowledge, goods and services".

The single definition covers all advanced biotechnology yet in addition numerous traditional or borderline activities. Consequently, the OECD suggests that the list based definition should at all times accompany a single definition. The list-based definition operationalizes the definition for estimation purposes. The list of biotechnology technique works as an interpretative rule to the single definition. The list is demonstrative as opposed to exhaustive and is required to change after some time as data collection and biotechnology related activities advance. In 2008, member nations of OECD chose to start work on amending and updating the list based on definition. The techniques include:-

- DNA/RNA
- Proteins and other molecules
- Cell and tissue culture and engineering:
- Process biotechnology te Gene and RNA vectors
- Bioinformatics
- Nanobiotechnology

Nearly eighteen of the OECD member countries and two of the non-member countries employ these definitions in their surveys. OECD Biotechnology Statistics 2009 (Brigitte van Beuzekom and Anthony Arundel)

Cartagena Protocol on Biosafety to the Convention on Biological Diversity was adopted in 2000.

The Cartagena Protocol on Biosafety to the Convention on Biological Diversity in contemporary international law has proclaimed one of the strongest references to the precautionary principle. The protocol is one of its kind which expanded the precautionary principle outside its ambit which is the preamble i.e., outline the principle in its operational titles. As a result of this, the Protocol has been attributed with "driving the precautionary principle to the front of international environmental law". Article 15(3) of the Protocol incorporates that parties may request the exporters to do the essential risk assessments. This is to allow the developing nations to proclaim measures formed on the precautionary principle, even in a circumstance where they don't have the administrative equipment to carry out the risk evaluation themselves. Despite the fact that the Protocol does not necessitate scientific knowledge and consensus to take a precautionary action, this should not be taken as the presence or absence of a risk. Despite such articulation present in the protocol, risk evaluations are to be carried out on a case-by-case basis and in a way that fits in with the standards and laws of the associated science. (Bhuvan Bhaskar Jha & Ashutosh Shankar)

UNESCO Declarations

The United Nations Convention on Biological Diversity (Convention or CBD) ended at the Earth Summit in Rio de Janeiro in the year 1992. It has 3 principal goals:

- The preservation of biological diversity
- The sustainable utilization of components of biological diversity.
- The reasonable and equitable sharing of the advantages emerging out of the usage of resources which are genetic.

The Convention on Biological Diversity is devoted to advancing sustainable development. Considered as a pragmatic instrument in bringing the standards of Agenda 21 into reality, the Convention perceives that biological diversity is more than plants, animals, microorganisms and environment – it is about individuals and our requirement for food security, medicines, clean air and water, shelter, and a safe environment in which to live.

Regulatory Environment in India

India does not have an express statute, unlike many other countries, to regulate Biotechnology in our food and farming. There are some statutes which govern the biotechnology in India. These are:-

1. Environment (Protection) Act, 1986 The central legislative policy for biosafety regulations is the nation is ostensibly the Environment (Protection) Act 1986. The Sections 6, 8 and 25 of the Act mutually frame the preamble through which all the at present existing biosafety regulations run in India. Section 6 of the Act gives the power to the Central Government to frame the fundamental guidelines on the standard methods, execute safeguards and put the vital limitations for treatment of hazardous substances and restrict the others. Then again, Section 8 of the Act forces a disallowance on a man from dealing with any hazardous substance unless acted in accordance with the procedures and safeguards. The last section i.e. Section 25 of the Act puts the obligation on the Central Government to stipulate the rules with respect to the procedures and protections for taking care of hazardous substances. As an immediate outcome of this, in the Indian Judicial System, it is agreed that the Biosafety rules are statutory in nature as their genesis is based on the aforementioned provisions of the Environment (Protection) Act. These aforementioned mentioned provisions have additionally prompted the Ministry of Environment and Forests to enact 1989 Biosafety Rules. (Bhuvan Bhaskar Jha & Ashutosh Shankar)

2. Biosafety Rules, 1989 They are applicable to the products prepared by using genetically engineered micro-organisms and other technology produce genetically created and manages their, production, storage and import. These rules likewise include the pre-release aspect of genetically modified organisms, specifically their research and development work other than the expansive scale applications and trials.1989 Biosafety Rules also includes hazardous organisms. The Rule 8 of the statute orders the prerequisite consent to be taken by the administrative bodies before the release or even the generation of genetically modified organisms and cells. The Rules no. 10 and 11 imposes the prerequisite of an consent for any such substances that contain genetically engineered organisms or even cells. In any case, the Rule 9 of this statute is the chief important as it explicitly bans the intentional/ or accidental release of genetically modified organisms (for test purposes) contained in its schedule, notwithstanding a circumstance where it has been confirmed as a 'special case' by the suitable authority. The aforementioned schedule is an element of 1989 Biosafety Rules which characterizes human and pathogens with respect to their risk profiles. (Bhuvan Bhaskar Jha & Ashutosh Shankar)

3. **Biotechnology Safety Guidelines, 1998** The Biotechnology safety guidelines are the outcome of Rule 4(2) of the 1989 Biosafety Rules which orders the need of guidelines manuals. These are to be laid down by the Review Committee on Genetic Manipulation. These guidelines are related to the evaluation of biosafety levels of which it conveys a detailed study. It also contains a detailed admonishment on recombinant DNA or rDNA activities, shipments, experiments and quality control delivered by genetic engineering. After passed by the Department of biotechnology in the year 1990 and before achieving its present form The Biotechnology safety guidelines were modified and corrected twice lastly modified in the year 1998 as per the progressive steps made in the field of rDNA research. (Bhuvan Bhaskar Jha & Ashutosh Shankar)

4. The National Biotechnology and Biosafety Bill, 2012: This bill is a crucial milestone to attain a functional and efficient legal framework for biotechnology, it contains conflicting provisions that should be looked at before it becomes a law. The bill is little narrow as it applies only to research and general discharge of genetically modified organisms and does not specify the full scope of Genetically Modified Organisms (GMO) activities that need regulation. The bill should clearly manage the full scope of activities which comprises of research, use, confined field trials, import, export and the general discharge of GMO. The bill additionally expresses that the IBC will be consisted of three members having knowledge on biosafety but the bill does not specify the manner of composition of the committee. Furthermore, it does not give the option to the public for participating in the decision-making process. (Barbara Ntambirweki Karugonjo)

5. **Biotechnology Regulatory Authority of India Bill, 2013** The Government of India in consonance with the provisions of the Cartagena Protocol, of which it is a member, recommended promulgating the National Biotechnology Regulatory Authority through the Biotechnology Regulatory Authority of India Bill. This will after its creation, be the chief authority on regulations and policies that come with the genetically modified organisms. The parliament is still left to pass the Bill which

proposes BRAI. In any case, it is faced with extreme resistance from the farmers and NGOs such as Greenpeace India because of a few of its faulty provisions that infringe the constitutional and legal rights of the agriculturists and the consumers. It is to be noted that these clashing provisions of the Bill should be altered and measures should be taken to guarantee the protection of such legal rights. (Bhuvan Bhaskar Jha & Ashutosh Shankar)

International & Regional Organizations in Biosafety

International Organisations

At International Level, there is no single comprehensive legal instrument that covers all aspects of biotechnology& Biosafety. Nevertheless, there are many agreements that cover the issues & constituted International Organisations.

The International organizations include the People

1. Codex Alimentarius,
2. World Health Organization
3. United Nations Food and Agriculture Organization (FAO),
4. United Nations Environmental Programme (UNEP),
5. United Nations Educational, Scientific and Cultural Organization (UNESCO)
6. United Nations Industrial Development Organization (UNIDO), etc

Organisation in India

The expansion of agreements & Organisations at international level has created various standard and rule relating to biotechnology that is a significant assistance to many countries. Article 26.1 of the Cartagena Protocol on Biosafety left open the possibility for member countries to include in their biosafety regulatory processes the assessment of socio-economic considerations (Falck-Zepeda & Zambrano, 2011).

In India, the Government enacted the Environment (Protection) Act in 1986 and thereafter, notified Rules & Procedures (Rules) for handling GMOs and hazardous organisms through a Gazette Notification from the Union Ministry of Environment & Forests. There are various statutory bodies to regulate the biosafety issues in Green Biotechnology. A six-level structure was set up which included these components

i. Recombinant DNA Advisory Committee,
ii. Review Committee on Genetic Manipulation
iii. Institutional Biosafety Committee
iv. Genetic Engineering Approval Committee
v. State Biotechnology Co-ordination Committee and
vi. District Level Committee

These six bodies were intended to cover the whole process related to decision making with respect to biotechnology including research, utilization and application.

The first three Committees work under the Department of Biotechnology while the rest are associated to the Ministry of Environment and Forests. The RDAC oversees advancement in GMOs not only at the national but at the international level too and proposes suitable directions. In the interim, trials based on research on the transgenic material are managed by the RCGM. A newly constituted which aids the RCGM assesses the transgenic crops and oversees biosafety data collection. All the institutions which perform research on the transgenic material are expected to form an IBSC, which will account to the RCGM. In the meantime, substantial scale and commercial discharge of GMOs should be cleared by the GEAC. The GEAC is aided by the SBCC and the DLC that supervise the safe utilization of GMOs. (Biswajit Dhar)

Regulatory Issues & Challenges in India

Modern biotechnology-the controversial manipulation of genes in living organisms-has far-reaching implications for agriculture, human health, trade and the environment (Bail, Falkner and Marquard, 2003). The insufficiencies in India's regulatory structure were in this way starkly uncovered by the Gujarat episode, which likewise drew out the inherent complexities in the biosafety policy and its execution. Apparently, there are apprehensions about the effectiveness and especially the preparedness of the nation in managing such a large scale development of GMOs and the dangers emerging from them. Lack of coordination, the gap in communication between the state and centre government and lack of monitoring authorities were a few glaring shortcomings found in the current framework. For example, the GEAC gave permission to use BT cotton in Andhra Pradesh, though both the State Biotechnology Coordination Committee (BCC) and the District Level Committee (DLC) were absent. Both the BCC and the DLC were created to administer the execution of the regulation and additionally to keep the check on the performance of GM crop. Despite in the field trials of MAHYCO's BT cotton, BCCs were not set up in the many states where trials were conducted; few state authorities were not even mindful of transgenics being tried on their ground. The authorities likewise disclosed their incapability to manage the uncontrolled and extensive utilization of illicit GM crops. The GEAC agreed to the inadequacies of the administrative authorities of the state and additionally of the centre. Today, there is a lack of trained manpower both at the centre and state levels. Devices to find and identify GMOs are not present in the quarantine or any other agency. Additionally, it would be troublesome for the agencies in ports or other passage to identify GMO in agricultural items that are foreign. Regulations are executed by ad hoc committees which consist mainly of people having scientific knowledge which have an absence of members from social science background or from people of the public. So, there is a lack of a policy which is coherent for GM crops. Guidelines and rules are consequently required to ensure imports of GM made food in the nation to stop India from turning into a dumping ground for GM food. (Lianchawii)

Conclusion

It seems that biotechnology is evolving at a pace at which technological steps in the field would seldom be able to be managed through credible biosafety standards.

These tensions have contributed to the developing scientific and popular response against GMOs, whose potential hazard keeps to be a matter of controversy around the world. The chief reason behind such doubts on genetic transfers has frequently been contended, comes from the largely anticipatory behaviour of biosafety governance. Considering such solid reservations among the popular scientific community, the export and use of such biotechnology, has likewise fuelled the need for an international regulatory framework as a biosafety protocol. Probably, an efficient administrative structure could avoid the probability of conflicts amongst nations, with respect to international trade in GMOs, and the dangers linked to biodiversity.

India is obligated to have a strong national biosafety policy in place as a signatory to the Cartagena protocol. Some of the crucial constraints are explicit in the Indian biosafety policy which is stipulated in the EPA, 1986. The treatment of India's first GM crop– Bt cotton, demonstrate serious shortcomings in the national regulatory framework. These constraints are obvious within the regulatory structure and its execution. The authorities faced serious criticism for their lack of transparency while giving approval to the Bt cotton. Reforms of decision making which includes participation from the general public could be one of the key factors that add to an effective biosafety regime. Moreover, for efficient execution and implementation of the regulation, it is necessary to strengthen the institutional framework. All said and done to build up a regulatory framework is one thing and its successful execution is another thing in which the real test lies.

References

Vaghasiya, K., K, & Shiroya, J., A.A Review Green biotechnology- A help to the environment.https://www.pharmatutor.org/articles/review-green-biotechnology-help-environment

Lianchawii. (2005). Biosafety in India Rethinking: GMO Regulation Economic and Political Weekly.40 (39), pp. 4284. https://www.researchgate.net/publication/262125715_Biosafety_in_India_Rethinking_GMO_Regulation

Keetch, P. D, Makinde D, Weebadde K, C., Maredia, M., K. (2014). Biosafety issues in food and agricultural systems in Africa, p. 9 https://www.researchgate.net/publication/262125715_Biosafety_in_India_Rethinking_GMO_Regulation

Bhatla, SC. Biosafety concerns in Plant Biotechnology, pp.15,18 https://www.mobt3ath.com/uplode/book/book-7844.pdf

Beuzekom, B., & Arundel. A. (2009).OECD Biotechnology Statistics 2009, p.8-9. https://www.oecd.org/sti/42833898.pdf

Bail, C., Falkner, R., & Marquard, H. (2003). The Cartegena Protocol on Biosafety. Reconciling Trade in Biotechnology with Environment and Development? Edited by C. Bail, R. Falkner and H. Marquard. London: Earthscan Publications Ltd and the Royal Institute of International Affairs (2002), pp. 578, £45.00. ISBN 1-85383-840-3. Experimental Agriculture, 39(1), 110-110. http://dx.doi.org/10.1017/s0014479702261050

Chatterjee, A., & Ghose, A. (2010). Genetically Modified Crops: Global and Indian Perspective. *Asian Development Review Biotechnology*, 12(2), 69-78. Retrieved from http://ris.org.in/sites/default/files/abdr%20july10.pdf

Dhar. Regulating Biotechnology in India. https://www.researchgate.net/publication/282327941_Regulating_Biotechnology_in_India

Falck-Zepeda, J., & Zambrano, P. (2011). Socio-economic Considerations in Biosafety and Biotechnology Decision Making: The Cartagena Protocol and National Biosafety Frameworks. *Review of Policy Research*, 28(2), 171-195. http://dx.doi.org/10.1111/j.1541-1338.2011.00488.x

Jha, B., & Shankar, A.(2017). Evaluating the Law on Regulation of Genetically Modified Crops in India. *Jamia law Journal*, 2, pp. 121.

Karugonjo, B. (2014). **Review of the National Biotechnology and Biosafety Bill 2012.** http://www.acode-u.org/Files/Publications/infosheet_24.pdf

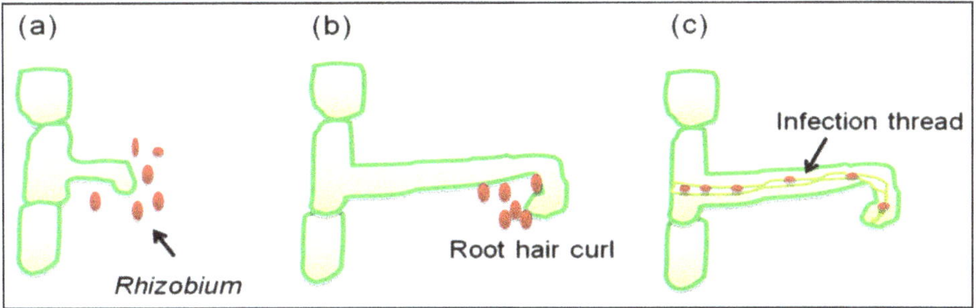

Figure 2.3: The Nodulation Process (a) Interaction and Attachment of *Rhizobium* with Root Cells of Host (b) Excretion of Nod Factors by Rhizobia Causes Root Hair Curling (c) Formation of Infection Thread and Nodule Formation (Adapted from [31]). (p.16)

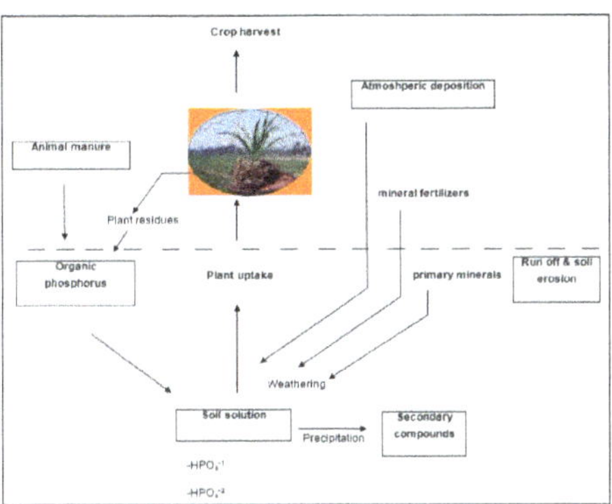

Figure 2.4: Phosphorous Mobilization is Soil (Adapted from [31]). (p. 19)

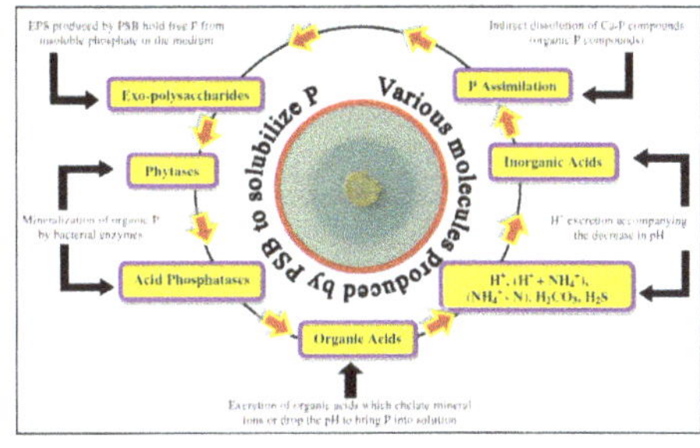

Figure 2.5: Various Mechanisms of PSB (Phosphate Solubilizing Bacteria) for Providing P to Plants (Adapted from [31]). (p. 19)

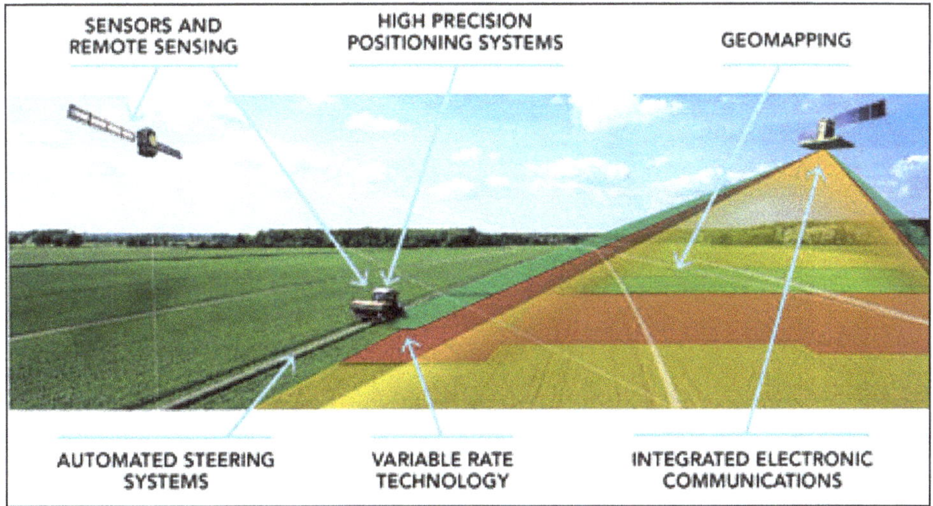

Figure 3.1: Basic Techniques Involved in Precision Farming Practice[4]. (p. 43)

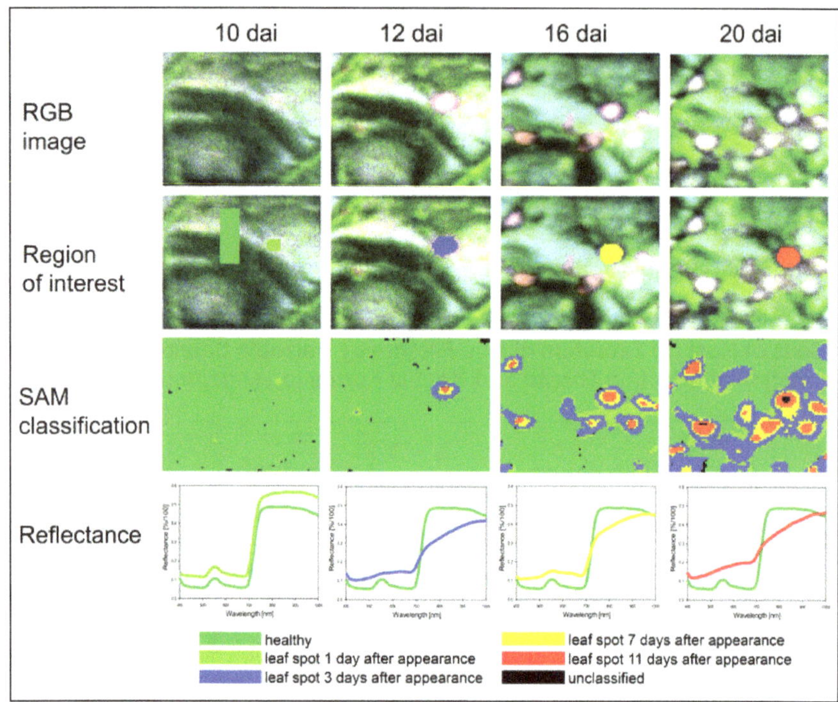

Figure 3.3: Hyper Spectral Imaging of *Cercospora* Leaf Spots Developed Post Fungal Infection.[11] (p. 46)

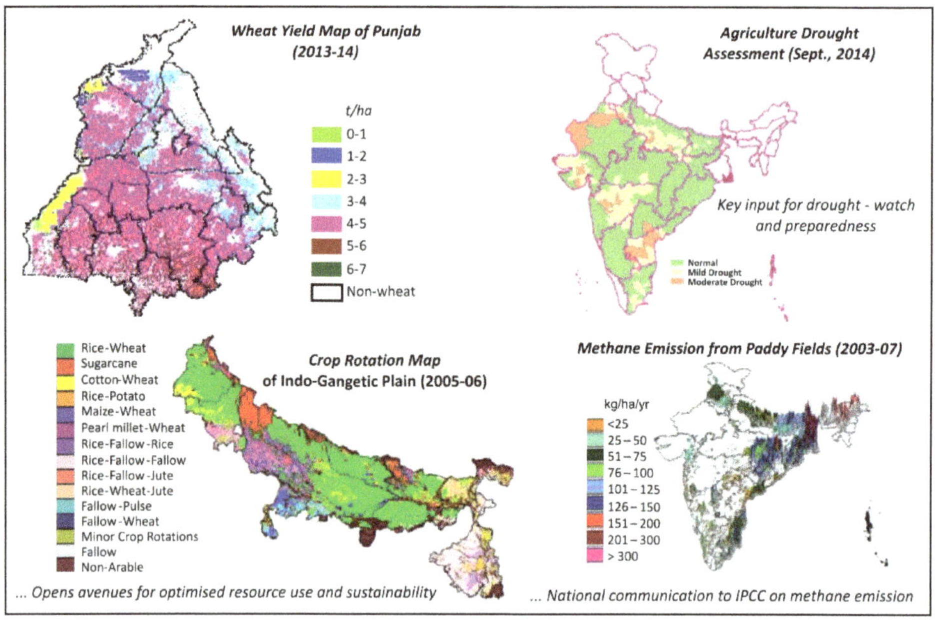

Figure 3.4: Information Obtained through the Remote Sensing Satellites that May Help in the Development of PA in in India (*Source*: website of National Remote sensing Centre, ISRO). (p. 50)

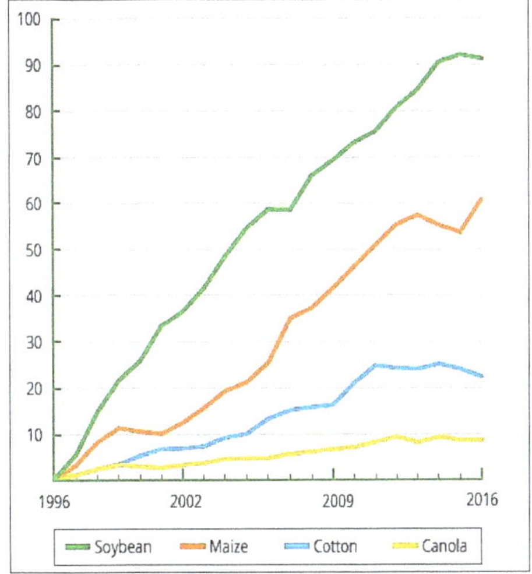

Figure 4.4: Global Area of Biotech Crops, 1996 to 2016 by Crop (Million Hectares).[6] (p. 67)

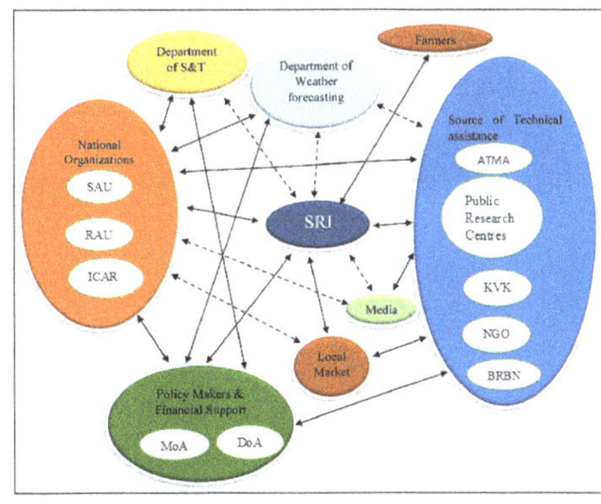

Figure 5.2: Actors of Policy Networks to Promote SRI Innovation (*Source*: Prepared by Author, 2017). (p. 82)

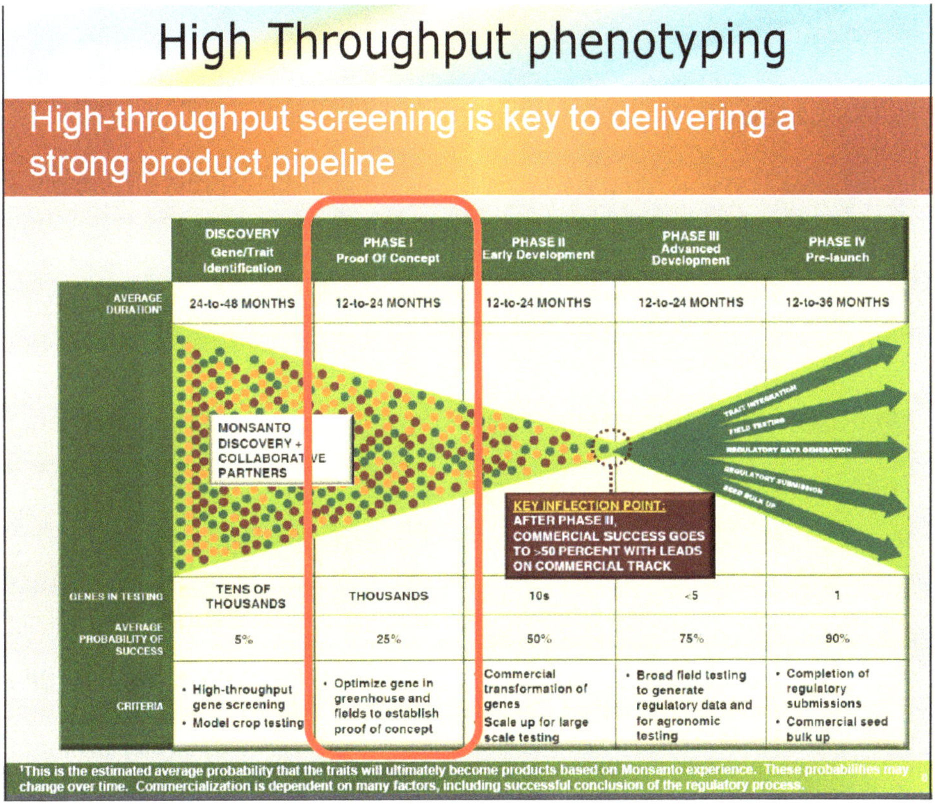

High Throughput phenotyping

High-throughput screening is key to delivering a strong product pipeline

	DISCOVERY Gene/Trait Identification	PHASE I Proof Of Concept	PHASE II Early Development	PHASE III Advanced Development	PHASE IV Pre-launch
AVERAGE DURATION	24-to-48 MONTHS	12-to-24 MONTHS	12-to-24 MONTHS	12-to-24 MONTHS	12-to-36 MONTHS
GENES IN TESTING	TENS OF THOUSANDS	THOUSANDS	10s	<5	1
AVERAGE PROBABILITY OF SUCCESS[1]	5%	25%	50%	75%	90%
CRITERIA	• High-throughput gene screening • Model crop testing	• Optimize gene in greenhouse and fields to establish proof of concept	Commercial transformation of genes Scale up for large scale testing	• Broad field testing to generate regulatory data and for agronomic testing	• Completion of regulatory submissions • Commercial seed bulk up

MONSANTO DISCOVERY + COLLABORATIVE PARTNERS

KEY INFLECTION POINT: AFTER PHASE II, COMMERCIAL SUCCESS GOES TO >50 PERCENT WITH LEADS ON COMMERCIAL TRACK

TRAIT INTEGRATION
FIELD TESTING
REGULATORY DATA GENERATION
REGULATORY SUBMISSION
SEED BULK UP

[1]This is the estimated average probability that the traits will ultimately become products based on Monsanto experience. These probabilities may change over time. Commercialization is dependent on many factors, including successful conclusion of the regulatory process.

(p. 100)

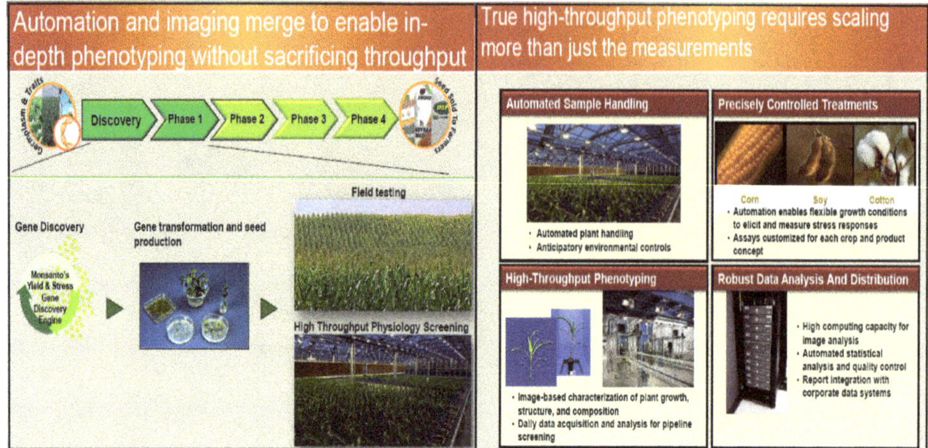

(p. 101)

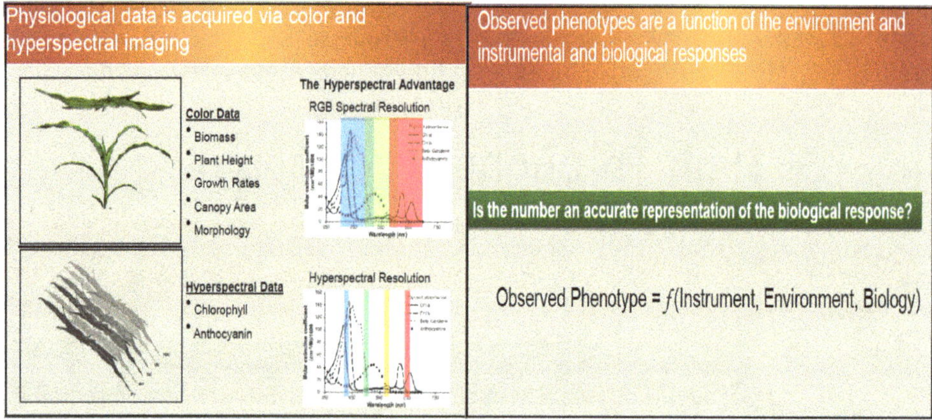

(p. 101)

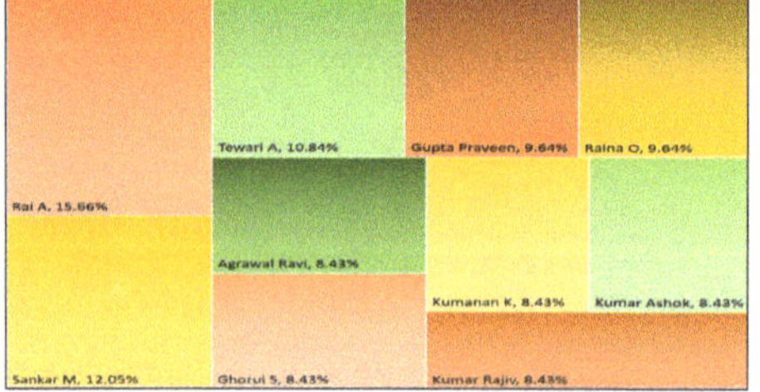

Figure 8.4: Top Authors on the Sector "Cloning" identified from Indian Citation Index (2004-17). (p. 124)

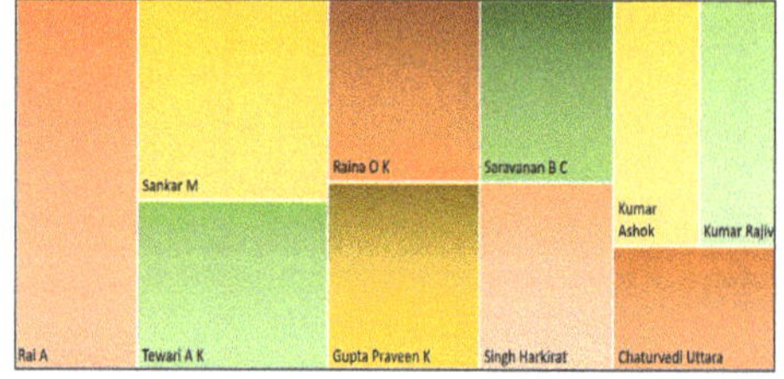

Figure 8.5: Top Ten Authors from UP on "Cloning" (2004-17). (p. 126)

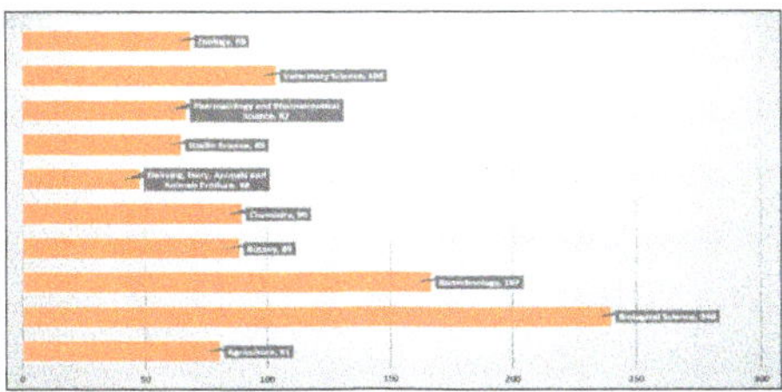

Figure 8.7: Categorization of the Work Related to "Cloning" from Year 2004-17 in Subject Category Derived from Indian Citation Index. (p. 130)

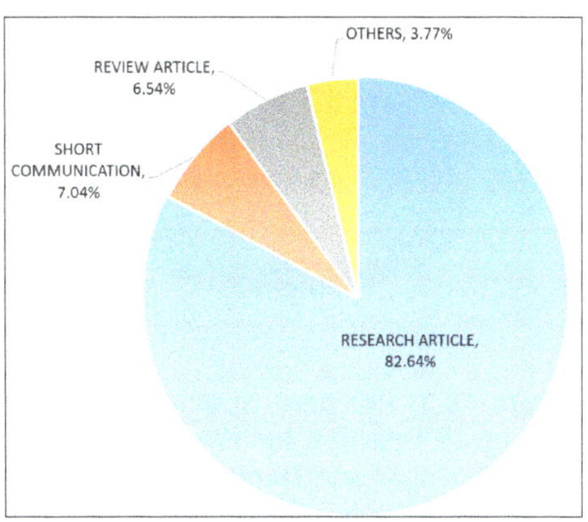

Figure 8.8: Per cent Proposition of Types of Documents on "Cloning" Prepared Based on Indian Citation Index (2004-17). (p. 130)

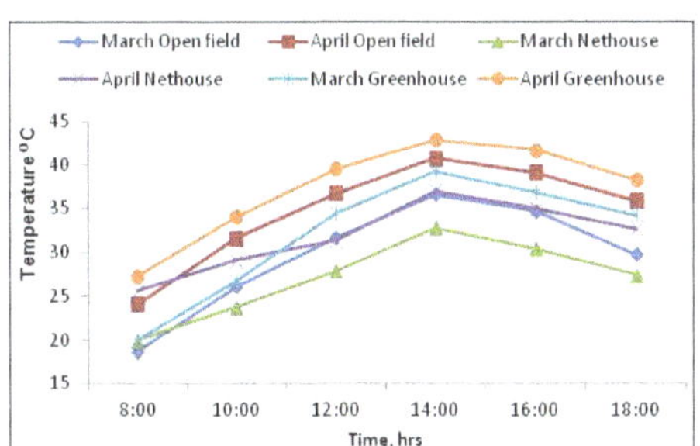

Figure 9.2: Diurnal Variation of Temperature in Greenhouse, Black Shade Net House and Open Field for March and April Month. (p. 138)

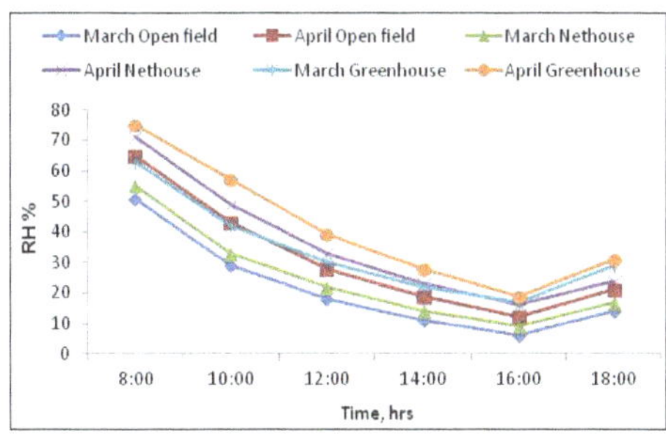

Figure 9.3: Diurnal Variation of Relative Humidity in Greenhouse, Black Shade Net House and Open Field of March and April Month. (p. 139)

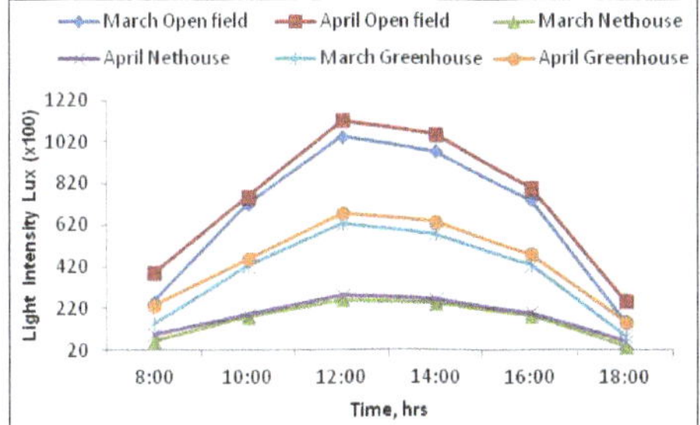

Figure 9.4: Diurnal Variation of Light Intensity Lux(x100) in Greenhouse, Black Shade Net House and Open Field of March and April Month. (p. 140)

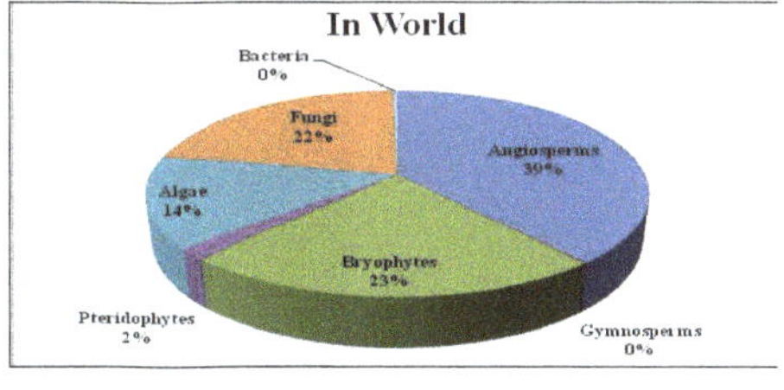

Figure 10.3: Per cent Species Identified among all Species for World, India and Gujarat (Nagar and Daniel, 2010). (p. 155)

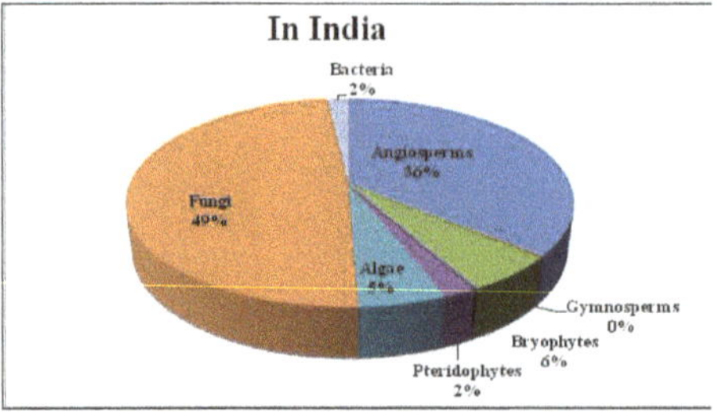

Figure 10.3: Per cent Species Identified among all Species for World, India and Gujarat (Nagar and Daniel, 2010). (p. 155)

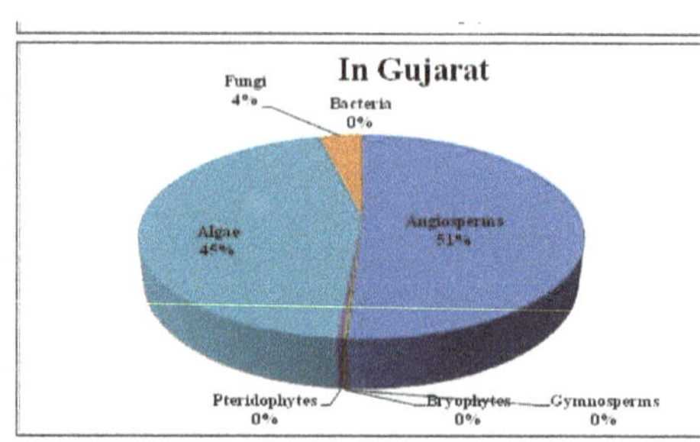

Figure 10.3: Per cent Species Identified among all Species for World, India and Gujarat (Nagar and Daniel, 2010). (p. 155)

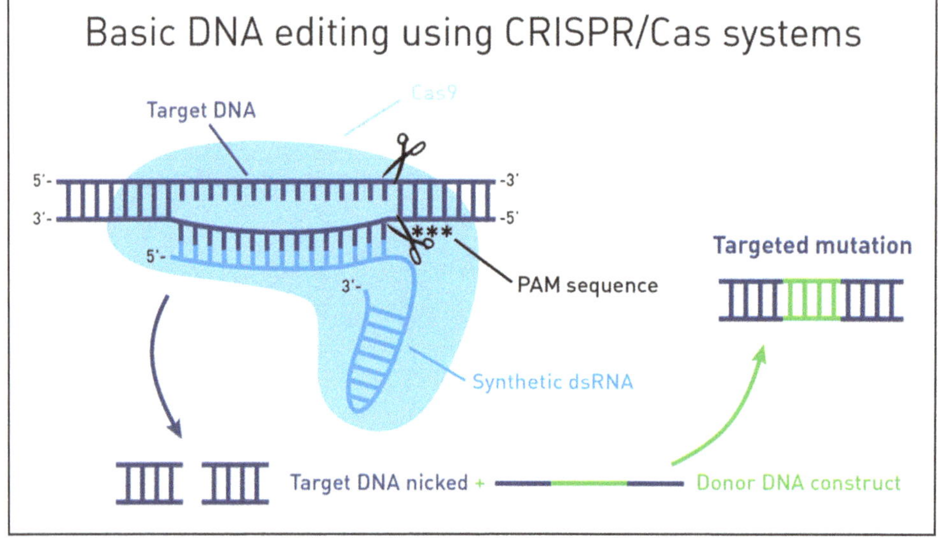

Figure 13.1: General Mechanism of CRISPR-Cas (https://www.jax.org/news-and-insights/jax-blog/2014/march/pros-and-cons-of-znfs-talens-and-crispr-cas). (p. 203)

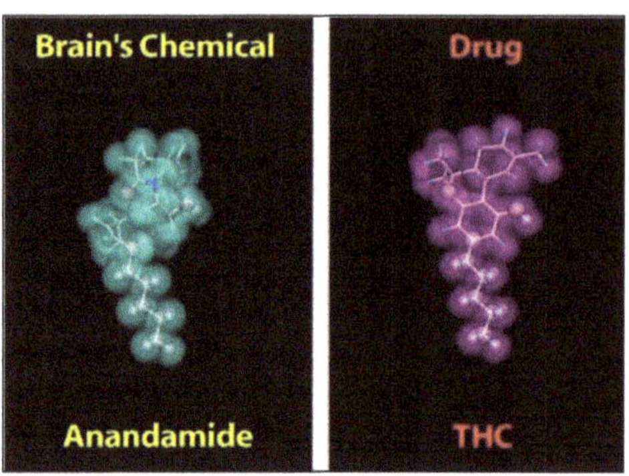

Figure 14.2: Structure of Anandamide and THC[20]. (p. 211)

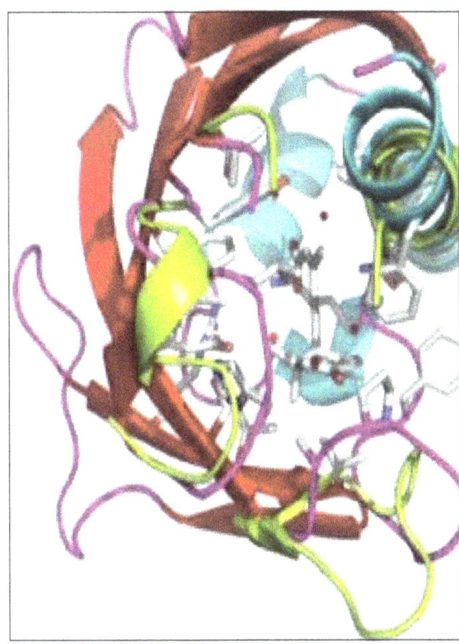

Figure 16.1: Structure of PYR1 Protein. (p. 237)

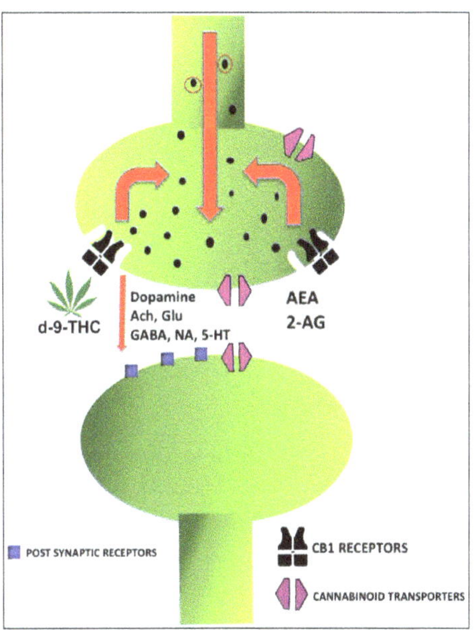

Figure 14.3: CB1 Receptors: Effects of Endocannabinoids and d-9-THC Release of Anandamide (AEA) and 2-arachidonoylglycerol (2-AG) to inhibit glutamate (Glu), Gamma-aminobutyric acid (GABA), acetylcholine (Ach), dopamine, noradrenaline (NA) and serotonin (5-HT)[27]. (p. 212)

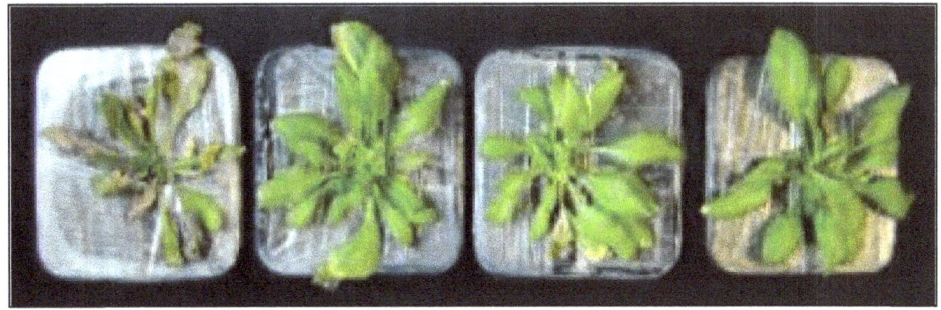

Figure 16.2: Condition of the Plant (Source: Rodriguez *et al.,* 1998). (p.238)

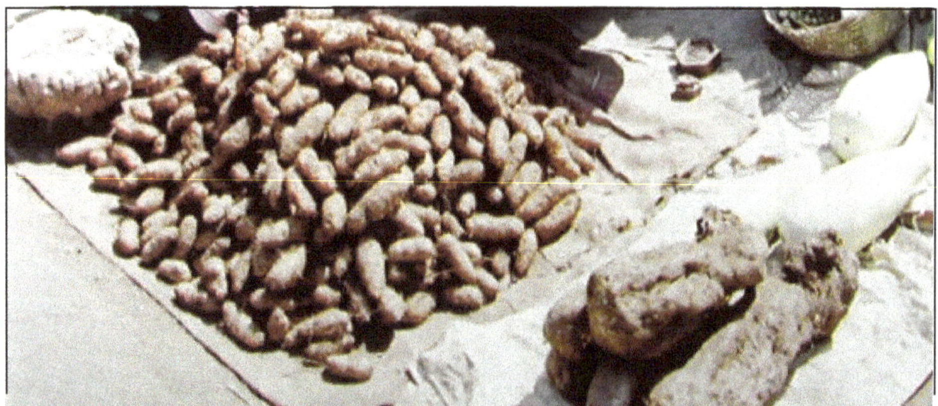

Figure 19.4: Wild Edible Tubers Consumed by Tribal Communities–Photo by Author Dr. D.K. Kulkarni. (p. 283)

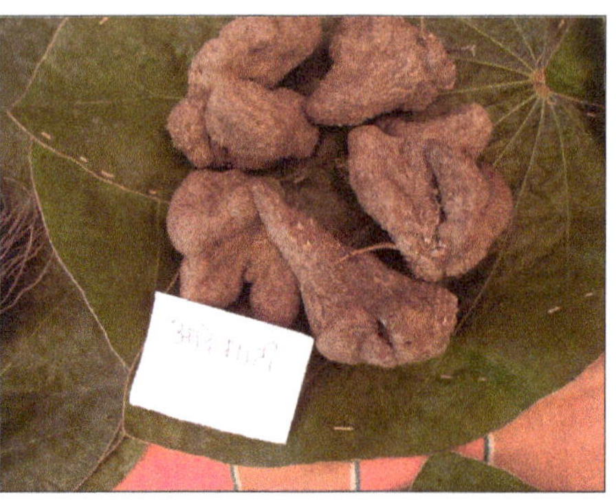

Figure 19.5: *Vigna vexillata* Tubers Consumed by Tribal Communities Photo by Dr. D.K. Kulkarni. (p. 285)

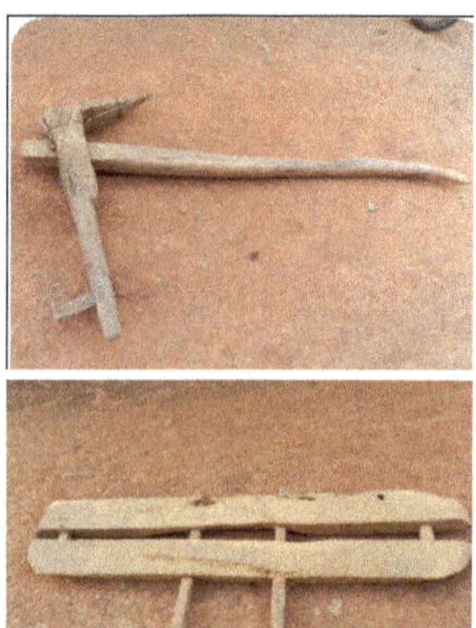

Figure 19.6: The Plow is the most Sacred Essential Implement. Petari used for crushing soil boulders-Photo by author Dr. K. Kulkarni. (p. 288)

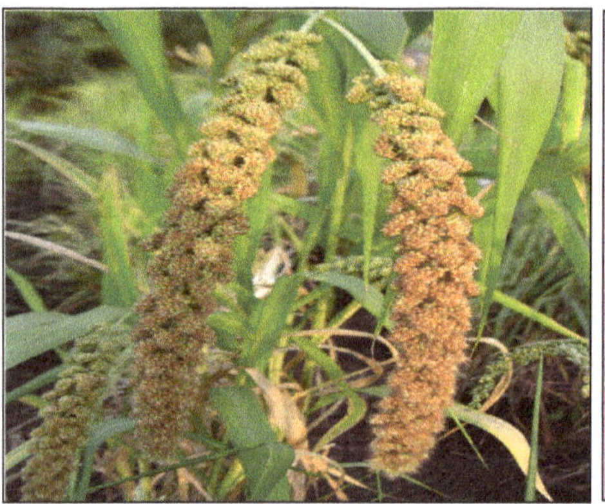

Figure 19.7: Foxtail Millets
Photo by Mr. Sanjay Patil. (p. 289)

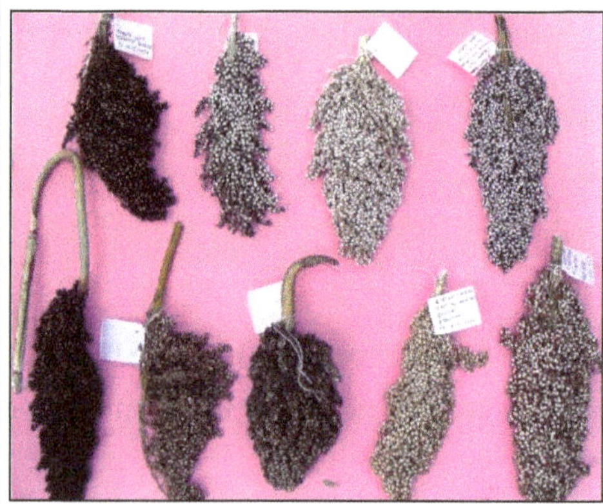

Sorghum Diversity (p. 289)

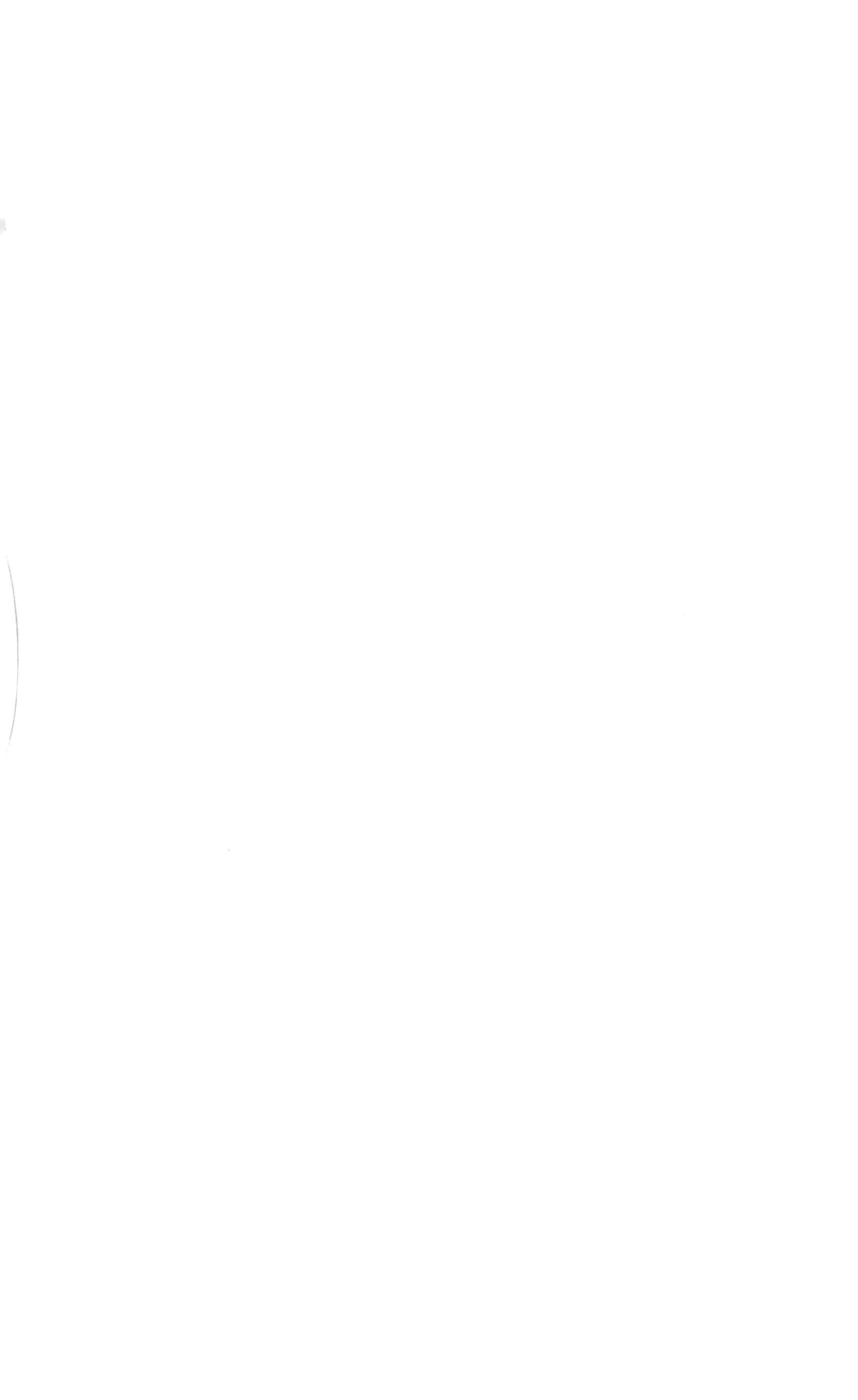

www.ingramcontent.com/pod-product-compliance
Ingram Content Group UK Ltd.
Pitfield, Milton Keynes, MK11 3LW, UK
UKHW021009290726
14059UKWH00001BA/44

9 789388 173926